Critical Perspectives in Public Health

Critical Perspectives in Public Health explores the concept of 'critical' public health, at a point when many of its core concerns appear to have moved to the mainstream of health policy. Issues such as addressing health inequalities and their socio-economic determinants, and the inclusion of public voices in policy-making, are now emerging as key policy aims for health systems across Europe and North America.

Combining analytical introductory chapters, edited versions of influential articles from the journal *Critical Public Health* and specially commissioned review articles, this volume examines the contemporary roles of 'critical voices' in public health research and practice from a range of disciplines and contexts. The book covers many of the pressing concerns for public health practitioners and researchers, including:

- the implications of new genetic technologies for public health;
- the impact of globalisation on local practice;
- the politics of citizen participation in health programmes;
- the impact of car-centred transport systems on health;
- the ethics of evaluation methods and the persistence of health inequalities.

Critical Perspectives in Public Health is organised into sections covering four key themes in public health: social inequalities; evidence for practice; globalisation; and technologies and the environments. With contributions from a range of countries including the United States, Canada, the UK, Australia and South Africa, it provides an accessible overview for students, practitioners and researchers in public health, health promotion, health policy and related fields.

Judith Green is Reader in Sociology of Health at the London School of Hygiene and Tropical Medicine, UK. Her research interests include the sociology of accidents, the organisation of healthcare and public understanding of health.

Ronald Labonté is Canada Research Chair in Globalisation and Health Equity at the University of Ottawa, Canada. Prior to joining academia, he worked for twenty-five years in health promotion and community health development.

Critical Perspectives in Public Health

Edited by Judith Green
and Ronald Labonté

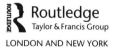
Routledge
Taylor & Francis Group

LONDON AND NEW YORK

First published 2008
by Routledge
2 Park Square, Milton Park, Abingdon, Oxon OX14 4RN

Simultaneously published in the USA and Canada
by Routledge
270 Madison Ave, New York, NY 10016

Routledge is an imprint of the Taylor & Francis Group, an informa business

© 2008 Judith Green and Ronald Labonté, selection and editorial matter;
individual chapters, the contributors

Typeset in Baskerville by
Keystroke, 28 High Street, Tettenhall, Wolverhampton
Printed and bound in Great Britain by
TJ International Ltd, Padstow, Cornwall

British Library Cataloguing in Publication Data
A catalogue record for this book is available from the British Library

Library of Congress Cataloging in Publication Data
Critical perspectives in public health / edited by Judith Green
and Ronald Labonté.
   p. ; cm.
   Includes revised articles from the journal Critical public health.
   Includes bibliographical references and index.
   1. Public health—Social aspects. 2. Social medicine. 3. Equality—
Health aspects. 4. Globalization—Health aspects. I. Green, Judith,
1961– II. Labonte, Ronald N. III. Critical public health.
   [DNLM: 1. Public Health—ethics. 2. Consumer Participation.
3. Health Policy. 4. Health Services Accessibility. 5. World Health.
WA 100 C934 2007]
   RA418.C72 2007
   362.1—dc22
                              2007011521

ISBN10: 0–415–40951–9 (hbk)
ISBN10: 0–415–40952–7 (pbk)
ISBN10: 0–203–93898–4 (ebk)

ISBN13: 978–0–415–40951–3 (hbk)
ISBN13: 978–0–415–40952–0 (pbk)
ISBN13: 978–0–203–93898–0 (ebk)

Contents

List of illustrations

Figures

Tables

Contributors

Pascale Allotey, Centre for Public Health Research, Brunel University, London, UK

Linda Bauld, Department of Social and Policy Sciences, University of Bath, UK

Chris Bonell, Department of Public Health and Policy, London School of Hygiene and Tropical Medicine, London, UK

Robin Bunton, School of Social Sciences and Law, University of Teesside, Middlesbrough, UK

Mickey Chopra, Health Systems Research Unit, Medical Research Council, South Africa and School of Public Health, University of the Western Cape, South Africa

George Davey Smith, Department of Social Medicine, University of Bristol, UK

Erica Di Ruggiero, Canadian Institutes of Health Research – Institute of Population and Public Health, Department of Public Health Services, University of Toronto, Canada

John Frank, Canadian Institutes of Health Research – Institute of Population and Public Health, Department of Public Health Services, University of Toronto, Canada

Peter Freund, Montclair State University, New Jersey, USA

Judith Green, Department of Public Health and Policy, London School of Hygiene and Tropical Medicine, UK

Sonia Grover, Paediatric and Adolescent Gynaecology, Royal Children's Hospital and University of Melbourne, Australia

Charlotte Humphrey, Division of Health and Social Care, King's College, London, UK

Ken Judge, School for Health, University of Bath, UK

Agnieszka Kosny, Institute of Work and Health, Toronto, Ontario, Canada

Nancy Krieger, Department of Society, Human Development, and Health, Harvard School of Public Health, Harvard University, USA

Ronald Labonté, Institute of Population Health and Faculty of Medicine, University of Ottawa, Ontario, Canada

Lori Lambert (Abenaki/Mi'kmaq), Salish Kootenai Tribal College, Montana, USA

Maureen Larkin (Maire Ni Lorcain) is retired and now resides in the Republic of Ireland

John Lynch, Institute for Social Research, University of Michigan, USA

Lenore Manderson, School of Psychology, Psychiatry and Psychological Medicine, Monash University, Victoria, Australia

George Martin, Montclair State University, New Jersey, USA

Tom McIntosh, Political Science, University of Regina, Regina, Saskatchewan, Canada

Carles Muntaner, Department of Behavioural and Community Health, School of Nursing, and Department of Epidemiology and Preventive Medicine, School of Medicine, University of Maryland–Baltimore, USA

Martin O'Neill, Centre for Lifelong Learning, University of Glamorgan, Wales, UK

Alan Petersen, School of Law and Social Science, University of Plymouth, UK

Michael Polanyi, KAIROS: Canadian Ecumenical Justice Initiatives, Toronto, Ontario, Canada

Renée C. Torgerson, Health Network, Canadian Policy Research Networks/Réseaux Canadiens de Recherche en Politiques Publiques, Canada

Joost Van Loon, Institute for Cultural Analysis, Nottingham Trent University, UK

Nina Wallerstein, Department of Family and Community Medicine, University of New Mexico, USA

Eberhard Wenzel, deceased, formerly with the School of Public Health, Griffith University, Brisbane, Australia

Gareth Williams, School of Social Sciences, Cardiff University, Wales, UK

David G. Whiteis, health policy analyst and freelance writer, Chicago, USA

Sally Zierler, Department of Community Health, Brown University, Providence, RI, USA

Preface: public health as social activism

A slightly abashed hagiography

In 1847, the Prussian province of Silesia was ravaged by a typhoid epidemic. The government hired a young pathologist, Rudolf Virchow, to investigate the problem. Virchow spent three weeks in early 1848, not studying disembodied statistics or bureaucratic reports, but living with the miners and their families. Typhoid, he pointed out in what has since become a classical work in social medicine, was only one of several diseases afflicting the coal miners, prime among the others being dysentery, measles and tuberculosis. Virchow named these diseases 'artificial' to emphasise that their prevalence was embedded in the poor housing, working conditions, diet and lack of sanitation among the coal miners. For Virchow, the answer to the question of how to prevent typhoid outbreaks in Silesia was quite simple: 'we must begin to promote the advancement of the entire population, and to stimulate a general common effort. A population will never achieve full education, freedom and prosperity in the form of a gift from the outside' (Virchow 2006: 92).

Virchow's short-term prescription was to form a committee of lay people and professionals to monitor the spread of typhoid and other diseases and to organise agricultural cooperatives to ensure the people had sufficient food to eat. His long-term solutions were more radical: improved occupational health and safety, better wages, decreased working hours and strong local and regional self-government. Virchow argued for progressive tax reform, removing the burden from the working poor and placing it on 'the plutocracy, which drew very large amounts from the Upper Silesian mines, did not recognise the Upper Silesians as human beings, but only as tools' (Virchow 2006: 90). He advocated democratic forms of industrial development, and even suggested hiring temporarily unemployed miners to build roadways, making it easier to transport fresh produce during the winter.

These recommendations were not quite what the Prussian government had in mind. They had not hired Virchow to call into question the economics of industrial capitalism. He was thanked for his report and promptly fired.[1] One week later, on his return to Berlin, Virchow joined with others erecting barricades and demonstrating passionately for political changes that they hoped would bring the democracy that Virchow believed was essential for health. He went on to establish a radical magazine titled *Medical Reform* in which full employment, adequate income, housing and nutrition were debated for their importance in creating health. A decade later, still believing that political action was necessary for health, Virchow became a member of the Berlin Municipal Council and eventually of the Prussian Parliament. Over his eighty years of work, he saw no distinction between being a health professional and a social activist.

'All disease has two causes,' Virchow allegedly once wrote, 'one pathological and the other political' (Bierman and Dunn 2006: 99).

Howard Waitzkin (2006: 10), in writing of the need to reassert Virchow's social criticism in public health, notes:

> The social origins of illness are not mysterious. Yet, more than a century and a half after Virchow's analysis first appeared, these problems remain with us. Public health generally has adopted the medical model of etiology. In this model, social conditions may increase susceptibility or exacerbate disease, but they are not primary causes like microbial agents or disturbances of normal physiology. Since investigation has not clarified the causes of illness within social structure, political strategy – both within and outside medicine – seldom has addressed the roots of disease in society.

It is to this task, in both investigation and action, and to the inspiration of Rudolf Virchow and scores more critical public health activists, past and present, that this book is dedicated.

Note

1 The same happened to one of the editors of this book, who, like Virchow, can attest that critical public health is not without its risks, and that if one is to be fired for it, better earlier than later in one's career.

References

Bierman, Arlene S. and Dunn, James R. (2006) 'Swimming upstream: access, health outcomes, and the social determinants of health', *Journal of General Internal Medicine*, 21(1): 99–100.

Virchow, R. (2006) 'Report on the typhus epidemic in upper Silesia', *Social Medicine*, 1: 11–98. (Translation and reprint of his 1848 report.)

Waitzkin, H. (2006) 'One and a half centuries of forgetting and rediscovering: Virchow's lasting contributions to social medicine', *Social Medicine*, 1: 5–10.

Acknowledgements

We would first of all like to thank the Editorial Board of *Critical Public Health* for their encouragement to publish a collection based on some of the excellent contributions to the journal in recent years. Particular thanks to Alex Scott-Samuel, for his continued inspirational support; Robin Bunton and Jane Wills, the current editors of the journal; and Jo Campling, the board chairperson. Jo sadly died while this book was being completed, but this project was one of the many that she had been instrumental in encouraging and facilitating, and we would like to record our debt to her commitment and enthusiasm. Finally, we owe a huge thanks to Joelle Walker and Shannon Warznak, for help in preparing the manuscript.

Introduction: from critique to engagement

Why critical public health matters

Judith Green and Ronald Labonté

The journal *Critical Public Health* started life as *Radical Community Medicine*, a partial honorific to Rudolf Virchow's own century-earlier journal titled *Radical Medicine*. Edited in Liverpool in the UK by Alex Scott-Samuel and resembling more a newsletter than an academic serial, the publication gave first voice to what would become identified as 'critical' in public health. One issue of *Radical Community Medicine*, devoted to debate about the future of public health in the UK, illustrated well the demands of the critical public health movement of the time (*RCM* 1986). Contributors covered the debate about professional power in medicine; demands for participative democracy and active community engagement in public health; and calls for action on the determinants of health. Articles urged public health practitioners to become activists around those issues that are core to providing health for all, such as maternity rights, housing and tobacco control. A small selection of its covers, crafted in the woodblock tradition of activist artists by Cliff Harper (to some resembling at times, if still elegantly, the socialist realism then prominent in radical aesthetics), captures the headlines of many of these debates.

Some twenty years later, it has become a common refrain wherever public health practitioners, academics and activists meet that these concerns have largely moved to the mainstream, at least in high-income countries. International and national public agendas now apparently espouse precisely those aims that once seemed marginal. Public health has become a broader church, less dominated by a medical elite, and one in which the contributions of not only other health professionals and community activists but those from education, leisure, welfare, environment, policing and other arenas are actively recruited: it has become everybody's business. While 'everybody's business' can easily become nobody's business (who leads, who follows and how is the intersectoral dance orchestrated?) broadly and deeply defined social determinants of health have become widely recognised within and beyond the health sectors of most countries. As Tony McMichael and Robert Beaglehole (2003: 2) put it, public health in its 'fullest sense . . . must include the lessening of social inequalities', an evidence-informed ethic that is reflected in the national health policies of many developed countries. In the UK, for instance, the Labour government, in rolling back the excesses of neoliberalism, focused on the impacts of inequalities in health (DoH 2003), and the mission of New Zealand's framework

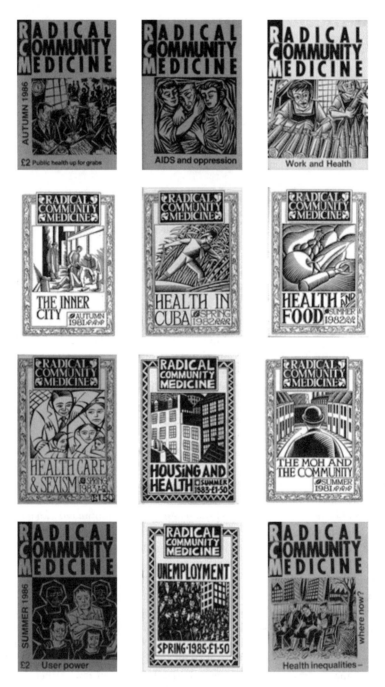

Figure I.1 Covers from issues of *Radical Community Medicine*, with artwork by Cliff Harper, as commissioned for *RCM* by Alex Scott-Samuel

for public health action is 'To reduce inequalities and improve overall health status' (MoH 2003: 27). Public participation has also become a central plank of governance in many democratic states, with governments increasingly encouraging such participation in policy-making and demanding that researchers consider the 'researched' as stakeholders in the process.

Many public health practitioners and researchers today, like Virchow, do see themselves as activists rather than neutral gatherers of public health information for the state. The gains of the public health community on tobacco control illustrate some of the successes of this advocacy, as activists became political campaigners, taking on the tobacco companies, developing lobbying skills and learning to use mass media to shape opinion (de Beyer and Waverley Brigden 2003). Partnerships beyond the traditional health sector ones have been crucial to success. In discussing the tobacco control successes in Bangladesh, for instance, Debra Efroymson and Saifuddin Ahmed (2003) note the importance of moving the debate away from a narrow one on health and locating it as one of poverty and social justice, in a country where money spent on tobacco products could make a significant difference to children's nutrition.

Mission unaccomplished

At first sight, then, critical public health has apparently done its job. What is the role of the critic once the radical agenda becomes accepted as mainstream? It is, perhaps, at one level invidious to distinguish 'critical' and 'mainstream' approaches in public health. Public health in general, as practice and academic endeavour, has traditionally been at the margins of both health policy and the academy, and the public health movement has had to position itself throughout its history as both new and radical. By the 1980s public health was already rebranding itself as the 'new public health' in the UK and elsewhere, with John Ashton and Howard Seymour (1988) calling for a turn towards the social and economic 'upstream' determinants of health and away from the dominance of therapeutic, curative medicine. For Fran Baum (1998), the new public health in Australia was marked by not only a renewed concern with the social determinants of health, but by an emphasis on social justice, healthy public policy and a globalising vision that took account of international inequalities. Internationally, this shift was recognised by the 1986 World Health Organization *Ottawa Charter for Health Promotion* (subtitled 'Towards a new public health'), which addressed health as a goal for which disease reduction was simply one of many means of achievement (that 'positive' health or well-being is influenced by the presence of disease and disability does not make the experiences synonymous). In many parts of the world, public health may retain a marginal position in healthcare systems (McKee and Zatonski 2003), but it has enjoyed a resurgence in most high-income countries that is now globalising through such instruments as the 2005 *Bangkok Charter on Health Promotion* (the formulation of which involved countries from around the world) and the WHO's 2005–8 Commission on the Social Determinants of Health, which aims to create greater policy attention in every country to the social causes of disease.

Why, then, claim a special role for a 'critical' voice in public health? With both national governments and international bodies accepting health as a priority, and calling for both equity and social justice, surely not only has public health become a critical endeavour, but its work has largely been done. Not so. Consider the more recent global concern over cross-border pandemics such as avian flu, multiple-drug-resistant tuberculosis or even the socially communicable spread of chronic diseases into poorer countries still coping with the burden of infectious ills. Does this concern lead to analyses of and actions on the social contexts? Or does it reposition public health away from its critical praxis and into a 'core business' of selective, cost-effective interventions that may reduce disease prevalence rates, but do little to alter the political conditions that give rise to them in the first place? Therein lies the heart of contemporary public health debate, and the reason for this book.

In publishing this volume, we clearly identify the ongoing vital role for critical voices. Indeed, we would argue a more urgent need than ever for a critical perspective in public health. This role is a double one of offering a critical voice *for* public health, but also, less comfortably, at times offering a critique of public health. The two are not incompatible: a critique *of* public health provides an essential reflexive role, ensuring that multiple voices are heard (something highlighted in several of this book's chapters), that the unintended effects of healthy public policy are noted and examined, and that public health does not suffer an excess of orthodoxy.

Becoming critical

What do we mean by 'critical'? A critical perspective in public health, like that in other disciplines, is one of, in Lee Harvey's (1990: 32) words, 'deconstructing taken-for-granted concepts and theoretical relationships by asking how these taken-for-granted elements actually relate to wider oppressive structures and how these structures legitimate and conceal their oppressive mechanisms'.

As Ronald Labonté and his colleagues have argued (Labonté *et al.* 2005), the implications of this for a public health project are twofold. First is the obligation to uncover how specific social structures, in their political and historical contexts, both construct and recreate conditions that threaten the health of populations, or particular groups within those populations. Second, though, is the praxis. A critical project is not merely an academic one which documents those structures, but one which challenges them and seeks the 'reconstruction of social, economic and political relations along emancipatory lines' (Labonté *et al.* 2005: 10). Critical public health is not a disinterested academic discipline, but one that engages with structures of power to challenge as well as describe them. It is a normative project, which explicitly 'takes sides'. As Nancy Krieger (2000: 287–8) puts it:

> [W]e must practise a passionate epistemology, a way of knowing that is at once critical, rigorous, humble and partisan, on the side of all who are burdened by premature mortality, preventable disease, and psychic or somatic trauma, on the side of all who would live in a world guided by love, not greed.

There are multiple ways of doing this and, as the range of readings in this volume demonstrates, critical voices in public health do not necessarily speak in unison. Structures of power are multiple and complex, and rarely are hierarchies clear cut. If we are championing community interests, there are inevitably questions of which parts of the community, and who is marginalised. There is considerable debate about not only the aims and legitimate questions for critical public health, but the proper 'tools of the trade', in terms of how we develop appropriate research methodologies for investigating health in ways which respect the different (and sometimes conflicting) perspectives of those with whom we are working. Within these necessary debates, though, are a number of potential roles for critical public health.

First are the obvious ones of 'keeping up the pressure' in ensuring that those issues that affect the public's health are high on the agenda, and acting as advocates for health when other values might conflict. On issues such as tobacco control, obesity and workplace health and safety, the vested interests of business mean that we still have to campaign to prioritise health over other interests. Inequality, poverty, social justice and participation may be part of mainstream international and national agendas, but the work of achieving progress has hardly been begun in a world where life expectancies range from thirty-six for women in Sierra Leone to eighty-five for women in Japan (WHO 2003), and within countries, mortality and morbidity are still marked by disparities of income, gender, geography and ethnicity. Too often national health policies accept the need to address inequities in health outcome, for instance, but shy away from addressing their underlying causes in social inequality (Wilkinson 1996), and instead simply 'target' the most vulnerable, as if the cause were their behaviour, rather than structural inequality itself. We see this in the differing constructions of risk: risk factors (which locate the problem within the body), risk groups (who have a significantly higher prevalence of risk factors) and risk conditions (the social contexts in which risk factors and groups are embedded). Even when we understand this embeddedness, the discourse of 'targeting' high-risk groups ineluctably locates the level of change within attributes of the group, which just as ineluctably reduces to their individual risk factors.

The issue of injury provides one example (Green 2006). Despite huge gains in reducing mortality from injuries in many developed countries, there are still shameful inequalities: one recent analysis of mortality data from the UK found that children of unemployed parents had thirteen times the risk of dying from an injury than did those born to parents in professional or higher managerial occupations (Edwards *et al.* 2006). Globally, of the 1.2 million people who die each year from road traffic injuries, around 85 per cent are in low- and middle-income countries (WHO 2004) – and many of them did not own motor vehicles but were simply poor rural pedestrians walking at night along poorly maintained roads increasingly populated by poorly maintained trucks moving about the raw resources that are the base of our integrating global economy. These inequalities are structural – the poorest are more exposed to risk. Yet still the majority of health promotion activity is orientated towards individualistic behavioural interventions, such as teaching children to cross the road safely, or equipping rural Africans with reflective arm-bands for their evening perambulations, which, however immediately helpful to some individuals, make the vulnerable responsible for keeping themselves safe in environments which endanger their health.

Playing the role of the advocate and learning the arts of politics are legitimate roles for public health activists, but critical voices also need to be penetrating, rather than unquestioningly championing those policies which appear to be 'good things'. So a second role for critical public health is asking the difficult questions about the successes and failures of public health, and constantly questioning our own 'taken-for-granted' assumptions. A good example is the fate of inter-sectoral alliances such as the WHO Healthy Cities projects. These encapsulate well both the promise and the failure of the new public health. With a recognition that the determinants of health lay outside the remit of the health service, the Healthy Cities projects were designed as a practical implementation of *Ottawa Charter* principles. However, tensions were evident from the outset. Although stressing community action and participation, they relied on 'top down' leadership (Stern and Green 2005). Developing healthy public policy around issues such as road safety or hazardous waste removal requires the collaboration of public statutory organisations, voluntary organisations and the private sector, yet public health is still delivered within 'modernist' organisations, obsessed with 'scientific explanations and techno-rational "fixes"' (Petersen and Lupton 1996: 144). The role of organisations and communities from outside the formal sector was always going to be problematic, invited in on terms and conditions set out by those in power. As David Craig (Craig and Porter 2006) points out in his analysis of partnership programmes in Waitakere, New Zealand, the costs of such participation are high. While professionals benefited from the networking and meetings to establish inter-sectoral partnerships (the emergence of what Craig calls the 'muffin economy'), community activists faced both the problems of credible representation (which sections of a community do leaders speak for and what is their legitimacy to do so?) and the limits of voluntarism, with little to show in terms of outputs (such as impact on poverty), except at the margins. The findings from studies of Healthy City and other inter-agency programmes in general point to the tensions of emphasising community participation as a simple route to emancipatory practice. Rather than uncritically supporting recent attempts to reinvigorate local democracy through increasing public participation, we should ask: in whose interests is such participation, and what effects might it have? Simplistic calls for community participation risk eliding and obscuring the difficulties and social inequalities of the multiple communities and social identities that exist within any city.

This is problematic for a number of reasons. First, public health's romantic infatuation with localism risks becoming a form of 'community-blaming' in which the higher-order levels of economic and political decision-making that ultimately determine the fate of whole communities or nations are given short shrift (Labonte 1993). The most invidious form of this is the 'targeting' of poor communities advocated by much contemporary inequalities policy. Apart from the intrinsic inappropriateness of the metaphor of 'targeting' (Green 2005) (which means 'to be the object of attack or abuse'), such policies focus the responsibility for solving the problem of inequality on exactly those most vulnerable to its effects and least able to change the structural determinants of health in their localities. The UK's strategy on health inequalities, for instance, explicitly 'encompasses local solutions for local health inequality problems given that local planners, front line staff and communities know best what their problems are, and how to deal with them' (DoH 2003: 5). It goes on to identify some of those who will be 'targeted' by specific interventions, including vulnerable older people, black and other minority ethnic groups, homeless people and asylum-seekers (DoH 2003: 10).

But what should ethnic minority communities do about the racist structures and cultures that impact on employment prospects, housing choices and interpersonal experiences, which in turn shape health outcomes? Presumably be more conscientious in taking hypertension medication, turning up for screening and providing wholesome fruit and vegetables for their families. And what about 'vulnerable elderly people', whose mobility is restricted by busy roads laid out for commuters with no time to waste, and inadequate funding for accessible public transport? Presumably be careful to remove risky 'trip hazards' from their homes, and wear hip protectors in case they should fall. It is, of course, essential that local voices are heard in the design and planning of public health programmes, but all too often those voices are asked only to comment on an agenda already defined by professionals, and to contribute to the individualistic health promotion interventions that attempt to ameliorate the effects of inequalities, rather than genuinely being included in participatory processes that would challenge the political processes that value fast roads over sustainable local communities, or economic structures that lead to the stigmatisation of asylum-seekers or refugees.

Turning the gaze inwards

If this process of challenging the taken-for-granted assumptions of public policy is part of the role of a critical public health, there is also the task of critiquing public health itself. Those speaking from the margins have the essential, if uncomfortable, obligation to look unflinchingly at their own practice, and identify how those policies and practices intended to improve health or reduce inequalities may also have other unintended social and cultural effects. It is the role of the critic to ask who benefits and who does not, and what the broader implications of shifts in practice are.

Alan Petersen and Deborah Lupton (1996) expand on this argument in their post-structuralist analysis of the new public health as 'a new morality', with its exercise of a particular form of power. Their critique of both the epistemological base of the 'new public health' and its implementation, in initiatives such as Healthy Cities, addresses the ways in which its discursive practices construct particular kinds of subjective individuals. Despite the emancipatory and egalitarian rhetoric, public health practice still delineates the normal and abnormal, the healthy and unhealthy. It is part of the apparatus of the modern state, and has a key role in governing the populace. Drawing on Foucault's work on 'governmentality', a number of commentators have begun to unpack the contours of this governance, in terms of its implications for the kinds of subjectivities we can experience in late modern societies, and the kinds of political processes which are made more or less possible.

Alan Petersen (1997), for instance, discusses the importance of Robert Castel's (1991) argument that preventative public policy has moved from a discourse of 'dangerousness' to one of 'risk', in which the emphasis has shifted from the control and confinement of dangerous individuals to one of anticipating and controlling risks in the abstract, identified through population statistics. This multiplies the possibilities for intervention, most obviously in techniques such as the preventative clinics of modern medical practice, which identify all those with risk factors for coronary heart disease, for instance, for preventative therapeutic action. At one level, there are potential critiques in terms of the costs of this escalation in surveillance, such as those of iatrogenic harm through mass medication, or the generation of anxiety. More fundamentally, this shift is one facet of contemporary political rationalities which are typical of neoliberal societies. Petersen (1997: 194) characterises this governance as: 'A form of rule involves creating a sphere of freedom for subjects so that they are able to exercise a regulated autonomy . . . [It] calls upon the individual to enter into the process of his or her own self-governance through processes of endless self-examination, self-care and self-improvement.'

Increasingly, the state's role in safeguarding the health of its population is reduced, as the individual is obliged to take care of himself. As ever more risk factors for disease and propensity to disease are identified, ever more aspects of our daily lives potentially come under the umbrella of state agencies to monitor and set targets for, but with a corresponding privatisation of responsibility for managing and minimising those risks. Food policy is one example. Alizon Draper and Judith Green (2002) outline shifts in the state's responsibility for food safety, beginning with concerns with adulteration and combating fraud and malfeasance for an emergent 'consumer society' which framed the public as largely passive and ignorant. By the end of the nineteenth century, with the growth of technologies for testing bacteriological contamination, negligence was added as a concern, with a concomitant set of responsibilities for those providing and selling food to prevent risk, rather than merely not cause danger. By the end of the twentieth century, the consumer had been framed as an active citizen, with responsibilities for not only making safe and nutritious choices for herself and her family, but engaging in a raft of 'consultative' exercises, organised in communities and schools around healthy eating and how it could be encouraged. The modern subject has responsibilities not just towards the self, but to the political body, as a new kind of citizenship emerges, with its emphasis on engagement and empowerment. To be healthy is now to be agential and self-motivated, yet the engagement required is usually a self-directed one. Community participation and empowerment become obligations on citizens to conduct themselves as self-caring individuals, orientated towards their own health rather than the social network.

These perspectives on governmentality have been fruitful ones for a critique of public health, at both the level of examining broader questions of health policy (for instance, delineating why some issues get on the agenda as 'health' issues, and how they are framed) and the more micro-concerns of subjectivities, and how individuals respond as 'risky selves'. One issue that has been emphasised in both national and international health policies agendas, for example, is that of social capital. Carles

Muntaner and his colleagues (see Chapter 2 of this volume) have noted the rise of social capital in public health discourse since the mid-1990s, despite the under-theorised conceptualisation in most of the usage and the tendency of public health to adopt more communitarian and psychological conceptualisations of the term. Their argument – that the concept has been useful in part because of its 'fit' with political ideologies of the EU and the USA which emphasise civic organisation and the minimisation of the state, and focus on local community action rather than structural divisions as a route to ameliorating inequalities – is one that takes into account the ways in which public health discourse is intricately linked to political rationality. We cannot make sense of public health purely in its own terms. It also nuances the critique of governmentality by acknowledging implicitly the state as a co-creator of social capital – or at least of its potential – and as a site of healthy and empowering social contestation rather than of singular repression. If public health is partly about regulating the social for some collective good, which is how Virchow viewed it, what is 'good' and how it is to be governed into existence remain the problematic of its practice.

About the collection

The articles collected here, all first appearing in *Critical Public Health*, illustrate well these kinds of contribution to a critical analysis for healthy public policy as well as an analysis of it. It would be impossible to provide a comprehensive collection on critical public health, and we have not attempted to do so. There are some obvious omissions. There is nothing, for example, on children's health and the focus on early childhood development, which is becoming a global campaign and not merely one of high-income countries with the wealth to afford stimulating environments. There remains little empirical doubt that early life experiences can embed physiological health pathways effects that do not manifest until much later. There is also the argument that it is easier to create cross-class generosity towards rectifying inequities facing 'innocent children' than those experienced by adults who are seen (in varying ideological degrees) as less-deserving architects of their own fates. Yet, as Nazeem Muhajarine and others have pointed out, 'If healthy families produce healthy children, the societal milieu with its structures, norms and values is the fundamental platform upon which lasting change must occur' (Muhajarine *et al.* 2006). The challenge for public health is to ensure the children's health agenda is a wedge in the doorway to a larger social health agenda.

Nor is there much about the positive health gains made in many parts of the world through the campaigns led by civil society organisations, often involving public health workers. Indeed, some readers might also consider that this book omits 'practical advice'. It does, and deliberately so. A critical public health practice is built upon moral, theoretical, empirical and experiential knowledge and reflection. It does not arise from a list of 'how tos'. The technical–rational world this implies actually runs counter to the demand for ongoing reflexivity by practitioners, and acceptance of the dynamic contingencies of what and where they find themselves located in their work. This does not deny that there are generalisations about practice that should and can be made. But such generalisations should arise from the entwining spirals of theory, evidence (in all its plural forms), analysis, action and reflection. That is the legacy of public health activists past, and the path of critical public health practice future.

Finally, the readings are inextricably tied to time and place; many of them are highly contextualised and at times the data they cite are decidedly dated. But that should not be of concern since what is important from a critical public vantage is *how* the authors have attempted to probe 'beneath the water line' of what the data and discourse of their time and place reveal in more generalised fashion about the power and practices that give rise to the problems. This is what sets a critical public health approach apart from the more conventional (though not unimportant) descriptive and monitoring functions of public health. In simple terms, a critical approach resembles the childlike endless querying of each stated fact, 'But why?' In more complex terms, it not only probes continuously deeper; it is fundamentally concerned with the social practices of power and how these practices (political, economic, engendered, cultural) work to stratify individuals into hierarchies, and so stratify their risk, vulnerability and access to resources for health.

References

Ashton, J. and Seymour, H. (1988) *The New Public Health*, Milton Keynes: Open University Press.

Baum, F. (1998) *The New Public Health: An Australian Perspective*, Oxford: Oxford University Press.

Beaglehole, R. (ed.) (2003) *Global Public Health: A New Era*, Oxford: Oxford University Press.

Castel, R. (1991) 'From dangerousness to risk', in G. Burchell, C. Gordon and P. Miller (eds), *The Foucault Effect: Studies in Governmentality*, Hemel Hempstead: Harvester Wheatsheaf.

Craig, D. and Porter, D. (2006) *Development beyond Neoliberalism? Governance, Poverty and Political Economy*, London: Routledge.

de Beyer, J. and Waverley Brigden, L. (eds) (2003) *Tobacco Control Policy: Strategies, Successes and Setbacks*, Washington, DC: World Bank/RITC.

DoH (Department of Health) (2003) *Tackling Health Inequalities: A Programme for Action*, London: DoH.

Draper, A. and Green, J. (2002) 'Food safety and consumers: constructions of choice and risk', *Social Policy and Administration*, 36: 610–25.

Edwards, P., Green, J., Roberts, I. and Lutchman, S. (2006) 'Deaths from injury in children and employment status in family: analysis of trends in class specific death rates', *British Medical Journal*, 333: 119–21.

Efroymson, D. and Ahmed, S. (2003) 'Building momentum for tobacco control: the case of Bangladesh' in J. de Beyer and L. Waverley Brigden (eds), *Tobacco Control Policy: Strategies, Successes and Setbacks*, Washington, DC: World Bank/RITC.

Green, J. (2005) 'Professions and community', *New Zealand Sociology*, 20: 122–41.

—— (2006) 'What role for critical public health?', *Critical Public Health*, 16: 171–3.

Harvey, L. (1990) *Critical Social Research*, London: Unwin Hyman.

Krieger, N. (2000) 'Passionate epistemology, critical advocacy, and public health: doing our profession proud', *Critical Public Health*, 10: 287–94.

Labonte, R. (1993) 'Partnerships and participation in community health', *Canadian Journal of Public Health*, 84: 237–40.

Labonté, R., Polanyi, M., Muhajarine, N., McIntosh, T. and Williams, A. (2005) 'Beyond the divides: towards critical population health research', *Critical Public Health*, 15: 5–17.

McKee, M. and Zatonski, W. (2003) 'Public health in Eastern Europe and the former Soviet Union', in R. Beaglehole (ed.), *Global Public Health: A New Era*, Oxford: Oxford University Press.

McMichael, A.J. and Beaglehole, R. (2003) 'The global context of public health', in R. Beaglehole (ed.), *Global Public Health: A New Era*, Oxford: Oxford University Press.

MoH (Ministry of Health) (2003) *Achieving Health for All People / Whakatutuki te oranga hauora mo ngā tāngata katoa: A Framework of Public Health Action for the New Zealand Health Strategy*, Wellington, NZ: Ministry of Health.

Muhajarine, N., Vu, L. and Labonté, R. (2006) 'Social contexts and children's health outcomes: researching across the boundaries', *Critical Public Health*, 16: 205–18.

Petersen, A. (1997) 'Risk, governance and the new public health', in A. Petersen and R. Bunton (eds), *Foucault, Health and Medicine*, London: Routledge.

Petersen, A. and Lupton, D. (1996) *The New Public Health: Health and Self in the Age of Risk*, London: Sage.

RCM (1986) 'Public health up for grabs?', *Radical Community Medicine*, 27, Autumn.

Stern, R. and Green, J. (2005) 'Boundary workers and the management of frustration: a case study of two Healthy City partnerships', *Health Promotion International*, 20: 269–78.

WHO (World Health Organization) (2003) *Facts and Figures: The World Health Report 2003*, Geneva: WHO.

—— (2004) *World Report on Road Traffic Injury Prevention*, Geneva: WHO.

Wilkinson, R.G. (1996) *Unhealthy Societies: The Afflictions of Inequality*, London: Routledge.

Part I

Unfair cases: social inequalities in health

Introduction

Ronald Labonté, John Frank and Erica Di Ruggiero

> When inequalities become too great, the idea of community becomes impossible.
> (Attributed to Raymond Aron)

Neither inequalities in health nor policy and practice attention to their causes and consequences are new. In recent Western history this attention has flared brightest when social inequalities have been greatest: the Industrial Revolution of the nineteenth century (during which Rudolf Virchow, whose hagiography introduced this book, was but one of many radical health reformers), the cyclic crises of capitalism leading to severe economic recession or depression such as the 'Dirty 30s' (when texts on poverty and health were commonplace), and the worldwide irruptions caused by rapid economic globalisation beginning in the 1980s, accelerated by the collapse of the Soviet Union. Often this attention distils to a patronising concern for the poor, fomenting ideologically driven debates about whether poverty should be considered in absolute or relative terms (empirical evidence supports the importance of both notions although 'absolute' poverty elides most closely with the welfare minimalism of today's free marketers) or what amount of inequality is good or bad for society or the economy as a whole (too much inequality can cause social disintegration and costly policing intervention, too little can dampen entrepreneurial incentives, leading to slower rates of growth; Anderson and O'Neil 2006), though how much growth is environmentally sustainable is a different and vastly more important question usually bracketed in such debates. David Woodward and Andrew Simms of the UK-based New Economics Foundation, as exceptions to this rule, calculate that during 1990–2001, only 0.6 per cent of global economic growth contributed to poverty reduction, compared with 2.2 per cent in the previous decade. Most of the benefits of growth were captured by elites in wealthier countries, yet the environmental costs of that growth were, and continue to be, borne disproportionately by the world's poor. The evidence, they conclude, firmly establishes wealth redistribution, rather than continued growth, as the most important means for 'levelling up' health equity via poverty reduction (Woodward and Simms 2006).

From inequality to inequity

Woodward's and Simms' conclusion has compelling moral argument as well as evidence behind it, but in appraising both we need first to distinguish between *inequality* and *inequity*. The former is a stochastic measure of sameness or difference; the latter is a normative valuation of whether the difference is fair or morally acceptable. Health equity is not the same as health equality, since some health inequalities cannot reasonably be described as unfair (e.g., genetic variation, biological sex differences), and some are neither preventable nor remediable, at least given the state of current knowledge. In public health discourse, health equity generally refers to the absence of avoidable or remediable differences in health among populations or groups defined socially, economically, demographically or geographically (Solar and Irwin 2005).

There are many models of equity. One of the simplest distinguishes horizontal from vertical equity. Horizontal equity means that equals are treated the same. For example, as citizens with equal entitlements, all Canadians have the right to access publicly insured health services without financial barriers. They also share equality before the law (though the value of the legal advice they might purchase remains an inequitably allocated market commodity), and the right to cast one, and only one, ballot in an election. Popularised under the rubric 'equality of oppor-tunity', horizontal equity pays little attention to gradients of inequality (preferring instead a minimal avoidance of absolute deprivation), and ignores that equal opportunity is only morally justified when individuals have equal pre-existing endowments (which they never do). In real-life conditions, equal opportunity produces increasingly unequal outcomes by positively discriminating in favour of those who already have more resources. Vertical equity, in contrast, enriches horizontal equity (which remains important despite its limitations) by stating that unequals are treated differently. Poorer Canadians suffer poorer health; therefore their average use of health services should be proportionately greater (unequal) than for wealthier Canadians, reversing the well-documented 'inverse care law' first noted by Julian Tudor Hart in the UK to describe how the wealthier and healthier consume a disproportionate amount of publicly financed services (Hart 1971). An example of combined horizontal and vertical equity exists in the risk-pooled cross-subsidisation principles for fairness in healthcare financing: the rich and healthy, through taxes or premiums, subsidise the poor and sick (World Health Organization 2000).

Beneath these principles of equity lie arguments rooted in ethics. The public health literature has been substantially enriched in recent years by an expansion of ethics theories that move beyond the individual and biomedical level (with its axioms of beneficence, non-maleficence, autonomy and dignity) to the social and political economy level (where human rights conventions and theories of capabilities, cosmopolitanism and relational justice, to name a few of the more dominant ones, create a messier terrain of social duties or obligations). A rights-based approach bases itself on various legally binding but unenforceable human rights treaties, although such treaties become judiciable when written into national laws (Hunt *et al.* 2002). Several of these treaties impose obligations on states with respect to health and most of its underlying social determinants (e.g., food, housing, water and environmental and working conditions). Importantly, these treaties do not guarantee a right to health *per se*; rather, they obligate states and other actors to ensure that all people have fair access to the resources required for health.

In this respect, the rights-based approach resembles the 'capabilities' argument advanced by such writers as the Nobel economist Amartya Sen (1999) and the feminist ethicist Martha Nussbaum (1992). This argument urges provision of a number of capabilities essential for people to be healthy. The list of these capabilities reads similarly to the conditions defined under human rights treaties (e.g., reproductive health, adequate nourishment and shelter, adequate education), but with a few novelties: the ability to use one's imagination, engage in meaningful relationships, emotional development, self-respect/dignity, the ability to play, and control over one's political and material environments (Nussbaum 2000: 78–80). What people do with these capabilities resides in their freedom of choice. Inequalities in health may arise from these choices, but inequities in health are firmly instantiated in unequal access to these capabilities (or, more accurately, to the social basis of these capabilities, which represent the duties of governments and their citizenry). As Nussbaum (2000) comments: 'The capabilities approach insists that this requires a great deal to make up for differences in starting point that are caused by natural endowment or by power' – that is, levelling up to compensate for historic inequalities. ('Levelling up' refers to lifting the bottom nearer to the top, since improving health equity by levelling those with better health *down*, towards a median, is both unethical and unlikely.)

Cosmopolitanism extends the fair provision of these capabilities across national borders, positing that 'principles of justice apply to all persons regardless of wherever they are in the cosmos; and varies from strong demands for fair terms of cooperation on a global scale to at a minimum adherence to the no harm principle' (Ruger 2006: 999). This directs attention to global asymmetries in wealth and power, and a major weakness in our current social order described in the reading by Labonté and Torgerson in Chapter 10: that economic power is global while political power – at least in its formal *government* rather than *governance* sense – remains national. Thomas Pogge's theory of relational justice offers perhaps the most comprehensive synthesis of political economy and philosophical reasoning for consideration at both national and global levels. He argues that a concern with the social distribution (and hence equitable provision) of the prerequisites (or capabilities) for health is insufficient in itself. These inequities did not arise from nothing; they were socially created and are socially maintained. Individuals therefore have a moral obligation to be concerned with their own role in creating and maintaining these inequities through interrogation of evidence and argument about their causal patterns. The stronger an individual's (or nation's or other population aggregate of individuals') involvement in bringing about adverse health outcomes, the greater is their moral obligation to redress them (Anand and Peter 2004: 6).

> By avoidably producing severe poverty, economic institutions substantially contribute to the incidence of many medical conditions. Persons materially

involved in upholding such institutions are then materially involved in the causation of such medical conditions.

(Pogge 2004: 137)

From society to health

Ethics may tell us *why* we have obligations to act on health inequities, apart from invoking the instrumental argument that unfairly sick people eventually threaten the health and well-being of the more affluent well. They do not necessarily inform us about how societies create health inequities in the first place. Here there is no shortage of models or frameworks that chart the relationships between social organisation and health outcomes. A recent, and compellingly simple, model posits that societies create health inequities in at least four different ways:

1   Differential stratification: where one sits in social hierarchies of wealth, authority or privilege, and how those hierarchies are structured by age, sex, ethnicity and geography, exerts a powerful influence on health outcomes.
2   Differential exposure to risk: one's social position influences exposure to unhealthy conditions in the workplace or living environments.
3   Differential vulnerabilities: how both of the above, over the course of life, affect one's physical susceptibility to disease.
4   Differential consequences: how being sick affects one's social stratification via impacts on employment and income; and the degree to which access to health services or other ameliorating social programmes or benefits (the prerequisites to health or capabilities) is commensurate with need (adapted from Diderichsen *et al.* 2001).

The veracity of these social pathways of health inequities has been codified in recent years in the epidemiological construct of 'the gradient': in most societies, for most measures of social stratification, for most diseases and certainly for life expectancy, there is a clear step-wise increase in morbidity and mortality as one slides down the hierarchy. Materialist, psychosocial and behavioural theories, in turn, have competed to explain this phenomenon, the first claiming a lack of sufficient material resources or control over one's environment for well-being (akin to the absolute poverty thesis), the second arguing that negative social comparison and loss of perceived control or self-worth underpins part of the difference (akin to the relative poverty thesis), and the third relating both to unhealthy behavioural adaptations (e.g., smoking, addiction, obesity). Increasingly, these three dominant explanatory models are seen as interrelated rather than separate (Marmot 2006) but limitations in their critical unpacking persist – that smoking is more common among lower social classes (at least in high-income countries) should not lead us to ask only how social class increases the risk of smoking; we need also to ask how societies and their economies create and stratify people by social class (Labonte 1997). Or, as another example, debate persists – though less vigorously than ten or twenty years ago – over the reverse causality problem. Does poverty make people sick, or does sickness create poverty? Framed uncritically as such, the question ignores the fact that social organisation creates both outcomes – sickness-inducing poverty (whether measured absolutely or relatively) and poverty-inducing sickness (through lack of equitable access to tax-funded ameliorative services, including income replacement or other forms of social protection when needed).

From describing to understanding

Each of these four pathways of social difference (in stratification, exposure, vulnerability and consequences) by which health inequities are created and maintained imply different forms of intervention. Each of the chapters in this part speaks to these implications, often focusing on the persisting need for new knowledge/research. We use the heuristic of three simple hypotheses as means to introduce the chapters that follow.

Social ordering of health status across time and in multiple societies provides critical insights about how human health is determined

Consistent with the imperative to reduce social inequalities and resulting health inequities, this field of research has focused much-needed policy attention on the nature of health gradients by socioeconomic status. It has also forcefully demonstrated how social factors influence our health, via processes that are mediated by high-level physiological regulatory systems in our bodies. Thus, these phenomena provide important insights into understanding windows of vulnerability to exposures, particularly affecting specific segments of the population. Much of this thinking has been arrived at through longitudinal studies over the life-course, conducted in developed country contexts.

As Mickey Chopra in his chapter points out, however, research into what produces health inequities in developing countries has been eclipsed by the persistence of the burden of infectious, nutrition- and reproductive-related disease largely explained by absolute poverty, and exacerbated by profound environmental hazards. This field of enquiry has also been limited by the paucity of high-quality health and healthcare data available in developing countries and routinely collected over time. Chopra makes a compelling case for why the study of inequities in health must be pursued, in spite of the logistical barriers faced in collecting data in resource-poor contexts, in order to highlight the social, structural and other factors at the root cause of these inequalities. Continuous public exposure of these explanatory contextual factors has the potential to provide some of the necessary evidence for policy and political action systematically to address the plight of the poor. As noted at the outset, knowledge about how societies create health inequities is not new; but the policy prescription to remedy them grates against the interests of those who benefit by sitting atop the social hierarchies. They need continuous recreation bolstered by social activism. Chopra also goes on to explain that the description of the multi-pathway causes of inequities, while critical, is insufficient to inform the needs of policy-makers even once they have been made to listen. More emphasis must therefore be placed – not only in developing countries but globally – on the study of the effectiveness of interventions to reduce inequities, at both the population level and the community level. Greater investment into the study of multi-level interventions would be further enabled by the use of mixed methods, participatory approaches to working with communities and the engagement of multiple disciplines – social scientists, social policy experts, epidemiologists, political scientists, and so on. (The importance of intervention research and what a critical stance on its undertaking implies for practitioners is the topic of this book's next part.)

Social environments – the places in which we live, work, play and learn – help to determine our health through social and economic structures across the life-course

Social environments operate at the individual, family, household, neighbourhood, community, region, society or nation-state level, and are influenced by policy and programmes intended to improve the quality of these environments as well as those with the opposite effects. Population and public health research needs to be geared towards a multi-level understanding of these environments, their relative contributions and the interactions between them, in terms of human health. As Sally Zierler and Nancy Krieger's chapter notes, a critical approach to understanding the social context through the lenses of multiple conceptual frameworks is essential to tracing the pathways to social inequalities for such risks as HIV infection among poor women in both rich and poor countries. Such an approach not only probes root causes more deeply; it is fundamentally concerned with the social practices of power and how these practices (political, economic, cultural, gendered) work to stratify individuals into hierarchies, and so stratify their risk, vulnerability and access to resources for health and well-being. While the data in this chapter is not current (an inevitability when living through a pandemic of the scale and pace of HIV), the authors' thoughtful analysis exemplifies an analytic approach to examining empirical findings in the light of social theories of stratification and exclusion that, in turn, create disease risk and vulnerability. It is this location of descriptive health inequities within analytical social theories that sets a critical public health approach apart from its more conventional practice. That conventional practice, however, continues to predominate – a gap analysis of income and health research in Canada found that fully two-thirds of 241 recently published studies failed to offer any model or theory of why income should be correlated with poorer health outcomes, much less why income inequalities exist in the first place (Raphael *et al.* 2005).

The extent of inequalities in income / wealth / education and political power may affect the overall average level of health in a society, beyond individual personal characteristics and 'lifestyle choices' influencing health

The study of income inequality, characterised through comparative analyses of whole societies, has been a current thrust in population and public health research, replacing decades of earlier concern with income poverty. Some have also turned their attention to whether and how social capital and other proposed correlates of the social distribution of income and wealth equality help to determine overall health status. Such psychosocial constructs as social capital have emerged to help characterise the ties between individuals, communities and social networks, and their links to health. More recent applications of social capital in public health suggest that the construct is being used alternatively to explain much of what has been attributed to economically redistributive policies and party politics. The record decline in health status in the former Soviet Union, for example, is sometimes attributed more to the absence of social capital that was the fault of command-control state centrism to engender the bonds of reciprocity and trust within civil society relations than to the adoption of unfettered market capitalism and the consequent collapse of social programmes and huge surge in poverty and inequality.

As Carles Muntaner, John Lynch and George Davey Smith aptly point out in their contribution, this misappropriated application of the 'social capital' concept comes at the expense of explicating what actually produces structural inequalities in whole societies. Other discerning critics have also concluded that the misuse of the 'social capital' concept in public health has led to a measurement of all that is good in a community, thereby consolidating the cultural, economic and political dimensions of community under one unwieldy and anodyne construct. Without proper interrogation through various sociological and economic lenses, issues of class, race, gender and other determinants fail to be properly elucidated in terms of their impacts on health inequalities. Further, as the authors state, communities which lose social capital may be seen as agents of their own demise, which leads to blaming the community (or, in the case of the former Soviet Union, its political system). Finally, political institutions may actually be further exacerbating health inequalities by their neoliberal policy-making, and by devolving responsibility from an already weakened state to the community, in the name of 'strengthening social capital'. Their assertions are a cautionary tale about the need to be critical in applying social theory to public health research. The task at hand is to explore and measure further what characterises these connections between individuals and groups, and how these connections among people have the potential to influence population health outcomes. That said, the authors conclude that the opportunity conferred by current attention on social capital in public health is to 'integrate sociology and economics' further to inform the study of socially produced inequalities in health.

One of these authors takes up that challenge in a later article in *Critical Public Health*, in which Carles Muntaner and his colleague Marisela Gomez examine how social capital (a term they adopt only by popular usage, preferring the concepts of social cohesion or integration) affects the relationship between urban redevelopment and neighbourhood health in an American city (Gomez and Muntaner 2005). Their study is notable for its emphasis on 'institutional social capital' in contrast to 'communitarian social capital'. The latter represents the networks of relationships (and their study) that are presumed to exist independent of class, caste, structure or state. The former, however, draws attention to the 'politics and power of the community or civil society in negotiating its demands with the local government and private institutions within a framework of government intervention' (Gomez and Muntaner 2005: 86). Stated simply, social capital – the structure and nature of social networks – is embedded within the structure and nature of social power relations. This later study is also exemplary for its application of mixed methods, in which administrative health data is combined with interviews, focus groups, surveys and in-depth key informant interviews to present a data-rich portrait of how strong 'bonding' and 'bridging' forms of social capital between select community leaders, private developers and local government had the effect of weakening these forms of social capital among other people in the community.

This weakening is also an artefact of the capture of ever more of the economic gains by an ever diminishing number of elites, at least in the more market-driven Anglo-American capitalist countries. In the words of Canadian health economist Bob Evans (2006: 14),

> income has since 1980 been increasingly concentrated in the hands of the top 0.01% of earners – a sort of corporate kleptocracy . . . Most of these top earners have seen the greatest gains in productivity over this time. The resources and political influence of the super-rich underlie the growing prominence of the 'elite' agenda: lower taxes, smaller government and privatization or shrinkage of social programmes. The marketing of this agenda may explain much of the nonsense that contaminates health policy debates.

This nonsense is grist for David Whiteis' exploration of how political and economic policies favour corporate power at the peril of the socially and politically marginalised. His depiction of disenfranchised citizens in the USA who are not able to leave the 'rotting cores' of inner cities – the product of diminishing tax bases, persistent racial and economic segregation, among other factors – calls for greater emphasis in the public discourse on the pathogenic impact of such political and economic policies. These 'upstream' political, social, cultural, economic and technological forces (which are inherently global in nature, as Part III of this book points out) have contributed to patterns of exploitation by the corporate sector to seek out new markets, resulting in affordable-housing shortages, a lack of investment in social, health and healthcare services, the displacement of employment opportunities and ultimately urban neighbourhood declines. According to Whiteis, explicitly linking economic injustice, public health and the privatisation of public services can serve to expose the perverse corporate interests that are being promulgated on the backs of society's most vulnerable. Economic and social justice must be central to health policy if we are to tackle the public health problems affecting the poor in our cities.

In summary, a vast body of interdisciplinary literature has accumulated over recent decades in an effort to characterise what produces inequities in health within and between countries. Most research has not sought, however, to generate the kind of policy and practice evidence to inform how best to reduce these inequities practically. In some instances, the lack of political will has been the root cause of ignoring useful evidence on what *can* reduce inequities in specific segments of the population. The authors in Part I have attempted to probe 'beneath the water line' of what the data and discourse of their time and place reveal, in more generalised fashion, about the power and practices that give rise to these challenges. This is what sets a critical public health approach apart from the more conventional (though still important) descriptive and monitoring functions of public health. In simple terms, a critical approach continues to probe 'the causes of the causes', as the WHO Commission on the Social Determinants of Health (Solar and Irwin 2005) recently expresses. Robust epidemiological and policy evidence must be complemented by concerted and effective political action in the name of social and economic justice if we are ever to tackle global inequalities in health effectively. The world's most disadvantaged populations deserve no less.

References

Anand, S. and Peter, F. (2004) 'Introduction', in S. Anand, F. Peter and A. Sen (eds), *Public Health, Ethics, and Equity*, New York: Oxford University Press.

Anderson, E. and O'Neil, T. (2006) *A New Equity Agenda? Reflections on the 2006 World Development Report, the 2005 Human Development Report and the 2005 Report on the World Social Situation* (Rep. No. 265), London: Overseas Development Institute.

Diderichsen, F., Evans, T. and Whitehead, M. (2001) 'The social basis of disparities in health', in M. Whitehead, T. Evans, F. Diderichsen, A. Bhuiya and M. Wirth (eds), *Challenging Inequities in Health: From Ethics to Action*, New York: Oxford University Press.

Evans, Robert G. (2006) 'From world war to class war: the rebound of the rich', *Healthcare Policy/Politiques de santé*, 2(1): 14–24.

Gomez, M.B. and Muntaner, C. (2005) 'Urban redevelopment and neighbourhood health in East Baltimore, Maryland: the role of communitarian and institutional social capital', *Critical Public Health*, 15: 83–102.

Hart, J.T. (1971) 'The inverse care law', *Lancet*, 1: 405–12.

Hunt, P., Nowak, M. and Osmani, S. (2002) *Draft Guidelines: A Human Rights Approach to Poverty Reduction Strategies*, Geneva: United Nations Office of the High Commissioner for Human Rights.

Labonte, R. (1997) 'The population health/health promotion debate in Canada: the politics of explanation, economics and action', *Critical Public Health*, 7: 7–27.

Marmot, M. (2006) 'Health in an unequal world', *Lancet*, 368: 2081–94.

Nussbaum, M. (1992) 'Human functioning and social justice: in defense of Aristotelian Essentialism', *Political Theory*, 29: 202–46.

——— (2000) *Women and Human Development: The Capabilities Approach*, Cambridge: Cambridge University Press.

Pogge, T.W. (2004) 'Relational conceptions of justice: responsibilities for health outcomes', in S. Anand, F. Peter and A. Sen (eds), *Public Health, Ethics, and Equity*, New York: Oxford University Press.

Raphael, D., Macdonald, J., Colman, R., Labonte, R., Hayward, K. and Torgerson, R. (2005) 'Researching income and income distribution as determinants of health in Canada: gaps between theoretical knowledge, research practice, and policy implementation', *Health Policy*, 72: 217–32.

Ruger, J.P. (2006) 'Ethics and governance of global health inequalities', *Journal of Epidemiology and Community Health*, 60: 998–1002.

Sen, A. (1999) *Development as Freedom*, Oxford: Oxford University Press.

Solar, O. and Irwin, A. (2005) *Towards a Conceptual Framework for Analysis and Action on the Social Determinants of Health: Discussion Paper for the Commission on Social Determinants of Health*, Geneva: World Health Organization.

Woodward, D. and Simms, A. (2006) *Growth Is Failing the Poor: The Unbalanced Distribution of the Benefits and Costs of Global Economic Growth* (Rep. No. 20), New York: United Nations Department of Economic and Social Affairs.

World Health Organization (2000) *World Health Report 2000: Health Systems*, Geneva: World Health Organization.

1 Inequalities in health in developing countries

Challenges for public health research[1]

Mickey Chopra

Introduction

There has been a significant increase in research and commentary on inequalities in health in the last two decades (Kennedy *et al.* 1998; Whitehead 1988; Wilkinson 1996). However, in the main, this has been restricted to the more developed countries. This is partly due to the continuing importance of the burden of disease caused by absolute poverty in developing countries. But research in these countries is also hampered by the lack of good-quality routine data on health status or healthcare disparities between different socioeconomic or ethnic groups. This is often exacerbated by the paucity of historical data, or well-established longitudinal survey data, to compare changes over time. This chapter will state the case for more systematic research and policy attention to be given to differences in health status between different social groups within developing countries. It will then go on to identify some of the approaches researchers in these countries could take in trying to provide evidence to inform policy interventions in light of the information constraints they face.

Why should we care about health inequalities in developing countries? First, there is increasing evidence that there are wide gaps in accessing healthcare and health outcomes between different social and income groups within poorer countries. Even in middle-income countries such as Mexico differences of up to nine years in life expectancy have been observed between rich and poor counties (Lozano *et al.* 2001). In these countries there is also alarming evidence that non-communicable diseases, which have traditionally been associated with growing affluence, are impacting most among the poorer sections of society. For example, in Brazil obesity among the poor and middle class far exceeds that among the rich (Monteiro *et al.* 2000). There is also good evidence that inequalities are increasing with the impact of globalisation (United Nations Development Programme 1997). This has been exacerbated in many poor countries by structural adjustment programmes that have included reducing public spending, reductions in import tariffs, depreciation of currencies and introduction of user fees that have discriminated against the poorest. In the Congo, for instance, the 1994 devaluation, prescribed by its adjustment programme, resulted in increasing food prices and a subsequent negative impact on the nutritional status of the poorest children (Martin-Prevel *et al.* 2000).

Second, there is a greater recognition of the economic rationale for improving the health of all members of society. This is happening not only at a conceptual level through the work of Nobel prize-winner Amartya Sen's work (Sen 1999) but through accumulating empirical work measuring the increased productivity of better-nourished and healthy workers. For example, one econometric study has estimated that approximately half of the economic growth achieved by the UK and a number of Western European countries between 1790 and 1980 was attributable to better nutrition and improved health and sanitation conditions and health investments (Fogel 1994).

Third, on more pragmatic health grounds, the universal presence of poorer workers in rich households, such as nannies, cleaners, gardeners, etc., in most poor countries is a potent reminder of the pathways of uncontrolled infectious diseases from the poor to the rich.

Finally, a holistic approach to the study of causes of inequality can expose the underlying structural factors that lead to a more radical approach towards addressing the needs of the poor.

Tackling health inequalities is obviously an ambitious task. This is especially so at a time when the policy options for national policy-makers are being increasingly narrowed by further integration into the global economic system and the need to abide by the rules and regulations of global trade organisations (Chopra 2002). A critical challenge for public health researchers in developing countries is therefore to provide policy-makers with relevant information that will assist them to make appropriate policy decisions to reduce the wide disparities in health and to evaluate such policy measures. This requires different types of evidence and studies, as outlined below.

Description of health inequality

There is a long history of descriptions of inequalities in health. Starting with crude estimates of differences in mortality between different spatial groups, descriptive studies have now moved on to measuring the distribution of health outcomes by household income, race/ethnicity and gender (Kennedy *et al.* 1998). Obviously limitations with the quality of routine data make this a more difficult task in poorer countries, but that should not deter efforts to improve or establish good-quality routine information systems. Nevertheless, in nearly all settings it is possible to use existing survey data.

International surveys such as the Living Standards Measurement Survey and Demographic Health Survey have allowed researchers to capture inequalities in child health and nutritional status by socioeconomic status for many low-income countries (Wagstaff 2000; Wagstaff and Watanabe 2000). The lack of direct information concerning income in some of these surveys can be circumvented through the use of measurements of key assets, items of expenditure and/or household types to classify households in different socioeconomic strata (Gwatkin 2001). For example, this approach has been used to show inequalities in malnutrition and incidence of diarrhoea and acute respiratory infections by wealth in many low-income countries (Gwatkin *et al.* 2000). These findings can be used by groups to advocate for greater equity in resource distribution. Descriptive data can also be used to show policy-makers that health inequities are reversible and suggest policy interventions. For instance, health inequalities between different socioeconomic groups in Sweden had almost disappeared by the mid-1960s (Whitehead *et al.* 2000). Whitehead *et al.* (2000) have also compared changes in health inequalities between Sweden and the UK over the last twenty years and shown the effect that Swedish welfare policies have in ameliorating increases in inequity.

The Rockefeller Foundation and the Swedish International Development Agency (SIDA) have recently launched an international 'equity gauge' project that is focusing upon building capacity within countries to use descriptions of health and healthcare inequity for advocacy and increased community participation in policy-making (GEGA 2003).

Explanatory studies

While descriptive studies play an important role in uncovering inequalities and demonstrating that inequality can be reduced, they do not provide enough information to inform policy-makers fully about the mechanisms through which economic inequalities affect health and hence suggest effective interventions. Gwatkin (2001: 722) puts this forcefully:

> This is a notable missing element in the work recently undertaken by epidemi-ologists and other researchers increasingly concerned with health equity and the health of the poor. The work to date has produced significant increases in knowledge about the magnitude and nature of health inequalities, and has resulted in valuable conceptual frameworks for approaching these issues. But it has not yet reached the heart of the matter: the identification of measures that can effectively deal with the inequalities that have been uncovered.

For this we must move on to either intervention studies or more sophisticated study designs that offer possible causal explanations.

Intervention studies provide the most compelling evidence for policy-makers. However, there is scant evidence of interventions that reduce inequalities on a large scale (Macintyre *et al.* 2001). This is partly because the optimal design for intervention studies is the randomised control trial. This sort of trial is suited to interventions that focus upon modifying individual risk behaviour such as cigarette smoking or changing diet. There is little evidence that such interventions are effective at a population level, especially for individuals from poor or disadvantaged backgrounds. This should not undermine the importance of evaluating interventions in a rigorous manner and of using an evidence-based approach in designing interventions. With greater foresight and advocacy, public health researchers can integrate rigorous evaluation designs, such as plausibility (Habicht *et al.* 1999) and randomised control designs, when new large-scale policies are being introduced (Macintyre 2003). Presently there are too few of these intervention studies, especially in middle- and low-income countries, for policy-makers to be able to design a comprehensive approach towards tackling inequalities in health. To compensate we must turn to research that attempts to show the consistent relationships between different factors and inequalities in health outcomes. If it can be established that these relationships are causal in nature then there is a basis for interventions to be designed.

Numerous conceptual frameworks that situate the various factors contributing to health inequalities have been developed (Whitehead *et al.* 2001). Most attention has been paid to the proximal factors, such as risky behaviours or public health service utilisation and provision. However, greater attention is now being paid to broader determinants, such as the environment, class and social factors (Berkman *et al.* 2000). But too often these are conceived as 'noise' in the analysis of individual factors that must be controlled for, and so they are usually either not measured or neutralised during the analysis phase (Krieger 2000). Graham (2001: 231) has pointed out that there is now a need to 'join up' epidemiological research on individual factors with sociological research that explores the wider changes in society: 'health is fashioned by: risk exposures across the life course within pathways shaped by the broader changes in the social-economic structure'.

Understanding the impact of the broader social structure on health and health inequities requires the incorporation of insights from such social sciences as sociology and social policy studies. The challenge for researchers is to highlight the multiple pathways that lead to health inequalities – participatory and qualitative method-ologies can play an important role, especially in low- and middle-income countries.

Clustering of risk factors

There is an accumulation of health hazards and risk factors for those in less advantaged socioeconomic groups, so that, for example, the people who live in the poorest housing and have the least safe working conditions are also the people who have the greatest risk of unemployment and have restricted access to healthcare when ill.

For example, in South Africa, black children growing up in rural areas are eight times less likely to have access to either a flush toilet or latrines and four times less likely to have access to tap water than their urban counterparts; and they are twice as likely to be malnourished (Labadarios 2000). Poorer people are also almost fifteen times more likely to be exposed to smoky domestic fuels (Bradshaw and Steyn 2001) and more likely to be the victims of road accidents, being shot dead or dying as a result of domestic violence in South Africa (Bradshaw *et al.* 2003).

Qualitative research can provide insights into the linkages that produce systematic differentials in exposure to health hazards and risk conditions in the population. An analysis of transport statistics combined with interviews with various role-players allowed researchers in Kenya to reveal the connections between the unregulated matatu (bus) system, the struggle for livelihoods of the drivers and the pervasive corruption among traffic officials all leading to far greater road traffic mortality among poorer people who have to use the matatu or travel as pedestrians (Nantulya and Muli-Musiime 2001).

Risky behaviour

Not only are poorer groups exposed to a greater number of risk factors, but they also tend to adopt more health-damaging behaviour in terms of smoking, diet, lack of exercise in leisure time, and lower uptake of preventive healthcare services. For example, in South Africa, men in the poorest quintile of the population are two and half times more likely to be smokers than those in the richest quintile and nearly twice as likely to be alcohol dependent (Bradshaw and Steyn 2001). Jha *et al.* (2002) report a similar gradient for smoking in other low-income countries. Understanding the reasons for this is important for designing interventions. Studies have pointed to the barriers and constraints that poor socioeconomic conditions place on the choice of a healthier way of life. Careful qualitative research, for instance, has been carried out to increase understanding of why poor people continue to smoke and in so doing drain their financial resources still further. Low-income mothers in the UK have been found to use smoking to cope with the highly stressful conditions associated with caring for children in hardship. Having a cigarette may be the only accepted reason for taking a voluntary break from monotonous working conditions (Wakefield *et al.* 1993). Exploratory research in Cape Town strongly suggests that lack of money restricts food choice, with women selecting high-calorie, fatty foods that are cheaply available locally (Thandi Puoane, personal communication with author).

Healthcare provision and utilisation

Using a relatively simple measure of wealth, Schellenberg *et al.* (2003) were able to tabulate the findings on health status and service use by socioeconomic quintile in Tanzania. They show that even in an apparently homogeneously poor rural area there are socioeconomic differences in health status and that the main difference between the more and less poor in health is not in the likelihood of being ill but in the access to adequate treatment once ill. This is in keeping with other studies in Africa that have found access to health services to be a key difference between different socioeconomic groups (Gwatkin *et al.* 2000; Filmer 2002). Once again the 'inverse care law', first described by Tudor Hart (2000) in the UK, is at work with those with higher socioeconomic and health status accessing greater public healthcare resources. Victora *et al.* (2000) have recently taken this further in Brazil and suggested that new technologies are also preferentially taken up in areas with higher socio-economic status. A study of over forty countries reports that even those interventions generally thought to be especially 'pro-poor', such as oral rehydration therapy and immunisation, tend to attain better coverage among better-off groups than among disadvantaged ones (Gwatkin *et al.* 2000). The failure of health services to reach the poor in developing countries, despite their higher disease burden, is not just a matter of the better-off using their higher incomes to purchase care from the private sector. Poor people also benefit less from government subsidies to the health sector. For example, in Indonesia in 1990 only 12 per cent of government health expenditure was used by the poorest 20 per cent, while the richest 20 per cent consumed 29 per cent of government funding in the health sector (World Bank 1993).

Structural and temporal changes

While this is important information, it is still restricted to individual risk factors. The limitations of such an approach are illustrated by a WHO technical report, *Confronting the Tobacco Epidemic in an Era of Trade Liberalisation* (2001). Using a broad range of data, the report demonstrated a positive relationship between trade liberalisation and tobacco consumption, with the greatest correlation in low-income countries. Thus, the availability of cheaper cigarettes, intensive marketing and increased availability all play important roles in influencing consumption. A similar case has been made against the actions of multinational food companies and the aggressive promotion of refined high-fat foods in developing countries (Chopra *et al.* 2002). To design effective and comprehensive policies therefore requires that the structural and temporal influences on health are more explicitly studied.

Researchers in the UK and Scandinavia are beginning to use longitudinal studies from the 1950s to illustrate the pathways that lead to the accumulation and reproduction of poor health and poverty. For example, findings from the 1958 National Child Development Survey in the UK show that the lives of those born in the lower economic classes are characterised by low educational qualifications, unemployment, redundancy and receipt of means-tested benefits (Power *et al.* 2002). They tend to become parents earlier and, in the case of women, have an increased chance of being a single parent. These domestic pathways interact with the economic pathways, with early parenthood more likely to lead to earlier cessation of education and restrictions in employment. Unfortunately, such longitudinal studies are rare in developing countries. However, qualitative life histories provide powerful illustrations of similar pathways. These can be supported by smaller panel studies and relationships found in cross-sectional surveys. For example, here is a quote from a woman living in rural South Africa:

> I had my first baby when I was at school, I was quite glad actually because it made me a real woman and I got some respect from my friends . . . the principal would not let me back into school and so I did not finish my studies . . . I work three days a week as a domestic . . . it's OK work but not what I really wanted to do.
>
> (Quoted in Chopra and Ross 1995: 21)

Analysis of the South African Demographic and Health Survey shows that the commonest reason for young black women to drop out of school early was pregnancy, with more than a third becoming pregnant before completing schooling (Nadine Nannan, personal communication with author).

This illumination of the socioeconomic determinants of the life-course helps to contextualise epidemiological analyses. We are now in a better position to understand how health inequalities are reproduced over time and across generations. Being born into poverty brings with it exposure to the health effects of disadvantage, transmitted *in utero* and in the early years of life. This is compounded by circumstances that set children on educational pathways which direct them onto (un)employment trajectories in adulthood, which bring further exposure to health risks in later life (Graham 2002).

However, a research paradigm that just focuses upon the health consequences and the social determinants of life-course disadvantage is insufficient in the present context, in which many middle- and low-income countries are undergoing rapid social and economic change. Globalisation is leading to significant changes in occupational and social structure in nearly all developing countries. A defining feature seems to be an acceleration of the gap between rich and poor. This, along with increasing absolute levels of poverty, is leading to a breakdown of social structure and cohesion in many communities, especially in rapidly urbanising centres. Once again testimonies from the poor can illustrate the ways in which changes in the economy and society are widening inequities and destroying social cohesion, and can provide powerful evidence to policy-makers. In-depth qualitative case studies have allowed Ramphele (2002) to paint a rich picture of the family and community stresses and strains that the rapid changes accompanying the demise of apartheid are having in Cape Town. Here is another example, from an old man in Uganda:

> Poverty has always been with us in our communities. It was there in the past, long before Europeans came, and it affected many – perhaps all of us. But it was a different type of poverty. People were not helpless. They acted together and never allowed it to 'squeeze' any member of the community. They shared a lot of things together: hunting, grazing animals, harvesting, etc. There was enough for basic survival. But now things have changed. Each person is on their own. A few people who have acquired material wealth are very scared of sliding back into poverty. They do not want to look like us. So they acquire more land, marry more wives, and take all the young men to work for them on their farms and factories distilling gin. So we are left to fight this poverty ourselves. And yet we only understand a little of it. It is only its effects that we can see. The causes we cannot grasp.
>
> (Quoted in World Bank 2000: 64)

This sense of being caught in a maelstrom of change without being able to comprehend the forces behind such changes has historical and contemporary parallels from industrialising Europe in the nineteenth century and Eastern Europe in the last decade. Historical research from Sweden suggests that during similar periods of rapid transition and urbanisation it was young men who bore the brunt of feelings of alienation, distrust and hopelessness, with large increases in mortality that continued many decades after female and child mortality began to decline (Sundin and Willner 2004). This often manifested itself in increased alcohol consumption related to increases in violence and crime and a general breakdown in what has been called 'social cohesion' (Berkman 2000). Similar experiences are being reported from Russia (Walberg *et al.* 1998). Male life expectancy has fallen dramatically in many sub-Saharan countries chiefly as a result of the HIV/AIDS epidemic but also due to increasing levels of violence and trauma. Researchers are beginning to trace the links between these epidemics and a breakdown in trust and cohesion in these societies (Barnett *et al.* 2000).

Conclusion

Inequalities in health have important implications for overall well-being even in low- and middle-income countries. The paucity of reliable routine data should encourage public health researchers in these countries to stretch their methodological imagination to include qualitative insights. Such an approach should facilitate a more probing investigation that moves beyond describing inequalities and begins to describe how they are produced and reproduced.

Note

1   This chapter was first published in *Critical Public Health* (2005) 15: 19–26.

References

Barnett, T., Whiteside, A. and Decosas, J. (2000) 'The Jaipur paradigm: a conceptual framework for understanding social susceptibility and vulnerability to HIV', *South African Medical Journal*, 90: 1098–101.

Berkman, L.F. (2000) 'Social support, social networks, social cohesion and health', *Social Work and Health Care*, 31: 3–14.

Berkman, L.F., Glass, T., Brissette, I. and Seeman, T.E. (2000) 'From social integration to health: Durkheim in the new millennium', *Social Science and Medicine*, 51: 843–57.

Bradshaw, D., Groenewald, P., Laubscher, R., Nannan, N., Nojilana, B., Norman R. *et al.* (2003) *Initial Burden of Disease Estimates for South Africa*, Cape Town: South African Medical Research Council.

Bradshaw, D. and Steyn, K. (2001) *Poverty and Chronic Diseases*, Cape Town: Medical Research Council.

Chopra, M. (2002) *Diet and Globalisation*, Geneva: World Health Organization.

Chopra, M., Galbraith, S. and Darnton-Hill, I. (2002) 'A global response to a global problem: the epidemic of overnutrition', *Bulletin of the World Health Organization*, 80: 952–8.

Chopra, M. and Ross, F. (1995) *Perceptions of Causes of Undernutrition in Rural South Africa*, Durban: Health Systems Trust.

Filmer, D. (2002) *Fever and Its Treatment among the More and Less Poor in Sub-Saharan Africa*, World Bank Development Economics Research Group Working Paper No. 2789, Washington, DC: World Bank.

Fogel, R.W. (1994) 'Economic growth, population theory and physiology: the bearing of long-term processes on the making of economic policy', *American Economic Review*, 84: 369–95.

GEGA (2003) Available at: <http://www.gega.co.za> (accessed 3 February 2004).

Graham, H. (2001) 'Research into policy', in D. Leon and G. Walt (eds), *Poverty, Health and Inequality*, Oxford: Oxford University Press.

—— (2002) 'Building an inter-disciplinary science of health inequalities: the example of lifecourse research', *Social Science and Medicine*, 55: 2005–16.

Gwatkin, D., Rutstein, S., Johnson, K., Pande, R. and Wagstaff, A. (2000) *Socioeconomic Differences in Health, Nutrition and Population*, Washington, DC: World Bank.

Gwatkin, D.R. (2001) 'The need for equity-oriented health reforms', *International Journal of Epidemiology*, 30: 720–3.

Habicht, J.P., Victora, C.G. and Vaughan, J.P. (1999) 'Evaluation designs for adequacy, plausibility and probability of public health programme performance and impact', *International Journal of Epidemiology*, 28: 10–18.

Jha, P., Ranson, M.K., Nguyen, S.N. and Yach, D. (2002) 'Estimates of global and regional smoking prevalence in 1995, by age and sex', *American Journal of Public Health*, 92: 1002–6.

Kennedy, B.P., Kawachi, I., Prothrow-Smith, D., Lochner, K. and Gupta, V. (1998) 'Social capital, income inequality, and firearm violent crime', *Social Science and Medicine*, 47: 7–17.

Krieger, N. (2000) 'Epidemiology and social sciences: towards a critical reengagement in the 21st century', *Epidemiologic Reviews*, 22: 155–63.

Labadarios, D. (2000) *The National Food Consumption Survey: Children aged 1–9 Years in South Africa, 1999*, Pretoria: Department of Health.

Lozano, R., Zurita, B., Franco, F., Ramirez, T., Hernandez, P. and Torres, J.L. (2001) 'Mexico: marginality, need and resource allocation at the county level', in T. Evans, M. Whitehead, F. Diderischen, A. Bhuiya and M. Wirth (eds), *Challenging Inequities in Health: From Ethics to Action*, London: Oxford University Press.

Macintyre, S. (2003) 'Evidence based policy making', *British Medical Journal*, 326: 5–6.

Macintyre, S., Chalmers, I., Horton, R. and Smith, R. (2001) 'Using evidence to inform health policy: case study', *British Medical Journal*, 322: 222–5.

Martin-Prevel, Y., Delpeuch, F., Traissac, P., Massamba, J.P., Adoua-Oyila, G., Coudert, K. *et al.* (2000) 'Deterioration in the nutritional status of young children and their mothers in Brazzaville, Congo, following the 1994 devaluation of the CFA franc', *Bulletin of the World Health Organization*, 78: 108–18.

Monteiro, C.A., Benicio, M.H., Mondini, L. and Popkin, B.M. (2000) 'Shifting obesity trends in Brazil', *European Journal of Clinical Nutrition*, 54: 342–6.

Nantulya, K. and Muli-Musiime, F. (2001) 'Explaining differences in road traffic accidents in Kenya', in T. Evans, M. Whitehead and F. Diderichsen (eds), *Challenging Inequities in Health: From Ethics to Action*, London: Oxford University Press.

Power, C., Stansfeld, S.A., Matthews, S., Manor, O. and Hope, S. (2002) 'Childhood and adulthood risk factors for socio-economic differentials in psychological distress: evidence from the 1958 British birth cohort', *Social Science and Medicine*, 55: 1989–2004.

Ramphele, M. (2002) *Steering by the Stars: Being Young in South Africa*, Cape Town: Tafelberg.

Schellenberg, J.A., Victora, C.G., Mushi, A., de Savigny, D., Schellenberg, D., Mshinda, H. *et al.* (2003) 'Tanzania Integrated Management of Childhood Illness MCE Baseline Household Survey Study Group: inequities among the very poor: health care for children in rural southern Tanzania', *Lancet*, 361: 561–6.

Sen, A. (1999) *Development as Freedom*, New York: New Anchor.

Sundin, J. and Willner, S. (2004) *Health and Social Transitions: A Comparative Perspective*, Linkoping: Linkoping University Press.

Tudor Hart, J. (2000) 'Commentary: three decades of the inverse care law', *British Medical Journal*, 320: 18–19.

United Nations Development Programme (1997) *Population Report*, New York: UNDP.

Victora, C.G., Vaughan, J.P., Barros, F.C., Silva, A.C. and Tomasi, E. (2000) 'Explaining trends in inequities: evidence from Brazilian child health studies', *Lancet*, 356: 1093–8.

Wagstaff, A. (2000) 'Socioeconomic inequalities in child mortality: comparisons across nine developing countries', *Bulletin of the World Health Organization*, 78: 19–29.

Wagstaff, A. and Watanabe, N. (2000) *Socioeconomic Inequalities in Child Malnutrition in the Developing World*, Policy Research Working Paper No. 2434, Washington, DC: World Bank.

Wakefield, M., Gillies, P., Graham, H., Madeley, R. and Symonds, M. (1993) 'Characteristics associated with smoking cessation during pregnancy among working class women', *Addiction*, 88: 1423–30.

Walberg, P., McKee, M., Shkolnikov, V., Chenet, L. and Leon, D.A. (1998) 'Economic change, crime, and mortality crisis in Russia: regional analysis', *British Medical Journal*, 317: 312–18.

Whitehead, M. (1988) *The Health Divide*, London: Pelican.

Whitehead, M., Dahlgren, G. and Gilson, L. (2001) 'Developing policy responses to inequities in health: a global perspective', in T. Evans, M. Whitehead and F. Diderichsen (eds), *Challenging Inequities in Health: From Ethics to Action*, London: Oxford University Press.

Whitehead, M., Diderichsen, F. and Burstrom, B. (2000) 'Researching the impact of public policy on inequalities in health', in H. Graham (ed.), *Understanding Health Inequalities*, Buckingham: Open University Press.

Wilkinson, R. (1996) *Unhealthy Societies: The Afflictions of Inequalities*, London and New York: Routledge.

World Bank (1993) *World Development Report 1993: Investing in Health*, Washington, DC: World Bank.

——— (2000) *Listening to the Voices of the Poor*, Washington, DC: World Bank.

World Health Organization (2001) *Confronting the Tobacco Epidemic in an Era of Trade Liberalization*, Technical Report, Geneva: WHO.

2 Social capital and the third way in public health[1]

Carles Muntaner, John Lynch and George Davey Smith

Within the last few years, we have witnessed the rapid appearance of the concept of social capital in public health discourse. Before 1995, there was only one reference to the term 'social capital' in the Medline database and that was in regard to so-called 'family social capital' and its effect on educational and occupational aspirations (Marjoribanks 1999). Though the basic ideas encapsulated in the current use of social capital can be traced to the origins of classical sociology and political science, the appearance of the term itself in the mid-1990s was largely stimulated by Robert Putnam's work on civic participation and its effect on local governance (Putnam *et al.* 1993). He popularised this thesis by discussing the decline of social capital using the metaphor that America was 'Bowling alone' (Putnam 1995a) – a powerful image that propelled Putnam to an audience with President Clinton to discuss the fraying of the social fabric in America. Since then, the concept of social capital has also appeared in other fields, such as sociology (Portes 1998) and development economics (Grootaert 1997; Ostrom 1999). In these fields, there has been a good deal of debate about the definition, operationalisation, and the theoretical and practical utility of the concept for improving human welfare, especially in regard to alleviating poverty and stimulating economic growth in less industrialised countries (Collier 1998; Knack and Keefer 1997). Despite all this activity, one of the leading scholars in this field, Michael Woolcock, has argued that the concept of social capital 'risks trying to explain too much with too little' (Woolcock 1998: 155).

Social capital and its use in public health

The term has also slipped effortlessly into the public health lexicon as if there were a clear, shared understanding of its meaning and its relevance for improving public health. The term social capital and its close cousin, social cohesion, have been used as multipurpose descriptors for all types and levels of connections among individuals, within families, friendship networks, businesses and communities (Wilkinson 1996; Aneshensel and Sucoff 1996; Kawachi and Kennedy 1997; Kawachi *et al.* 1997a, b; Fullilove 1998; Baum 1997, 1999; Kennedy *et al.* 1999). It has been the subject of theme conferences (11th National Health Promotion Conference, Perth, Australia); government-sponsored discussion papers (Jenson 1998; Lavis and Stoddart 1999);

million-dollar calls for research proposals funded by the Centers for Disease Control in the USA; and proposed as an important avenue of public health intervention.

But what do we measure when we say 'social capital?' Hawe and Shiell (2000) have commented that the health-related applications of social capital have often involved measuring 'all that is good in a community'. Conflating the political, cultural and economic aspects of a community under the single umbrella of social capital may mask important conceptual distinctions as to the origins of those group resources and may obscure the fact that these dimensions are not necessarily equally important as determinants of health. Under this kind of undifferentiated approach, establishing an arts festival (the cultural dimension) and a job creation programme (the economic dimension) are both interventions to improve social capital. Are they likely to have an equal impact on public health? This in no way denies the importance of improving the cultural life of a community through programmes of arts and music. The question is whether tossing all these dimensions into the grab bag of social capital can inform strategies to improve public health.

The reasons for the uncritical acceptance of social capital into public health discourse are of interest in themselves. Discussion of the concept comes from at least three main sources: from those concerned with community-based health promotion (Baum 1999; Cooper *et al.* 1999); from those in the social support field (Cooper *et al.* 1999; Tijhuis *et al.* 1995); and from those who have claimed that social capital and social cohesion are the main mediators of the link between income inequality and population health (Wilkinson 1996; Kawachi *et al.* 1997a, b). What links these three is that they are all motivated by the underlying idea that there is something about the connections among individuals that is important for public health. This idea is not new (see Rose 1985) and there have been many critiques of an overly individualistic approach to public health research and intervention (Krieger 1994; Lynch *et al.* 1997; Muntaner and O'Campo 1993). The concept and language of social capital have perhaps been seen as offering a new and exciting way to invigorate supra-individual public health research and to provide support for a non-individualised, social science approach to improving public health (Baum 1999).

Public health and the connections among individuals

The goal of moving beyond individualistic theory and practice in public health is laudable. Populations are not just unrelated heaps of individuals, whose patterns of connections can be ignored. However, overly simplistic interpretations of the pattern of connections among people may mask, not reveal, determinants of population health. For example, strong links among individuals can both increase and decrease the risk of certain health outcomes. Tight connections among infants in a day-care centre may increase their risk of otitis-media. In one context, strong friendship networks of peers can increase the risk of smoking, drinking or use of illicit drugs, while in a different situation similar links may decrease the risk of suicide. Tight networks among the Mafia, neo-Nazi parties, or semi-clandestine business organisations such as the Trilateral Commission, the WTO or GATT increase health risks for other members of the population. Scratch beyond a superficial level and the public health consequences of how individuals and groups are connected rapidly become very complicated.

We are advocates of the idea that the way individuals and groups connect to form friendship networks, neighbourhoods and communities can be important for public health. We are less convinced that the under-theorised concept of social capital, in its present form, can provide an adequate basis to understand how these connections may be linked to population health.

Theoretical differences with social science

> 'When I use a word', Humpty Dumpty said, in a rather scornful tone, 'it means just what I choose it to mean – neither more nor less'. 'The question is', said Alice, 'whether you can make words mean so many different things'. 'The question is', said Humpty Dumpty, 'which is to be the master – that's all'.
>
> (Lewis Carroll, *Alice through the Looking Glass*)

Because the scant empirical literature on social capital and health has been accompanied by enthusiastic expectations about social capital's future relevance to public health (Kawachi *et al.* 1997a, b; Marmot 1998; Mustard 1996), social capital often conveys the authoritarian arbitrariness of Alice's famous exchange with Humpty Dumpty. Powerful institutions, actors and funding agencies have a lot to say about what a concept means and what concepts are considered legitimate for empirical research (Muntaner *et al.* 1997; Muntaner 1999a, b; Wing 1998). Nevertheless, because public health is a science, and thus has adjacent disciplines, we can examine the compatibility of its social capital construct with regard to the social capital theories that have been developed in contiguous disciplines (e.g., sociology, demography and international development).

Almost exclusively, the construct of social capital adopted by public health researchers has been the most psychological, the communitarian view (Putnam *et al.* 1993). This conception emphasises civic engagement, as in membership in local non-governmental organisations, or norms of reciprocity and trust among community members. Communitarians, who often favour minimal government and self-reliance (Etzioni and George 1999), present their position as a 'third way' between laissez-faire neoliberalism and social democracy (Etzioni and George 1999), and have been supported by the New Labour and New Democrat administrations in the UK and USA (Muntaner and Lynch 1999a). The 'small government' communitarian view, with its emphasis on civic organisations (third sector, not-for-profit institutions, and non-governmental organisations), undermines not only government intervention in the social democratic European welfare state but political representation, since national class-based parties that strive for state control are substituted with idealised notions of small-scale political organising at the community level (Muntaner and Lynch 1999a). Social capital may thus function as a health policy alternative to large-scale government redistribution (i.e., dismantling or reducing the post-Second World War welfare state) (Wainwright 1996; Muntaner and Lynch 1999a).

In social epidemiology, social capital presents a model of the social determinants of health that does not include any analysis of structural inequalities (e.g., class, gender or racial relations) in favour of a horizontal view of social relations based on distributive inequalities in income (Muntaner and Lynch 1999b). As a consequence, class-, race- or gender-based political movements are also ignored as explanations for reducing social inequalities in health (Muntaner and Lynch 1999a).

In social science, in particular in sociology, demography and developmental economics, social capital has at least two other conceptualisations that have a larger theoretical content: one is that of network analysis (Granovetter 1973; Portes 1998; Woolcock 1998). This view of social capital acknowledges the existence of stratification as well as the negative effects of strong networks for communities (e.g., in Mafia 'families'). For example, Granovetter showed the differences in the networks of professionals and non-professionals – weak ties among professionals facilitate access to information about job opportunities. Portes showed the conditions under which strong networks among immigrants have facilitated the enrichment of ethnic businessmen in the USA. Another sociological approach to social capital emphasises the role of institutions, including the state. This institutional approach considers both a community's social capital – its internal cohesion, ties and networks – as well as the type of relation that the state has with it (Szreter 1999). This 'embeddedness' or institutional support dictates how the state cooperates with civil society to foster economic development via interaction between private and public institutions, legal and democratic systems, and citizen rights (Woolcock 1998). This notion of social capital is the more encompassing and allows the greater explanatory potential and integration with other sociological traditions in social epidemiology and public health (e.g., the study of the health effects of class, gender and race relations).

Idealist social psychology – 'Bowling with de Tocqueville' and other exaggerations

Social capital in public health is coined in terms of a lay/commonsense social psychology that has great appeal in the USA and elsewhere (Cooper *et al.* 1999; Baum 1999; Kawachi *et al.* 1997a). Who would oppose the notion that civic participation, trust in communities or good neighbourly relations are good for health? In the USA, the 'mom and apple pie' idea that good community relations are desirable is part of the collective wisdom among communitarians, liberals and social conservatives alike (Putnam 1995a, b; Etzioni and George 1999). But behind this conventional aspiration for achieving 'healthy communities' also lies an idealised view of past community life that is seldom warranted (Lynch and Kaplan 1997).

Rather, multiple local interest group associations (or social capital) may be seen as both potential barriers and supports to creating public policies aimed to improve population health. For example, the failure of creating a broad working-class political party capable of establishing a strong welfare state, including the lack of universal access to healthcare (Navarro 1994), has been a barrier to improvements in public health in the USA. Furthermore, a recent analysis of voter participation data in American cities *circa* 1880 lends no support to the social capital perspective whereby civic associations would have beneficial impact on broad-based political participation (Kaufman 1999). Rather, these analyses reveal that civic associations functioned as powerful interest groups that lobbied for specific party platforms that were not necessarily in the broader public interest.

Another inaccuracy of the received wisdom is the uncritical acceptance of Putnam's 'Bowling alone' thesis on the decline of social capital in the USA (Kawachi *et al.* 1997b; Kawachi and Kennedy 1997; Kawachi *et al.* 1999; Wilkinson *et al.* 1998a, b). The available evidence in the USA suggests that there has not been a decline in associations over the last two decades (Smith 1997; Paxton 1999). Furthermore, older forms of civic participation that have perhaps declined have been transformed over time (Skocpol 1999). In addition, Putnam's analysis of social capital as the key factor underlying economic development in several Italian regions (e.g., Emilia-Romagna) has also been challenged (e.g., the neglect of class relations or nineteenth century socialist and Catholic political traditions in the creation of contemporary social capital; Warren 1994). The notion that social capital drives political and economic performance has been refuted with new analyses of data from Italian regions and other industrial democracies (Jackman *et al.* 1996). Our overall point here is that the discourse around social capital in public health has tended to focus on its upside. We believe a more complete reading of the literature relevant to understanding the likely health effects of social capital reveals that the concept has been portrayed narrowly and has focused on more optimistic appraisals of its relevance to population health.

Communitarians of the world unite! Ignoring the class, gender and race structure

Given the scant support for the social capital hypotheses reviewed above, one would expect that policy-makers and researchers alike would be more sanguine in their approach to the subject. At least, some acknowledgement of alternative mechanisms driving the political, economic and health performance of nations (e.g., political movements and class relations) might be expected from objective scholars; especially since in other areas of social science, social capital has been integrated with research on social inequalities (e.g., class, gender and race: Gould 1993; Brines 1999; Erikson 1996; Muntaner *et al.* 1999; Persell *et al.* 1992; Zweigenhaft 1993; Borjas 1992; Pattillo 1998; Schneider *et al.* 1997). Unfortunately, in the enthusiastic entourage of social capital, this is not the case (e.g., Kawachi *et al.* 1997a) and with few exceptions the mostly communitarian approach to social capital in public health shies away from these mechanisms (Muntaner and Lynch 1999a, b).

Familiar health policy implications – 'the importance of subjectivity'

One implication of social capital in public health is the role of individual subjectivity in mediating the relation between inequality and health (Wilkinson 1996, 1999). The breakdown in social cohesion occurs because individuals perceive their relative position in the social distribution of income, which creates anxiety and other psycho-social injuries which, in turn, affect health (Wilkinson 1999). As no explanations for the causes of income inequalities are provided, this psychosocial mechanism becomes the central explanation of social cohesion models in public health (Muntaner and Lynch 1999b). The move towards psychosocial explanations of the effects of social cohesion is rather surprising, as just a few years ago the field of social inequalities in health was still materialist (Kaplan 1995). Even researchers who had been relatively sympathetic to such materialist explanations as social class and working conditions (Marmot and Theorell 1988) seem suddenly convinced by social capital/psychosocial environment explanations for health inequalities (Marmot 1998).

The culture of inequality mechanism underlying the social capital-health association is not, however, all that innovative. For example, the culture of poverty hypothesis popularised by Oscar Lewis (1998 [1963]) is strikingly similar to the social capital/social cohesion formulations by Wilkinson and colleagues, albeit more psychologically reductionist and 'victim blaming' than the latter (Muntaner and Lynch 1999a). The culture of poverty states that some poor communities bring poverty upon themselves because of few community ties and little community heritage (i.e., social capital). Perceptions and subjectivity are all important, as it is not objective inequalities that ultimately determine the well-being of populations but the subjective response to those inequalities.

Another of the implications of the social capital/social cohesion hypothesis for public health is that communities may be seen as responsible for their crime rates (Sampson *et al.* 1997) or aggregated health rates, an idea that nicely justifies the privatisation of health services, such as managed care (Stoto 1999). Another possible direction for public health may be that we take a step back from the structural sources of health inequalities – after all, if they are not an integral part of our theories of health inequalities and are so difficult to change, then perhaps an achievable alternative is to retreat to mass psychotherapy for the poor to change their perceptions of place in the social hierarchy (e.g., Proudfoot and Guest 1997). Again, this idea is not new. In the 1960s the functionalist sociologist Warner (1960) revealed his hopes for his book *Social Class in America*:

> The lives of many are destroyed because they do not understand the workings of social class. It is the hope of the authors that this book will provide a corrective instrument which will permit men and women better to evaluate their social situations and thereby better adapt themselves to social reality and fit their dreams and aspirations to what is possible.

Elsewhere, we have labelled this new set of public health implications associated with the idea of a loss of social capital 'blaming the community' (Muntaner and Lynch 1999a). The problem with subjectivity as an explanation for health inequalities is not only that it has little empirical support but that it may yield anti-egalitarian public health policies (Muntaner and Lynch 1999a, b). Such anti-egalitarian public policy outcomes are not desired by any of the proponents of the social capital/

psychosocial environment approach to health inequalities, or, for that matter, anyone in the broader public health community. This is because social egalitarianism constitutes one of public health's core values (Muntaner 2000).

Can social capital be saved from shallowness?

Why now? Explaining the growing interest in social capital

The literature on different approaches to social capital (e.g., communitarian, network, institutional) has been growing for the last three decades. However, not until the 1990s has the concept of social capital/social cohesion gained popularity in public health (e.g., Wilkinson 1996) and development studies (Woolcock 1998).

To understand the timely emergence of social capital from a psychosocial construct in the sociology of education (Coleman 1990) to the next research 'paradigm' in developmental economics at the World Bank (Stiglitz 1996, 1997), we need to understand the difficult position of international lending institutions in the current decade. After the demise of the Soviet Union, the so-called Washington Consensus rhetoric of minimal governments, austerity measures, debt repayment and neo-classical (e.g., rational choice) economics pervaded unchallenged (Chomsky 1999). This economic 'logic' nevertheless had to be tempered once a series of economic crises, in part fuelled by International Monetary Fund and World Bank policies, started to appear around the globe (e.g., Mexico, Russia, Brazil and East Asia; Galbraith 1999). Criticism of IMF austerity policies escalated (Kolko 1999) even at World Bank headquarters, where the Bank's new chief economist began using a more social democratic language in which a positive role for governments was acknowledged, including references to social capital as a key factor in economic development (Stiglitz 1996, 1997). The Bank's interest in social capital thus marked a departure from economic imperialism, rational choice and public choice models, and a growing attention to integrating economics with sociology (Woolcock 1998; World Bank 1999a).

Sceptical observers argue that economic development happens precisely when countries do not follow IMF policies (Chomsky 1999); that countries that receive IMF and World Bank funding and advice suffer increases in social inequalities (Kentor 1998); and that social democracy has already been successfully tested in some European countries during part of the Second World War period, without need for social capital explanations. On close scrutiny, now that communism and big bureaucratic states cannot be blamed, social capital allows for a different kind of criticism of debtor countries (e.g., Woolcock 1998). It allows for the characterisation of countries as 'corrupt' or 'developmental' according to the character of the ties between state, private sector and civil society (Evans 1995). For example, after the crisis of 1997, South Korea, a country formerly praised for its Asian values and Confucian capitalism, became an example of 'crony' capitalism, while the role of the deregulation of Korean financial markets in the crisis was ignored (Galbraith 1999).

In the case of Russia, the economic policy dictated by Harvard and the IMF (Wedel 1998) are not to blame for its failure to develop; that has been caused by

Russian corruption ('Fuelling Russia's Economy' 1999). Thus, in the World Bank's post-Washington Consensus documents, the interpretation of what happened to Russia in the 1990s is thought of as capitalism without proper social capital (i.e., deficient governmental regulation), rather than communism's inevitable heritage (World Bank 1999a, b). Russian events such as the 30 per cent GDP decline and unregulated monopolies are explained as the outcome of a deliberate hurry to privatise before any institutional capability to regulate could be put in place. They are used as examples of social capital failure that provide a rationale for the World Bank's retreat from neoliberalism and its attempt to build a new development theory. Social capital is used to inform a supposedly new comprehensive and partici-patory approach to development, which avoids small government and authoritarian top-down neoliberalism (Stiglitz 1997; Woolcock 1998). The underlying notion is that with adequate levels of social capital (proper civil and state guidance and regulation), the internationalisation of markets and private property are optimal for the welfare of nations (World Bank 1999a, b).

What is not to be done: a 'Third Way' for comparative health research

Social capital has been explicitly associated with 'Third Way' social policies in the USA and EU (Szreter 1999). The Third Way, as developed in the New Labour and New Democrat governments and their intellectuals (Robert Reich, Anthony Giddens), has been associated with the reduced role of the state, privatisation of social services, labour market flexibility, non-governmental organisations, modern philanthropy and the demise of the welfare state (Muntaner and Lynch 1999a). Critics of the Third Way have argued that instead of representing a new set of policies by social democratic parties, it represents a capitulation to the political right that leads to greater social inequalities (Albo and Zuege 1999; Muntaner and Lynch 1999a, b). Albo and Zuege have argued that the failures of European social democracy in the seventies and early eighties sent them into a path of retreat, accommodation and confusion from which they still have to recover. The Third Way rhetoric, more often defined by what it is not than by what it is (Giddens 1994), would be part of a search for a 'big idea' that would ensure a durable political base for social democratic parties in the new European capitalism. It is this potential role for social capital in public health that we think should be avoided (Muntaner and Lynch 1999b).

   Within public health, rather than discarding structural inequalities such as gender, race and class as outmoded materialism, in favour of psychosocial constructs such as social cohesion (Wilkinson 1999), a much more fruitful strategy would be to seize the opportunity that social capital offers to integrate sociology and economics into the field of social inequalities in health. For example, the Marxian tradition of class inequality (Wright 1997) could be integrated with the Weberian tradition of institutional social capital (Evans 1995). The institutional view of social capital stresses how states operate: some states are efficient or inefficient, others are strong or weak. The role of political institutions such as parties, the judicial system, how the executive and legislative branches of governments operate (e.g., the rationalisation of state bureaucracies) become central to understanding how states are formed (Evans 1995). From a Marxian perspective, on the other hand, class inequality guides the analysis of the state. How does the capitalist class influence the legislative, administrative and executive branches of government? What are the class alliances (capitalist vs. working class) and splits among different segments of the capitalist class (financial vs. industrial) that affect government function or the relationship between the capitalist class and state elites (Kadushin 1995)? But then, as public health scholars and activists, should we place false hopes on initiatives heralded by institutions (Amin 1997) that have helped generate the health inequalities that we want to eliminate?

Note

1   This chapter was first published in *Critical Public Health* (2000) 10: 107–24.

References

Albo, G. and Zuege, A. (1999) 'European capitalism today: between the Euro and the third way', *Monthly Review*, 51: 100–19.

Amin, S. (1997) *Capitalism in the Age of Globalization: The Management of Contemporary Society*, Atlantic Highlands, NJ: Zed Books.

Aneshensel, C.S. and Sucoff, C.A. (1996) 'The neighbourhood context of adolescent mental health', *Journal of Health and Social Behaviour*, 37: 293–310.

Baum, F. (1997) 'Public health and civil society: understanding and valuing the connection', *Australian Journal of Public Health*, 21: 673–5.

—— (1999) 'Social capital: is it good for your health? Issues for a public health agenda', *Journal of Epidemiology and Community Health*, 53: 195–6.

Borjas, G.J. (1992) 'Ethnic capital and intergenerational mobility', *Quarterly Journal of Economics*, 107: 123–50.

Brines, J. (1999) 'The ties that bind: principles of cohesion in cohabitation and marriage', *American Sociological Review*, 64: 333–55.

Carroll, L. (1999) *The Complete Works of Lewis Carroll*, Harmondsworth: Penguin.

Chomsky, N. (1999) *Profit over People: Neoliberalism and Global Order*, New York: Seven Stories Press.

Coleman, J. (1990) *Foundations of Social Theory*, Cambridge, MA: Harvard University Press.

Collier, P. (1998) *Social Capital and Poverty*, Washington, DC: World Bank, Social Capital Initiative.

Cooper, H., Arber, S. and Ginn, J. (1999) *The Influence of Social Support and Social Capital on Health*, London: Health Education Authority.

Erikson, B.H. (1996) 'Culture, class and connections', *American Journal of Sociology*, 102: 217–51.

Etzioni, A. and George, R.P. (1999) 'Virtue and the state: a dialogue between a communitarian and a social conservative', *Responsive Community*, 9: 54–6.

Evans, P. (1995) *Embedded Autonomy*, Princeton, NJ: Princeton University Press.

'Fuelling Russia's Economy' (1999), *The Economist*. Accessed at: <http://www.economist.com/editorial/justforyou/19990828/1d6020.html>.

Fullilove, M.T. (1998) 'Promoting social cohesion to improve health', *Journal of the American Medical Women's Association*, 53: 72–6.

Galbraith, J.K. (1999) 'The crisis of globalization', *Dissent*, Spring: 13–19.

Giddens, A. (1994) *Beyond Left and Right*, Palo Alto, CA: Stanford University Press.

Gould, R.V. (1991) 'Multiple networks and mobilization in the Paris commune, 1871', *American Sociological Review*, 56: 716–29.

—— (1993) 'Trade cohesion, class unity, and urban insurrection', *American Journal of Sociology*, 98: 721–54.

Granovetter, M. (1973) 'The strength of weak ties', *American Journal of Sociology*, 78: 1360–80.

Grootaert, C. (1997) *Social Capital: The Missing Link? In Expanding the Measure of Wealth: Indicators of Environmentally Sustainable Development*, Environmentally Sustainable Development Studies and Monographs Series No. 7, Washington, DC: World Bank.

Hawe, P. and Shiell, A. (2000) 'Social capital and health promotion: a review', *Social Science and Medicine*, 51: 871–85.

Jackman, R.W. *et al.* (1996) 'A renaissance of political culture', *American Journal of Political Science*, 40: 632–59.

Jenson, J. (1998) *Mapping Social Cohesion: The State of Canadian Research*, Ottawa: Canadian Policy Research Networks.

Kadushin, C. (1995) 'Friendship among the French financial elite', *American Sociology Review*, 60: 202–21.

Kaplan, G.A. (1995) 'Where do shared pathways lead? Some reflections on a research agenda', *Psychosomatic Medicine*, 57: 208–12.

Kaufman, J. (1999) 'Three views of associationalism in 19th century America: an empirical examination', *American Journal of Sociology*, 104: 1296–345.

Kawachi, I. and Kennedy, B. (1997) 'Health and social cohesion: why care about income inequality?', *British Medical Journal*, 314: 1037–9.

Kawachi, I., Kennedy, B. and Lochner, K. (1997a) 'Long live community: social capital as public health', *American Prospect*, November–December: 56–9.

Kawachi, I., Kennedy, B. and Pothrow-Smith, D. (1997b) 'Social capital, income inequality, and mortality', *American Journal of Public Health*, 87: 1491–8.

Kawachi, I., Kennedy, B.P. and Wilkinson, G. (1999) 'Crime: social disorganization and relative deprivation', *Social Science and Medicine*, 48: 719–31.

Kennedy, B.P., Kawachi, I. and Brainerd, E. (1999) 'The role of social capital in the Russian mortality crisis', *World Development*, 26: 2029–43.

Kentor, J. (1998) 'The long-term effects of foreign investment dependence on economic growth, 1940–1990', *American Journal of Sociology*, 103: 1024–46.

Knack, S. and Keefer, P. (1997) 'Does social capital have an economic pay off? A cross-country investigation', *Quarterly Journal of Economics*, 112: 1251–88.

Kolko, G. (1999) 'Ravaging the poor: the international monetary fund indicted by its own data', *International Journal of Health Services*, 29: 51–7.

Krieger, N. (1994) 'Epidemiology and the web of causation: has anyone seen the spider?', *Social Science and Medicine*, 39: 887–903.

Lavis, J.N. and Stoddart, G.L. (1999) *Social Cohesion and Health*, Toronto: Canadian Institute for Advanced Research, Programmes in Population Health.

Lewis, O. (1998) 'The culture of poverty', *Society*, 35: 7–9.

Lynch, J.W. and Kaplan, G.A. (1997) 'Wither studies on the socioeconomic foundations of population health?', *American Journal of Public Health*, 87: 1409–11.

Lynch, J.W., Kaplan, G.A. and Salonen, J.T. (1997) 'Why do poor people behave poorly? Variations in adult health behaviour and psychosocial characteristics, by stage of the socioeconomic lifecourse', *Social Science and Medicine*, 44: 809–20.

Marjoribanks, K. (1999) 'Family human and social capital and young adults' educational attainment and occupational aspirations', *Psychological Reports*, 69: 237–8.

Marmot, M. (1998) 'Improvement of the social environment to improve health', *Lancet*, 351: 57–60.

Marmot, M. and Theorell T. (1988) 'Social class and cardiovascular disease: the contribution of work', *International Journal of Health Services*, 18: 659–74.

Muntaner, C. (1999a) 'Invited commentary: social mechanisms, race and social epidemiology', *American Journal of Epidemiology*, 150: 121–6.

—— (1999b) 'Teaching social inequalities in health: barriers and opportunities', *Scandinavian Journal of Public Health*, 27: 161–5.

—— (2000) 'Applied epidemiology', *Journal of Public Health Policy*, 21: 99–102.

Muntaner, C. and Lynch, J. (1999a) 'Income inequality and social cohesion versus class relations: a critique of Wilkinson's neo-Durkheimian research programmes', *International Journal of Health Services*, 29: 59–82.

Muntaner, C. and Lynch, J. (1999b) 'The social class determinants of income inequality and social cohesion Part I: further comments on Wilkinson's reply', *International Journal of Health Services*, 29: 699–715.

Muntaner, C., Nieto, J. and O'Campo, P. (1997) 'Additional clarification re: on race, social class, and epidemiologic research', *American Journal of Epidemiology*, 146: 607–8.

Muntaner, C., Oates, G. and Lynch, J. (1999) 'The social class determinants of income inequality and social cohesion Part 2: presentation of an alternative model', *International Journal of Health Services*, 29: 715–32.

Muntaner, C. and O'Campo, P. (1993) 'A critical appraisal of the Demand/Control model of the psychosocial work environment: epistemological, social, behavioural and class considerations', *Social Science and Medicine*, 36: 1509–17.

Mustard, J.F. (1996) *Health and Social Capital in Health and Social Organization: Towards a Health Policy for the 21st Century*, New York: Routledge.

Navarro, V. (1994) *The Politics of Health Policy*, Amityville, NY: Baywood.

Ostrom, E. (1999) 'Revisiting the commons: local lessons, global challenges', *Science*, 284: 278–82.

Pattillo, M.E. (1998) 'Sweet mothers and gangbangers: managing crime in a black middle-class neighbourhood', *Social Forces*, 76: 747–74.

Paxton, P. (1999) 'Is social capital declining in the United States? A multiple indicator assessment', *American Journal of Sociology*, 105: 88–127.

Persell, C.H., Catsambis, S. and Cookson, P.W. (1992) 'Differential asset conversion: class and gendered pathways to selective colleges', *Sociology of Education*, 65: 208–25.

Portes, A. (1998) 'Social capital: its origins and applications in contemporary sociology', *Annual Review of Sociology*, 24: 1–24.

Proudfoot, J. and Guest, D. (1997) 'Effect of cognitive-behavioural training on job-finding among long-term unemployed people', *Lancet*, 350: 96–100.

Putnam, R. (1995a) 'Bowling alone: America's declining social capital', *Journal of Democracy*, 6: 65–78.

Putnam, R. (1995b) 'The prosperous community: social capital and public life', *American Prospect*, Spring: 27–40.

Putnam, R., Leonardi, R. and Nanetti, R. (1993) *Making Democracy Work: Civic Traditions in Modern Italy*, Princeton, NJ: Princeton University Press.

Rose, G. (1985) 'Sick individuals and sick populations', *International Journal of Epidemiology*, 14: 32–8.

Sampson, R.J., Raudenbush, S.W. and Earls, F. (1997) 'Neighbourhoods and violent crime: a multilevel study of collective efficacy', *Science*, 277: 918–24.

Schneider, M. *et al.* (1997) 'Networks to nowhere: segregation and stratification in networks of information about schools', *American Journal of Political Science*, 41: 1201–23.

Skocpol, T. (1999) 'Associations without members', *American Prospect*, 45: 66–73.

Smith, T. (1997) 'Factors relating to misanthropy in contemporary American society', *Social Science Research*, 26: 170–96.

Stiglitz, J. (1996) 'Some lessons from the East Asian miracle', *World Bank Research Observer*, 11: 151–78.

—— (1997) 'An agenda for development for the twenty-first century', in B. Pleskovic and J. Stiglitz (eds), *Annual Bank Conference on Development Economics 1997*, Washington, DC: World Bank.

Stoto, M.A. (1999) 'Sharing responsibility for the public's health', *Public Health Reports*, 114: 231–5.

Szreter, S. (1999) 'A new political economy for New Labour – the importance of social capital', *Renewal*, 7: 30–44.

Tocqueville, A. de (1969 [1835]) *Democracy in America*, New York: Anchor.

Tijhuis, M.A., Flap, H.D., Foets, M. and Groenewegen, P.P. (1995) 'Social support and stressful events in two dimensions: life events and illness as an event', *Social Science and Medicine*, 40: 1513–26.

Wainwright, D. (1996) 'The political transformation of the health inequalities debate', *Critical Social Policy*, 16: 67–82.

Warner, W.L. (1960) *Social Class in America*, New York: Harper and Row.

Warren, M.R. (1994) 'Exploitation or cooperation? The political basis of regional variation in the Italian informal economy', *Politics and Society*, 22: 89.

Wedel, J.R. (1998) *Collision and Collusion: the Strange Case of Western Aid to Eastern Europe 1989–1998*, London: St Martin's Press.

Wilkinson, R.G. (1996) *Unhealthy Societies: The Afflictions of Inequality*, Routledge: London.

—— (1999) 'Income inequality, social cohesion, and health: clarifying the theory – a reply to Muntaner and Lynch', *International Journal of Health Services*, 29: 525–43.

Wilkinson R.G. Kawachi, I. and Kennedy, B. (1998a) 'Mortality, the social environment, crime and violence', *Sociology of Health and Illness*, 20: 578–97.

—— (1998b) 'Mortality, the social environment and violence', in M. Bartley, D. Blane and G. Davey Smith (eds), *The Sociology of Health Inequalities*, Oxford: Blackwell Publishers.

Wing, S. (1998) 'Whose epidemiology, whose health?', *International Journal of Health Services*, 28: 241–52.

Woolcock, M. (1998) 'Social capital and economic development: a critical review', *Theory and Society*, 27: 151–208.

World Bank Group (1999a) *Social Capital for Development*, Washington, DC: World Bank. Available at: <http://www.worldbank.org/poverty/scapital>.

—— (1999b) *World Bank Calls for a Narrowing of the Knowledge Gap between Rich and Poor*, Washington, DC: World Bank.

Wright, E.O. (1997) *Class Counts: Comparative Studies in Class Analysis*, New York: Cambridge University Press.

Zweigenhaft, R.L. (1993) 'Accumulation of cultural and social capital', *Social Spectrum*, 13: 365–76.

3 HIV infection in women

Social inequalities as determinants of risk[1]

Sally Zierler and Nancy Krieger

Introduction

In 1981, six women in the United States were noted to have an unexplained underlying cellular immune deficiency (Guinan and Hardy 1987). It was a description of the same phenomenon among five previously healthy young gay white men, however, that prompted the 1981 MMWR report now viewed as the first official recognition of AIDS (Centers for Disease Control 1981). A retrospective study of underlying causes of death suggested that forty-eight young women died of AIDS in the years 1980–1 (Chu *et al.* 1990). Although not described in that report, we imagine, based on what has been documented since then, that these women were young, between the ages of fifteen and forty-four years; their neighbourhoods were poor and so were they; if they could get work, they were rarely earning wages to meet basic needs for food, childcare, clothing and shelter; mostly they depended on public assistance and men for economic survival. Most were also likely to have been women of colour – African-American, Latina, Haitian, American Indian – who were raising young children. Unlike white gay men diagnosed with AIDS, sickness among these women was not unexpected. It was just a part of the ongoing, usual excess morbidity and mortality among the poor and racially oppressed.

Sixteen years later, in 1997, as the proportion of women among AIDS cases continues to rise – from 6 per cent in 1984 to 21 per cent in 1997 – the vast majority of women with AIDS in the United States are still poor women of colour (Centers for Disease Control and Prevention 1997). Globally, about 3.1 million new infections are estimated to have occurred during 1996, implying that between 3,000 and 4,000 women were infected each day. Most women infected were under twenty-five. As of December 1996, UNAIDS estimated that more than 8.4 million AIDS cases had occurred since the start of the epidemic (an estimate far larger than the official reports to WHO of 1.5 million). Whereas in the USA, about 20 per cent of AIDS cases are women, globally this estimate more than doubles (with women defined as greater than twelve years old) (Mann *et al.* 1994). In the USA, AIDS is the leading cause of death in black women between twenty-five and forty-four, and the rate of death is nine times that of white women of comparable age with AIDS (Centers for Disease Control and Prevention 1994).

What explains the vulnerability of these women to HIV? Why is it that economic deprivation and membership in groups defined, in part, by discrimination, are so interwoven with risk of AIDS among women? Or, more bluntly, how is it that women's relations with power in personal (as with sexual partners) and public (as with opportunities for earning a living wage) life shape the distribution of HIV in women?

Our central thesis is that the biology of transmission and infection – whether by sex or drugs – is inextricably bound to social and economic relations of power and control. And it is these relations that overwhelmingly account for which women are at risk for HIV infection. Thus, this article, drawing on a variety of theories concerned with health and social justice, reframes HIV occurrence among women as a function of social, economic and political conditions. Focusing on women in the USA, we briefly review empirical studies that bring to light underlying causes of risk and discuss how such reframing would affect surveillance and production of knowledge about what drives the epidemic among women. Our major premise is that the work of public health is not only to reduce human suffering, but to envision and create conditions of human health.

Social inequalities and HIV in US women: setting the context

> The pain in our shoulder comes
> You say, from the damp; and this is also the reason
> For the stain on the wall of our flat.
> So tell us:
> Where does the damp come from?
> > Bertolt Brecht (Brecht 1976)

How we explain and alter occurrence of HIV infection among women depends, in part, on conceptual frameworks that guide collection and interpretation of data, as well as design and implementation of policies and programmes. To date, much of the literature on women and HIV has relied upon what can be termed 'biomedical' (Fee and Krieger 1993; Lock and Gordon 1988; Tesh 1988), 'lifestyle' (Tesh 1988; Coreil *et al.* 1985; Terris 1980) and 'psychological' (Ajzen and Fishbein 1980; Bandura 1977; Becker 1974; Prochaska *et al.* 1992; Rosenstock *et al.* 1988) theories of disease causation (Table 3.1). By contrast, in this chapter we rely upon four alternative conceptual frameworks to guide our perspective of causes of HIV among US women. These frameworks (summarised in Table 3.2) are: feminist (Doyal 1994; Hubbard 1990; Thomas 1994; Treichler 1988), social production of disease/ political economy of health (Black *et al.* 1985; Doyal 1979; Farmer *et al.* 1996; Laurell 1989), ecosocial theory (Krieger 1994), and human rights (Mann *et al.* 1994; United Nations 1948). Overlapping yet distinct, these frameworks together make connections between disease and inequality on the one hand, and health and social justice on the other. Specifically, they guide us to enquire how inequalities structured in relation to class, gender, race/ethnicity and sexuality affect risk of and resistance to HIV infection. The frameworks in which we discuss HIV have utility throughout the world for women living in poor countries, particularly where resources are not shared, as well as poor women living in wealthy countries.

Fundamental to these four alternative frameworks is locating women socially and economically in US society around the time that AIDS emerged in the early 1980s. The deep recession in 1974–5, coupled with a decline in manufacturing jobs in cities, triggered urban fiscal crises that challenged city government's ability to provide services 'for increasingly poor, deteriorating, jobless and crime-ridden neighbourhoods' (Cluster and Rutter 1980). Poverty increased dramatically among residents of the five largest US cities: New York, Chicago, Los Angeles, Philadelphia, Detroit (Wilson 1987). Today, these five cities alone account for nearly a third of all US AIDS cases (Centers for Disease Control and Prevention 1997).

As summarised in Table 3.3, starting in the 1980s, three factors dramatically affected lives of women in ways that increased their susceptibility to HIV infection: enormous increases in military spending coupled with large cuts in taxation of the wealthy led to a ballooning federal fiscal deficit, used to justify drastic reductions in federal funds allocated to social programmes; persistent and growing economic inequalities, overall and along racial/ethnic lines; and a racially biased 'war on drugs' against a growing drug economy.

In a context of decreasing educational and economic opportunity within the legal labour market, the allure of the illegal drug economy as a source of income became more powerful during the early 1980s. Residents of neighbourhoods fraught with economic impoverishment, social disintegration and boredom were, and continue to be, susceptible to use of psychoactive drugs for relief and stimulation. Not surprisingly, higher prevalence of drug traffic and drug use occurs in such neighbourhoods, including drugs linked to risk of HIV infection, such as crack, cocaine and heroin (Lillie-Blanton *et al.* 1993; Lusane 1991; National Institute on Drug Abuse 1991; US Department of Health and Human Services 1985). Among people living there are economically poor women of colour and the families they support. Young men living in these communities also have been and remain at extremely high risk of violent death, unemployment and arrest.

The growing toll of drugs and the war on drugs on lives of women caught up in the drug economy is attested to by data on trends in arrests and incarceration. During the 1980s, most arrests among women had been for economic crimes linked to poverty and the drug economy (Bureau of Justice Statistics 1991). Racially selective enforcement of drug laws, ranging from reporting and arrest to sentencing and imprisonment, has also contributed to the disproportionately high percentage of black and Hispanic inmates (Lusane 1991; Bureau of Justice Statistics 1995; Lake 1993). Reflecting combined social forces driving risk of imprisonment and risk of HIV among women, HIV seroprevalence among incarcerated women across ten US correctional facilities in 1989 was estimated to be 2.5 to 14.7 per cent (Vlahov *et al.* 1991), 16.7 to 98 times the prevalence of HIV relative to the average prevalence of childbearing women measured in the CDC national survey (Gwinn *et al.* 1991; Steinberg *et al.* 1995).

Table 3.1 Individual-level frameworks for studies of occurrence and prevention of HIV infection among women

Framework	Key question	Major assumptions	Application of framework to studies
Biomedical	How do humans, as biological organisms, become ill?	• Knowledge based on scientific method viewed as objective, value free, without ideologic or political influence • Disease occurrence based on individual susceptibility to biologic, chemical or physical exposures • Population disease patterns are sums of affected individuals • Solutions emerge from basic/clinical sciences	• Relative efficiency of viral sexual transmission from men to women • Vaginal mucosal immunity to HIV infection • Female endocrine levels and HIV immunology • Female genital tract inflammation and susceptibility to infection • Female genital tract inflammation and HIV load • HIV vaccine development • Vaginal microbicides to prevent HIV infection • Reducing HIV viral load
Behavioural/Lifestyle	How do individual behavioural and cultural factors affect health and disease?	• Disease occurrence based on individual choices of ways of living • Population disease patterns are sums of these individual choices • Individuals voluntarily can alter these ways of living	• 'Mode of transmission' research, primarily sex with men and injection drug use • Prostitution as risk factor • Cultural factors attributed to membership in racial/ethnic groups

Psychological	What motivates individuals to change behaviours that increase risk for disease?		• Measure change/reduction in individual risk-taking with sex and injection drug use
• Health Belief Model		• Perceiving behaviour as detrimental to health will motivate change • Perception of personal susceptibility to disease, severity of disease, and social support influence change	
• Theory of Reasoned Action		• Intentions influence health behaviour • Social norms, attitudes and perceived control affect intentions and influence change	
• Social Cognitive Theory		• Health behaviour is function and social incentives, vicarious learning/expectation • Perceived self-efficacy in affecting change influences behaviour	
• Stages of Change		• Health behavioural change structured by predictable sequence of readiness: precontemplation, contemplation, decision, action, maintenance • Stage specific interventions stimulate change to next stage in sequence	

Table 3.2 Structural-level frameworks for studies of occurrence and prevention of HIV infection among women

Framework	Key question	Major assumptions	Application of framework to studies
Feminist	How do gender inequalities affect health of women (as well as men and children)?	• Women's position and experiences in society are determined by social roles and conventions, not by biology. • Relations of power between women and men affect health. • Interventions to alter distribution of disease include social policies that secure and protect women's economic, legal and physical/sexual autonomy.	• Gender disparities in power and sexual risk of HIV. • Gender-based patterns of injection drug sharing. • Gender differences in socially sanctioned sexual expression. • Sexual and physical violence against women as determinants of risk of HIV infection. • Reproductive autonomy and HIV testing among pregnant women.
Social production of disease; political economy of health	How do economic and social relations forged by society's economic, social and political structure affect health?	• Relative social and economic positioning shape behaviours. • Relations between subordinate–dominant groups affect patterns of disease through material and social inequalities. • Population-level interventions shift structural conditions that cause material and social deprivation, thus altering societal distribution of disease.	• Social welfare policy, economic dependence on men and risk of sexual HIV transmission to women. • Social class position and HIV infection in women. • Racism and onset of injection drug use among women at risk of HIV infection. • Reduction in municipal fire protection, destruction of housing, and HIV incidence among women.

Ecosocial	How do developmental and evolutionary biology interact with social, economic and political conditions to explain population patterns of health, disease and well-being?	• Social relations and ecologic conditions literally incorporate themselves into the body throughout the life-course.	• Thinness of peripubescent vaginal mucosal lining and vaginal susceptibility to HIV infection among girls who depend on older men economically, socially, and sexually. • Age-specific vaginal tract inflammation and HIV among women in relation to family history of activism in the Civil Rights Movement of the 1960s.
Human rights	How do violations of human rights drive population patterns of disease?	• Human dignity is a necessary condition for health. • Preconditions for human dignity imply good health. • Social, economic and political conditions that endanger people's health are human rights violations. • Solutions to violations lie in holding governments accountable for the well-being of their people.	• Effect of removing legal barriers to women's education on HIV incidence among women. • HIV incidence among drug dependent pregnant women who live in states that criminalise drug use in pregnancy. • Effect of enforcing domestic violence ordinances and marital rape laws on HIV incidence among women.

Table 3.3 Measuring* social inequalities in relation to HIV infection: examples for US women

Economics	Political/legal	Race/ethnicity and Racism	Gender
• Income and work	• Voter participation	• Self-identity vs. how perceived by others	• Uses of sex: social, economic
• Sources (legal and illegal)	• Awareness of legal rights	• Awareness of ancestry and family origins/roots	• Sexual identity
• Nature of work (doing what, with and for whom)	• Awareness of public officials	• Participation in Civil Rights movement (past and current racial justice work)	• Sexual fulfilment
• Number of people supported on income	• Neighbourhood/community work: awareness/involvement/activism	• Racial/ethnic pride	• Reproductive autonomy
• Amount/month	• Workplace organising/activism	• Cultural/ethnic social resources (community groups/churches)	• Awareness and use of services to support women's sexual and reproductive health
• Health insurance	• Lobbying/social advocacy work	• Racial/ethnic composition of neighbourhood/block-group	• Involvement in women's groups (political, social, health-related)
• Proportion of income for food, housing, drugs (illicit/prescribed)	• Awareness of eligibility for benefits/resources and how to access them	• Race/ethnicity of elected officials	• Parenting and other care-giving responsibilities
• Level of income in relation to poverty line and fluctuations	• Legal access to and use of clean needles/syringes	• Experience with racially motivated violence	• Gender-based violence: sexual, physical, verbal threats
• Experiences with hunger, homelessness, insufficient heat	• Interactions with police	*Networks*	• Gender-based control: economic and social
• Housing status: rent, own, none	• Arrest/incarceration experience	• Family, friends, sexual partners	• Gender-based discrimination
• Household crowding	*Violence*	• Spiritual	• Lesbian-based discrimination
• Use of public/private	• Exposure to street, workplace or public violence (witness, victim, participant)	• Work-related	• Marital/partner status
• Transport; own or access to car	• Gang membership	• Drug-related: distribution, use, recovery	
• Education credentials	• Own/carry gun or other weapon	• Turnover of network membership	
• Literacy level in primary language and English	• Nature of violence		
• Access to recreation and culture	• Response to violence		
• State-level: tax base; budget for education, housing, welfare and other social services, art/culture			

Note: *Pattern over life-course (childhood to present); at level of individual, household, network, neighbourhood, region

Source: adapted from Zierler and Krieger (1997)

Framing risk of HIV infection among US women: a review of the literature

Economic inequalities and HIV in women

Among the first public health articles to frame women's experience with HIV infection within the larger social and economic conditions in their lives was the *Health/PAC Bulletin*'s powerful commentary by Anastos and Marte (1989). The authors wrote not about drug use and sex, but rather about where women were situated geographically and socially: 'For many women, their address alone places them at risk . . . poor black and Latina women are at unduly high risk for infection, whatever their life-style, because poverty and lack of resources and opportunity keep them in areas of high HIV seroprevalence' (Anastos and Marte 1989).

Race/racism and HIV in women

How might racism affect HIV risk in women? Although no empirical studies on racism against women and HIV have been published to date, we hypothesise that both economic and non-economic forms of racism create conditions affecting women's risk. First, several commentaries on racial/ethnic disparities in AIDS have called attention to economic inequalities rooted in racial discrimination as a cause of HIV infection (Dalton 1989; Friedman *et al.* 1987; Thomas and Quinn 1991; Quinn 1993). Following a political economy of health framework, these commentaries emphasise that excess relative risk of AIDS among communities of colour, notably African-American, American Indian and Latina people, reflects underlying forces of discrimination in employment, housing, earning power and educational opportunity. Living amid such constraints, social and economic strategies for work, play and love may involve more risk for drug use, partnerships with drug users, and income-earning strategies that include sex and drugs than among people living free of constraints imposed by racial and class subordination.

Second, non-economic expressions of racism could increase risk of HIV infection among women. In response to daily assaults of racial prejudice (Essed 1991) and denial of dignity (Friedman 1991) women may turn to readily available mind-altering substances for relief as well as for self-medication from depression (Battle 1990; Cochran and Mays 1994), particularly if their lovers use drugs. Condom use is likely to be less of a priority in this context (Ickovics and Rodin 1992). Within the walls of residential hypersegregation, closed-in social networks harbour not only HIV, but other subclinical sexually transmitted diseases that may be co-factors for vaginal susceptibility to HIV infection (Mayer and Anderson 1995). Additionally, racism construed as a psychosocial stressor might increase biological susceptibility to infection, since studies have found that social stressors may impair immune function (Ickovics and Rodin 1992). Although studies have not yet measured how racism and resistance to racism may affect women's risk of infection, effects of racism on health in other contexts have begun to be measured and demonstrated in relation to elevated blood pressure (Williams 1992; Krieger and Zierler 1996) and impaired mental health (Cochran and Mays 1994; Dressler 1993; Neighbors *et al.* 1996).

Gender inequalities in relation to sex, violence and drugs

Women's risk of HIV infection may also be linked to both economic and non-economic forms of gender-based inequality, especially as these pertain to sex, violence and illicit drugs. As we will review, a number of studies have documented how socially constructed dependence translates into women being in the difficult position of having to risk loss of income for food, housing, transportation and pleasure to prevent HIV infection with men who may not be willing to use condoms. Before adulthood, young girls' vulnerability to experiences of gender-based violence, such as incestuous sexual and physical abuse, lays the groundwork for drug and alcohol addiction and dissociated sexuality in which women may not be aware of their right and capability to claim when, how and with whom they are sexual. And finally, gendered social roles play out in the social experience of drug use, just as they do in other aspects of women's everyday lives.

Gender inequality and sex

Women's experiences of sex with men may include unsafe sex with the possibility of HIV transmission within a context that is about mutual and loving expression of shared desire. However, when expressions of sexuality preclude condom use because of fear of loss of material support for women or their children, or because of beliefs that women should not make sexual demands of men, or because of fear that male sexual partners will react violently to discussions of low-risk sex, it is gender inequality that is driving women's risk of HIV infection. Studies of white, black and Hispanic women accordingly have shown that condom use is less frequent in couples where women are economically dependent upon men, feel powerless (Amaro 1995), or rely on men for social status (Pivnick 1993; Males 1995) or protection (e.g., among homeless women; Fisher *et al.* 1995).

Gender-based violence

As feminist and human rights analyses emphasise, girls and women can be victimised by men regardless of economic circumstances. Political economy of health and ecosocial approaches further contextualise these experiences by theorising how state-sponsored, public and private expressions of violence interact with material and social deprivation over women's life-course.

In the case of women and HIV infection, past and present experiences with violence can affect risk in several ways. First, childhood sexual abuse – noted repeatedly to have occurred in alarming prevalence among women currently infected as well as women living amid conditions of increasing risk for infection – has profound, long-term impacts on psychological and physical health. Most relevant to HIV risk are sequelae that include high-risk sex, prostitution, crack use, injection drug use, recurrent sexual assault, homelessness and incarceration (Fisher *et al.* 1995; James and Meyerding 1977; Paone *et al.* 1995; Zierler *et al.* 1991;

Zierler *et al.* 1996). Notably, among women living with HIV infection, nearly half report forced sexual experiences in childhood or teenage years (Zierler *et al.* 1996; Zierler 1997; Vlahov *et al.* 1996).

Second, numerous studies document how violence or fear of violence affects women's ability to protect themselves sexually (Zierler 1997; O'Campo *et al.* 1995). A study of Brazilian sex workers further found that 23 per cent of women reported fear of violence if they insisted that clients wear condoms and the prevalence of this concern tripled when requesting condom use with men whom they regarded as 'non clients' (Lurie *et al.* 1995). In the WIHS multi-site cohort study of HIV-infected women, 67 per cent reported sexual or physical violence by a current or past partner, and in nearly a third of women this occurred in the past year. Limited empirical data, moreover, indicate that women's disclosure of HIV infection itself may be a trigger for partner violence (Gielen *et al.* 1995).

A third connection between HIV experiences and violence emerges in a context of homelessness among women. Twenty-two to 86 per cent of homeless women cite domestic abuse as their reason for being homeless (Fisher *et al.* 1995; Mills and Ota 1989), and without a safe place to live, women face dangers of street life that include exposure to HIV from rape, sex for economic survival, and drugs.

In considering issues of gender-based violence in the lives of women at risk of or living with HIV infection, a political economy of health framework underscores that men inflicting this violence are also likely to be living amid conditions of economic and social hardship. Sharing with women positions of similar class and racial/ethnic inequalities, men additionally carry distinct gendered authority and social roles which, in a context of poverty, have limited room for healthy expression. As people who may use violence against women, these men also may have experienced assaults against their own humanity through physical displacement, racial discrimination, incarceration, economic impoverishment and the social alienation that accompanies these experiences. Thus, the brutally logical concurrence of violence and HIV happens within a larger structural control of social and economic resources and their distribution.

Gender inequalities and illicit drugs

Gender inequalities may affect social patterning of illicit drug use that has bearing on women's risk of HIV infection. This social patterning spans from onset to dependency and extends to drug treatment. A number of studies have observed that heterosexual teenage girls and women were more likely to begin and to continue drug use with boyfriends and male partners. Men, on the other hand, were more likely to begin and then continue to share drugs with male friends and associates (Amaro and Hardy-Fanta 1995; Paone *et al.* 1995; Dwyer *et al.* 1994; Rosenbaum 1979; Sotheran *et al.* 1992).

Sexual identity as a source of inequality in lesbian risk for HIV infection

To our knowledge, no studies have examined how sexual *identity* as lesbian may influence risk of HIV infection. The sparse data published or presented to date on lesbians and HIV infection suggest that apart from identity as lesbian and frequency of sex with men, lesbians share similar conditions of poverty, and gender and racial/ethnic subordination as women who identify as heterosexual and bisexual. Principal modes of infection of lesbians are the same as for heterosexual women: by injection drug use and sexual contact with men (Chu *et al.* 1992; Lemp *et al.* 1995). Only five cases have been reported in the medical literature of likely woman-to-woman sexual transmission (Marmor *et al.* 1986; Monzon and Capellan 1987; Perry *et al.* 1989; Rich *et al.* 1993; Sabatini *et al.* 1984). Because data on sexual identity were not included for most published studies on HIV infection in women, distinctions between identity (as lesbian, bisexual or heterosexual) and practice (sex with women, with men, or both) have been blurred. These distinctions may matter, since women who identify as lesbian may have experiences of social isolation and discrimination in addition to those resulting from class, gender and racial/ethnic position (Stevens 1993; Moore *et al.* 1997).

Shifting the public health paradigm of accountability

Returning to our initial question – what accounts for the distribution of HIV among women in the United States? – the data we have reviewed explain HIV incidence in relation to social inequalities. These inequalities and women's responses to them explain why women globally are most likely to become infected with HIV if they are living in poor countries or poor women living in countries with wealth. Globally, nearly two-thirds of women with AIDS live in sub-Saharan African, and in that area, more than half of the estimated fourteen million adults and children with HIV or AIDS are women. The prevalence of HIV/AIDS is believed to be more than five cases for every hundred residents. In the Caribbean, it is nearly two cases for every hundred residents. In absolute numbers, the next highest population of HIV/AIDS, after Africa, is in South and South East Asia, where the epidemic appeared most explosively nearly ten years after it was first observed in the USA and Africa. The next highest populations are in Latin America and North America, Western Europe, Australia and New Zealand. In Mumbai, prevalence has reached 50 per cent among sex workers, and 2.5 per cent among pregnant women attending prenatal care clinics. As a free market economy restructures conditions in Vietnam, HIV prevalence jumped recently from 9 to 38 per cent over a two-year period, and similar trends have been seen in Myanmar and Malaysia among women engaged in sex work for economic survival, or because they are forced to engage in this work by bosses. Further evidence of links between social disintegration and HIV spread are being documented in Eastern and Central Europe (Mann and Tarantola 1996).

What would it mean for epidemiologists and other public health researchers to draw upon social justice frameworks described earlier and in Table 3.2 to develop measurable surveillance tools and research questions? To begin, surveillance data on HIV and AIDS can be described according to characteristics of neighbourhoods or nations where infection is occurring. US Census data, for example, are accessible and rich in descriptors of social and economic conditions at the block-group level (a geographically contiguous area comprising around 1,000 people). Geocoding HIV/AIDS surveillance data to incorporate census-based socioeconomic information would permit characterising socioeconomic conditions of neighbourhoods and also of state economic areas and regional economies, in relation to trends in HIV incidence and AIDS diagnoses. One application would be to develop what one researcher has named 'AIDS impact statements', similar to the environmental impact statements required in the USA that address possible effects of economic policies on the environment (Friedman *et al.* 1987).

Social and economic reorganisation at the national and transnational level – as occurs, for example, as a result of World Bank lending policies, or multinational corporate labour practices – leads to migration and repositioning of populations in ways that spread HIV infection (Lurie *et al.* 1995; Farmer *et al.* 1993). Thus, Farmer and colleagues have tracked rising water from construction of a hydroelectric plant that dammed Haiti's largest river to spread of AIDS among families forced to relocate from their original farmlands to higher, less fertile ground. In a context of deepening poverty, they tell the story of women sharing sex with men who might offer women alternatives to destitution in their lives. Acephie Joseph, who later died of AIDS, said 'I looked around and saw how poor we all were, how the old people were finished . . . It was a way out, that's how I saw it' (quoted in Farmer *et al.* 1993). Political economy of health analyses of AIDS as a disease of development have linked spread of HIV to global economic interests structured by the World Bank and International Monetary Fund (Farmer *et al.* 1996; Lurie *et al.* 1995; Basset and Mihloyi 1994; Jochelson *et al.* 1994; Schoepf 1993). Schoepf, for example, has described how women in the Democratic Republic of Congo have survived amid macroeconomic conditions that underscore already pervasive gender inequality in the labour market and in childbearing decision-making. Strapped with responsibilities for childcare and wage-earning in extreme conditions of poverty, women 'engage in . . . activities in the informal sector', usually involving sex for material sustenance, sometimes at the request of their families for purchasing land or building materials or to repay debts. Men, less constrained by caring for children, have sought wages from jobs that involved travelling or living away from home for long periods of time. These labour migrations became a source of HIV infection among men as they sought sexual contact with women or men along their routes. Upon returning home, these men then introduced HIV into their families (Schoepf 1993). Analyses of women and AIDS in Zimbabwe (Basset and Mihloyi 1994) and South Africa (Jochelson *et al.* 1994) have reported comparable findings. Examples like these shift the public health paradigm of accountability of HIV transmission from individuals to policies that stimulate growth of the private and export sectors in developing countries by disruption of local control over rural and urban markets within these countries. Shifts in wealth and poverty in the USA in the 1980s and 1990s, redistribution of global power and increasing control by a market economy reflect political and economic decisions of people; these decisions – and the trends in AIDS they have fostered – are not immutable or inevitable.

Second, research studies, in part driven by descriptions emerging from expanded surveillance data, would require development of methodologies for valid measures of women's various experiences with discrimination and subordination, as well as experiences with creative responses and resistance to inequality. Examples of social determinants that are measurable for studies of occurrence of HIV infection among women are listed in Table 3.3. Highlighting resistance and adaptation strategies as well as subordination, these determinants pertain to women's experiences regarding: knowledge of and exercise of political and legal rights; racial/ethnic identity and racism; gender, sexual identity, and gender and sexual inequalities involving sex, violence and drug use; public and private violence; and social networks. Studies generating such data would provide public health professionals with empirical documentation to advance legislative and regulatory action to reduce HIV transmission.

Regulating policy at governmental and transnational corporate levels requires access to participation in policy decision-making that affects distribution of wealth, such as tax policy and living wage standards. Training of local organisations to monitor human rights violations holds governments accountable for conditions that impose HIV risk on populations within their borders. Global capitalism's use of humans for profit must follow regulations required of all human activity: the Universal Declaration of Human Rights (United Nations 1948).

It is likely that the moment of HIV transmission into women's bodies is a very private one. Yet the chosen or imposed action that facilitates transmission hardly measures the enormous public forces that culminate in this irrevocable transference of viral particles. This review, in offering theoretical frameworks that contextualise HIV infection among women within social, economic and political structures, calls for greater emphasis on naming and measuring the impact of these public sociopolitical forces.

Note

1 This chapter was first published in *Critical Public Health* (1998) 8: 13–32.

References

Ajzen, I. and Fishbein, M. (1980) *Understanding Attitudes and Predicting Social Behavior*, Engle-wood Cliffs, NJ: Prentice Hall.

Amaro, H. (1995) 'Love, sex and power', *American Psychology*, 50: 437–47.

Amaro, H. and Hardy-Fanta, C. (1995) 'Gender relations in addiction and recovery', *Journal of Psychoactive Drugs*, 27: 325–37.

Anastos, K. and Marte, C. (1989) 'Women – the missing persons in the AIDS epidemic', *Health/PAC Bulletin*, Winter: 6–15.

Bandura, A. (1977) 'Self-efficacy: toward a unifying theory of behavioral change', *Psychological Review*, 84: 191–215.

Basset, M. and Mihloyi, M. (1994) 'Women and AIDS in Zimbabwe: the making of an epidemic', in N. Krieger and G. Margo (eds), *AIDS: The Politics of Survival*, Amityville, NY: Baywood.

Battle, S. (1990) 'Moving targets: alcohol, crack and black women', in E.C. White (ed.), *The Black Women's Health Book: Speaking for Ourselves*, Seattle, WA: Seal Press.

Becker, M.H. (1974) 'The health belief model and sick role behavior', *Health Education Monographs*, 2: 409–19.

Black, D., Morris, J.N., Smith, C. and Townsend, P. (1985) *Inequalities in Health: The Black Report*, Harmondsworth: Penguin.

Brecht, B. (1976 [*c*. 1938]) 'A worker's speech to a doctor', in *Poems 1913–1965*, New York: Methuen.

Bureau of Justice Statistics (1991) *Women in Prison*, Washington, DC: US Department of Justice.

—— (1995) *Prisoners in 1994*, Washington, DC: US Department of Justice.

Centers for Disease Control (1981) 'Pneumocystis pneumonia – Los Angeles', *Morbidity and Mortality Weekly Report*, 30: 250–2.

Centers for Disease Control and Prevention (1994) 'Update: mortality attributable to HIV infection among persons aged 25–44 years – United States', *Morbidity and Mortality Weekly Report*, 45: 121–5.

—— (1997) *HIV/AIDS Surveillance Report*, midyear edition, Atlanta, GA: US Department of Health and Human Services, Public Health Service.

Chu, S.Y., Buehler, J.W. and Berkelman, R.L. (1990) 'Impact of the human immuno-deficiency virus epidemic on mortality in women of reproductive age, United States', *Journal of the American Medical Association*, 264: 225–9.

Chu S.Y., Hammett, T.A. and Buehler, J.W. (1992) 'Update: epidemiology of reported cases of AIDS in women who report sex only with other women, United States, 1980–1991', *AIDS*, 6: 518–19.

Cluster, D. and Rutter, N. (1980) *Shrinking Dollars, Vanishing Jobs*, Boston, MA: Beacon Press.

Cochran, S.D. and Mays, V.M. (1994) 'Depressive distress among homosexually active African-American men and women', *American Journal of Psychology*, 151: 524–9.

Coreil, J., Levin, J.S. and Jaco, E.G. (1985) 'Life style – an emergent concept in the socio-medical science', *Culture, Medicine and Psychiatry*, 9: 423–37.

Dalton, H.L. (1989) 'AIDS in blackface', *Daedalus*, 115: 205–27.

Doyal, L. (1979) *The Political Economy of Health*, London: Pluto Press.

—— (1994) 'HIV and AIDS: putting women on the global agenda', in L. Doyal, J. Naidoo and T. Wilton (eds), *AIDS: Setting a feminist agenda*, London: Taylor and Francis.

Dressler, W.W. (1993) 'Health in the African American community: accounting for health inequalities', *Medical Anthropology Quarterly*, 7: 325–45.

Dwyer, R., Richardson, D., Ross, M.W., Wodak, A., Miller, M.E. and Gold, J. (1994) 'A comparison of HIV risk between women and men who inject drugs', *AIDS Education and Prevention*, 6: 379–89.

Essed, P. (1991) *Understanding Everyday Racism: An Interdisciplinary Theory*, Newbury Park, CA: Sage.

Farmer, P., Conners, M. and Simmons, J. (1996) *Women, Poverty and AIDS*, Monroe, ME: Common Courage Press.

Farmer, P., Lindenbaum, S. and Good, M.J.D. (1993) 'Women, poverty and AIDS: an introduction', *Culture, Medicine and Psychiatry*, 17: 387–97.

Fee, E. and Krieger, N. (1993) 'Understanding AIDS: historical interpretations and the limits of biomedical individualism', *American Journal of Public Health*, 83: 1477–86.

Fisher, B., Hovell, M., Hofstetter, C.R. and Hough, R. (1995) 'Risks associated with long-term homelessness among women: battery, rape, and HIV infection', *International Journal of Health Services*, 25: 351–69.

Friedman, S.R. (1991) 'Alienated labor and dignity denial in capitalist society', in B. Berberoglu (ed.), *Critical Perspectives in Sociology*, Dubuque, IA: Kendall/Hunt.

Friedman, S.R., Sotheran, J.L., Abdul-Quader, A., Primm, B.J., Des Jarlais, D.C. *et al.* (1987) 'The AIDS epidemic among blacks and Hispanics', *Milbank Quarterly*, 65: 455–99.

Gielen, A.C., O'Campo, P., Faden, R. and Eke, A. (1995) *Women with HIV: Disclosure Concerns and Experiences*, presented at Women and HIV Infection Conference, Washington, DC (Abstr. TA1-88).

Guinan, M.E. and Hardy, A. (1987) 'Epidemiology of AIDS in women in the United States: 1981 through 1986', *Journal of the American Medical Association*, 257: 2039–42.

Gwinn, M., Pappaioanou, M., George, R. *et al.* (1991) 'Prevalence of HIV infection in childbearing women in the United States', *Journal of the American Medical Association*, 265: 1704–8.

Hubbard, R. (1990) *The Politics of Women's Biology*, New Brunswick, NJ: Rutgers University Press.

Ickovics, J.R. and Rodin, J. (1992) 'Women and AIDS in the United States: epidemiology, natural history, and mediating mechanisms', *Health Psychology*, 11: 1–16.

James, J. and Meyerding, J. (1977) 'Early sexual experience and prostitution', *American Journal of Psychiatry*, 134: 1381–5.

Jochelson, K., Mothibeli, M. and Leger, J.-P. (1994) 'Human immunodeficiency virus and migrant labor in South Africa', in N. Krieger and G. Margo (eds), *AIDS: The Politics of Survival*, Amityville, NY: Baywood.

Krieger, N. (1994) 'Epidemiology and the web of causation: has anyone seen the spider?', *Social Science and Medicine*, 39: 887–903.

Krieger, N. and Sidney, S. (1996) 'Racial discrimination and blood pressure: the CARDIA study of young black and white women and men', *American Journal of Public Health*, 86: 1370–8.

Krieger, N. and Zierler, S. (1996) 'Accounting for health of women', *Current Issues in Public Health*, 1: 251–6.

Lake, E.S. (1993) 'An exploration of the violent victim experiences of female offenders', *Violence and Victims*, 8: 41–51.

Laurell, A.C. (1989) 'Social analysis of collective health in Latin America', *Social Science and Medicine*, 28: 1183–91.

Lemp, G.F., Jones, M., Kellogg, T.A., Nieri, G.N., Anderson, L., Withum, D. and Katz, M. (1995) 'HIV seroprevalence and risk behaviors among lesbians and bisexual women in San Francisco and Berkeley, California', *American Journal of Public Health*, 85: 1549–52.

Lillie-Blanton, M., Anthony, J.C. and Schuster, C.R. (1993) 'Probing the meaning of racial/ethnic group comparisons in crack cocaine smoking', *Journal of the American Medical Association*, 269: 993–7.

Lock, M. and Gordon, D. (1988) *Biomedicine Examined*, Dordrecht: Kluwer Academic.

Lurie, P., Fernandes, M.E.L., Hughes, V., Arevalo, E.L., Hudes, E.S., Reingold, A., Hearst, N. and Instituto Adolfo Lutz Study Group (1995) 'Socioeconomic status and risk of HIV-1, syphilis and hepatitis B infection among sex workers in São Paulo State, Brazil', *AIDS*, 9: S31–S37.

Lurie, P., Hintzen, P. and Lowe, R.A. (1995) 'Socioeconomic obstacles to HIV prevention and treatment in developing countries: the roles of the International Monetary Fund and the World Bank', *AIDS*, 9: 539–46.

Lusane, C. (1991) *Pipe Dream Blues: Racism and the War on Drugs*, Boston, MA: South End Press.

Males, M.A. (1995) 'Adult involvement in teenage childbearing and STD', *Lancet*, 340: 64–5.

Mann, J. and Tarantola, D. (1996) *AIDS in the World II*, New York: Oxford University Press.

Mann, J.M., Gostin, L., Gruskin, S., Brennan, T., Lazzarini, Z. and Fineberg, H.V. (1994) 'Health and human rights', *Health and Human Rights*, 1: 6–23.

Marmor, M., Weiss, L.R. and Lyden, M. (1986) 'Possible female-to-female transmission of human immunodeficiency virus' (letter), *Annals of Internal Medicine*, 105: 969.

Mayer, K.H. and Anderson, D.J. (1995) 'Heterosexual HIV transmission', *Infectious Agents and Disease*, 4: 273–84.

Mills, C. and Ota, H. (1989) 'Homeless women with minor children in the Detroit metropolitan area', *Social Work*, 34: 185–9.

Monzon, O.T. and Capellan, J.M.B. (1987) 'Female-to-female transmission of HIV' (letter), *Lancet*, 2: 40–1.

Moore, J., Warren, D., Zierler, S., Schuman, P., Solomon, L., Schoenbaum, E. and Kennedy, M. (1997) 'Characteristics of HIV infected lesbians and bisexual women', *Women's Health: Research on Gender, Behavior, and Policy*, 2: 49–60.

National Institute on Drug Abuse (1991) *National Household Survey on Drug Abuse: Population Estimates*, Dept. of HHS Pub. no. 91–1732, Washington, DC: US Government Printing Office.

Neighbors, H.W., Jackson, J.S., Broman, C. and Thompson, E. (1996) 'Racism and the mental health of African Americans: the role of self and system blame', *Ethnicity and Disease*, 6: 167–75.

O'Campo, P., Gilen, A., Faden, R., Xue, X., Kass, N. and Wang, M. (1995) 'Violence by male partners against women during the childbearing year', *American Journal of Public Health*, 85: 1092–7.

Paone, D., Caloir, S., Shi, Q. and Des Jarlais, D.C. (1995) 'Sex, drugs, and syringe exchange in New York City: women's experiences', *Journal of the American Medical Women's Association*, 50: 109–14.

Paone, D., Chavkin, W., Willets, I., Friedmann, P. and Des Jarlais, D.C. (1992) 'The impact of sexual abuse: implications for drug treatment', *Journal of Women's Health*, 1: 149–53.

Perry, S., Jacobsberg, L. and Fogel, K. (1989) 'Orogenital transmission of HIV', *Annals of Internal Medicine*, 111: 951–2.

Pivnick, A. (1993) 'HIV infection and the meaning of condoms', *Culture, Medicine and Psychiatry*, 17: 431–53.

Prochaska, J., DiClemente, C. and Norcross, J. (1992) 'In search of how people change', *American Psychology*, 47: 1102–14.

Quinn, S.C. (1993) 'AIDS and the African American woman: the triple burden of race, class, and gender', *Health Education Quarterly*, 20: 305–20.

Rich, J.D., Buck, A., Tuomala, R.E. and Kazanjian, P.H. (1993) 'Transmission of human immunodeficiency virus infection presumed to have occurred via female homosexual contact', *Clinical Infectious Diseases*, 17: 1003–5.

Rosenbaum, M. (1979) 'Difficulties in taking care of business: women addicts as mothers', *American Journal of Drug and Alcohol Abuse*, 6: 431–46.

Rosenstock, I.M., Strecher, V. and Becker, M. (1988) 'Social learning theory and the health belief model', *Health Education Quarterly*, 15: 175–83.

Rothenberg, K.H. and Paskey, S.J. (1995) 'The risk of domestic violence and women with HIV infection: implications for partner notification policy, and the law', *American Journal of Public Health*, 85: 1569–76.

Sabatini, M.T., Patel, K. and Hirshman, R. (1984) 'Kaposi's sarcoma and T-cell lymphoma in an immunodeficient woman: a case report', *AIDS Research*, 1: 135–7.

Schoepf, B.G. (1993) 'Gender, development, and AIDS: a political economy and culture framework', *Women and International Development Annual*, 3: 53–85.

Sotheran, J.L., Wenston, J.A., Rockwell, R., Des Jarlais, D. and Friedman, S.R. (1992) *Injecting Drug users: Why Do Women Share Syringes More Often than Men?*, paper presented at American Public Health Association Conference, Washington, DC.

Steinberg, S., Davis, S. and Gwinn, M. (1995) *Prevalence of HIV among Childbearing Women in the United States, 1989–1993*, paper presented at HIV Infection in Women Conference, Washington, DC (Abstr. WE2–55).

Stevens, P.E. (1993) 'Lesbians and HIV: clinical, research, and policy issues', *American Journal of Orthopsychiatry*, 63: 289–94.

Terris, M. (1980) 'The lifestyle approach to prevention: editorial', *Journal of Public Health Policy*, 1: 5–9.

Tesh, S. (1988) *Hidden Arguments: Political Ideology and Disease Prevention Policy*, New Brunswick, NJ: Rutgers University Press.

Thomas, S.B. and Quinn, S.C. (1991) 'The Tuskegee Syphilis Study, 1932–1972: implications for HIV education and AIDS risk education programmes in the black community', *American Journal of Public Health*, 81: 1498–504.

Thomas, V.G. (1994) 'Using feminist and social structural analysis to focus on health of poor women', *Women and Health*, 22: 1–15.

Treichler, P.A. (1988) 'AIDS, gender, and biomedical discourse: current contests for meaning', in E. Fee and D.M. Fox (eds), *AIDS: The Burdens of History*, Berkeley, CA: University of California Press.

United Nations (1948) *Universal Declaration of Human Rights*, adopted and proclaimed by UN General Assembly Resolution 217A (III), 10 December.

US Department of Health and Human Services (1985) *Report of the Secretary's Task Force on Black and Minority Health*, Washington, DC: US Government Printing Office.

Vlahov, D., Brewer, T.F., Castro, K.G., Narkunas, J.P., Salive, M.E. *et al.* (1991) 'Prevalence of antibody to HIV-1 among entrants to US correctional facilities', *Journal of the American Medical Association*, 265: 1129–32.

Vlahov, D., Wientge, D., Moore, J., Flynn, C., Schuman, P. *et al.* (1996) *Violence among Women with or at Risk for HIV infection*, paper presented at the XI International AIDS Meeting, Vancouver, Canada.

Williams, D.R. (1992) 'Black–white differences in blood pressure: the role of social factors', *Ethnicity and Disease*, 2: 126–41.

Wilson, W.J. (1987) *The Truly Disadvantaged: The Inner-City, the Underclass, and Public Policy*, Chicago, IL: University of Chicago Press.

Worth, D., Paone, D. and Chavkin, W. (1993) 'From the private family domain to the public health forum: sexual abuse, women and risk for HIV infection', *SIECUS Report*, 21: 13–17.

Zierler, S. (1997) 'Hitting hard: HIV and violence against women', in J. Manlowe and N. Goldstein (eds), *Gender Politics of HIV*, New York: New York University Press.

Zierler, S., Feingold, L., Laufer, D., Velentgas, P., Kantrowitz-Gordon, I. and Mayer, K. (1991) 'Adult survivors of childhood sexual abuse and subsequent risk of HIV infection', *American Journal of Public Health*, 81: 572–5.

Zierler, S. and Krieger, N. (1997) 'Reframing women's risk: social inequalities and HIV infection', *Annual Reviews of Public Health*, 18: 401–36.

Zierler, S., Witbeck, B. and Mayer, K. (1996) 'Sexual violence and HIV in women', *American Journal of Preventive Medicine*, 12: 304–10.

4 Poverty, policy and pathogenesis

Economic justice and public health in the USA[1]

David G. Whiteis

Introduction: health gap or wealth gap? Social class, uneven development and public health

> Countries, regions, and peoples . . . may be involuntarily delinked from the world process of evolution or development . . . on terms that are not of their own choosing. The lemon is discarded after squeezing it dry . . . this new dualism is the result of the process of social and technological evolution, which others call 'development'. Moreover, this new dualism is between those who do and those who cannot participate in a world wide division of labor.
>
> (Frank 1996)

The social and economic crisis that currently threatens the health and survival of poor and minority communities in the USA is not a static or isolated phenomenon. It has deepened alongside an unprecedented consolidation of wealth in other regions and economic sectors – a consolidation that both exemplifies and stems from the growing corporate hegemony that has characterised Western economic development in recent years.

Despite a national annual per capita income of over $26,000, approximately 35.5 million Americans (13.3 per cent) live below the poverty level. This includes nearly one in five (19.9 per cent) of all US children under the age of eighteen (Mishel *et al.* 1999). The poverty rate among black children, as of 1997, was 37.2 per cent; among Hispanic children, 35.8 per cent (Sherman 1997). Among two-parent families headed by individuals under thirty, poverty rates increased by over 100 per cent between 1973 and 1994 (Collins *et al.* 1999a).

Between 1978 and 1993, the young child poverty rate (YCPR), defined as the percentage of children less than six years of age living below the federal poverty level, increased in the USA by 52 per cent, to 26.2 per cent of all young children. As of 1997, the YCPR was 22 per cent (National Center for Children in Poverty 1999). The 'underclass', defined as 'the most socially alienated and economically deprived Americans', currently constitutes between 5 and 10 per cent of all poor people in the USA. Chronic poverty, characterised by unemployment spanning several generations, is increasingly prevalent among underclass groups (Kliegman 1992).

Patterns of inequality have become especially evident in major cities. Between 1980 and 1990, in the 100 largest cities in the USA, the percentage of census tracts characterised as extreme poverty tracts (at least 40 per cent of all residents living below the federal poverty level) increased from 9.7 per cent to 13.7 per cent (Kasarda 1993). Between 1970 and 1990, the unevenness of the distribution of the poor throughout US metropolitan areas increased by 11 per cent (Abramson *et al*. 1995).

Meanwhile, beneficiaries of corporate growth have enjoyed concomitant advantages. Between 1983 and 1995, the wealthiest 1 per cent of US households experienced a 17 per cent gain in real net worth (assets minus debt); the poorest 40 per cent of US households suffered an 80 per cent decline. As of 1995, the top 20 per cent of US households controlled 93 per cent of the nation's total household wealth. Fully 85 per cent of the gains from the stock market boom that occurred between 1989 and 1997 were gleaned by the wealthiest 10 per cent of US households (Wolff 1998).

The implications of these trends for public and community health are severe. Across ages and demographic groups, exposure and susceptibility to disease are distributed according to social, political and economic patterns. Among infants and young children, for example, virtually all of the most prevalent mortalities and morbidities are associated with poverty and social neglect. Among these are perinatal drug use (Feldman *et al*. 1992); violence (Mason and Proctor 1992); lead poisoning (Fischer and Boyer 1993); and poor parental educational attainment (Schoendorf *et al*. 1992). Postnatal infectious diseases such as tuberculosis, HIV and AIDS (Snider and Roper 1992), and infantile diarrhoea (Ho *et al*. 1988) are likewise highly associated with poverty. Between 1973 and 1991, the proportion of adult mortality in the USA directly attributable to poverty increased from 16.1 per cent to 17.7 per cent (Hahn *et al*. 1995).

Due to entrenched patterns of racial and economic segregation, the association among socioeconomic status, disease and mortality is especially strong among populations of colour. Overall, US black mortality rates are 52 per cent higher than rates for whites. Black infant mortality is around twice as high as white infant mortality: black infant mortality rates average 14 deaths per 1,000 live births; white rates average 6 deaths per 1,000 (MacDorman and Atkinson 1998; Collins *et al*. 1999b). Over 60 per cent of the disparity between black/white infant mortality is accounted for by excess death rates among very low birthweight infants (Rowley 1995).

Among adults, black men have the lowest life expectancy of all Americans: sixty-six years; as opposed to seventy-four years for white men (National Center for Health Statistics 1999). Black women have longer life expectancy at birth than black men, but there remains a nearly six-year difference between life expectancy at birth for black women (seventy-four years) and white women (eighty years) (Collins *et al*. 1999b).

It is insufficient, moreover, to view the relationship between poverty and health as static. Inequality *between* social classes, rather than a low standard of living within any one class or group, represents the most significant predictor of health status across populations and geographic regions. A 1992 study of nine developed countries, including the USA, found that fully 75 per cent of the variation in life expectancy was accounted for by the proportion of income going to successive tenths of the population, ranked from poorest to richest (Wilkinson 1992). In the USA, income inequality both between and within states, rather than the median income level of a state or region, is associated with age-adjusted mortality rates, low birthweight, infant mortality, malignant neoplasms, homicide rates, and other indices of poor health (Kaplan *et al.* 1996; Kennedy *et al.* 1996).

These data show conclusively that excess morbidity and mortality among poor and minority populations are linked to variables that cannot adequately be addressed through mainstream ameliorative and preventive strategies, most of which focus primarily on personal risk reduction, behaviour change, and access to medical care. Contemporary health policy and reform debates, however, have virtually ignored the pathogenic role played by economic and social inequality in the etiology and dispersion patterns of disease. If public health work is successfully to confront the pathogenic effects associated with social and economic injustice, it must first address the root causes behind these conditions.

Poverty as process: the 'development of underdevelopment' in US cities

In the USA, where policy is driven primarily by the demands of capital, socio-economic inequalities are largely a function of longstanding historical processes of uneven economic growth and resource distribution. These processes are not merely an unintended consequence of capital accumulation; they have been directly produced by it. They are analogous to the 'development of underdevelopment' that policy analysts and economists have long noted in relationships between First and Third World countries (Frank 1988), and which represents 'the hallmark of the geography of capitalism' (Smith 1990: xii).

Capitalist development proliferates alongside underdevelopment; capital accumulation leaves economic breakdown in its wake. Systematic extraction of resources strips populations and regions of the means to attain economic and political autonomy, thus rendering them vulnerable to further exploitation (Amin 1996). Capital 'moves to where the rate of profit is highest . . . synchronized with the rhythm of accumulation and crisis' (Smith 1990: 148). This is a dynamic process, characterised by shifting geographic patterns of investment, disinvestment and reinvestment, with resultant disparities in wealth. Through this process, the political and economic abandonment of working-class and 'underclass' communities no longer deemed integral to capitalist development is linked to the parallel phenomena of *increased* investment and prosperity elsewhere.

In the late nineteenth century, the development of a factory-based, industrial mode of production facilitated the rise of the 'industrial city', in which central areas were sites of massive capital investment (Gordon 1984). Returns on this investment were sufficient to support an urban workforce that grew steadily in most cities during the early and middle years of the twentieth century; thus grew a core of working-class communities, adjacent to factories and other sites of production but socially and politically segregated from more affluent white-collar enclaves. Capitalist development, however, requires continued expansion and reinvestment. Localised investment and economic development, such as helped drive the growth of late nineteenth- and early twentieth-century industrial core cities, eventually prove to be self-limiting. As production increases, unemployment is reduced; wages and ground rents increase. Profit rates fall and competitive advantages begin to wane, necessitating strategies to lower production costs.

Primary among such cost-cutting mechanisms in the twentieth century has been relocation of capital into regions where raw materials and labour are less expensive (Feagin and Smith 1989). In the USA, the pattern of relocation initially extended primarily from the urban core to the urban periphery and nearby suburbs. Impelled by infrastructure improvements and technological advances such as highways and communications technology, the scope of dispersion widened significantly in the years following the Second World War, helping to facilitate the growth of 'exurbia', the resource-rich ring of outer suburbs that developed adjacent to older industrial cities such as New York, Detroit and Chicago (Jackson 1985). In recent decades the patterns of dispersal have continued to widen, spurred by further technological development and the perpetual need to exploit new resources and new markets. During the 1970s and early 1980s, non-unionised regions of the USA such as the Deep South and the Sun Belt were preferred targets for plant relocation. Since the mid-1980s the Third World has become more attractive: although data on the exact number of American jobs lost due to corporate relocations have been disputed, it is clear that the transfer has been substantial (Howland 1988; Browne and Sims 1993). Many of these jobs pay Third World workers one dollar an hour or less (Texas Employment Commission 1995). Through the use of sophisticated computer and telecommunications techniques, workers in these remote areas may now be closely monitored from corporate offices in 'post-industrial' US cities (Rich 1983; Whiteis 1997).

Privatised profits, socialised costs

As in earlier eras, however, costs have not been truly saved by such strategies; they have been redistributed downward. During the American economic 'recovery' of 1990–3, over four million workers were displaced from full-time jobs. Nearly 30 per cent of all new jobs created during this period were in the temporary-help industry; part-time jobs accounted for another 25.9 per cent. Virtually none of these jobs are unionised ('Displaced workers face rough road' 1994; 'The joyless recovery' 1994). As of 1997, nearly 30 per cent of all jobs in the USA were classified as 'nonstandard positions' – e.g., part-time, temporary, day labour, self-employed, independent contracting – the majority of which offered lower-than-average wages, fewer benefits (including health insurance), and less security than full-time employment (Mishel *et al.* 1999).

Also as before, these economic trends are reflected in urban geographic, political and social relations. Especially in older metropolitan regions, there has been a massive transformation from labour-intensive, production-based economic activity to capital-intensive, information-based corporate enterprise. The modern 'post-industrial' city is characterised by an affluent downtown filled mostly with corporate headquarters, favoured by lenient zoning and tax structures. Geographically close by, but economically and politically isolated, are decaying 'inner-city' communities, overwhelmingly populated by non-whites and increasingly bereft of services, finance capital or even commerce (Fasenfest 1989).

Again, however, it must be noted that these conditions under capitalism are not static. The shifting, cyclical pattern of uneven development continues to manifest itself: these long-neglected 'declining neighbourhoods' have become attractive to investors, as ground rent and real estate have become sufficiently devalued to attract speculation. The result is gentrification, in which 'inner-city' communities are marketed to professional-class populations returning from the suburbs. Thus does capital continue to express its internal contradictions geographically: development leads to saturation and attendant decline in profit, thus necessitating capital flight; resultant devaluation, in turn, eventually attracts reinvestment.

This 'revitalisation' does not, however, improve conditions for long-time residents, most of whom can no longer afford to remain in these newly lucrative real estate markets after rents and property tax rates increase. Depletion of affordable housing in the wake of redevelopment and gentrification has become a nationwide crisis. In the USA between 1985 and 1991, an average of 130,000 units of low-cost housing was lost annually; 64 per cent of this annual loss (83,000 units) occurred in central cities. A significant proportion of units have been lost to 'reverse filtering', or the upgrading from lower to higher rent status (Joint Center for Housing Studies 1995). The result has been a severe housing shortage for poor and moderate-income residents, especially in urban areas.

Uneven development and public policy: public resources, private gain

The corporate transformation of the modern urban landscape, along with the worsening conditions of inequality associated with it, has been, to a significant extent, publicly subsidised. This public subsidisation of private profit is fostered by an ideological framework, which has been labelled *recapitalisation* and legitimises the role of the public sector in facilitating capital growth (Tomaskovic-Devey and Miller 1983). Under this ideology, the 'bounds of the expressible', as delineated by the common self-interest between corporate and state power, seriously curtail the scope of policy discussion and debate (Herman and Chomsky 1988); corporate profit becomes the primary criterion by which regulatory and distributional policy is evaluated. Basic ideological assumptions – e.g., that the market is the appropriate arbiter of social relations and the legitimate mechanism for distributing goods, both public and private – are seldom questioned.

Recapitalisation strategies include reduction of corporate tax burdens; the contraction of the public sector, including the transformation of formerly public goods into market commodities (e.g., 'privatisation'); reductions in social spending (including massive cutbacks in federal, state and local public health and human services expenditures); deregulation of business and industry, including reductions in anti-trust action and labour law enforcement; promotion of research and development of technologies to rationalise production and increase economic efficiency; the weakening of unions and the hiring of non-unionised and part-time workers; reliance on money supply, rather than macro-level intervention, to stabilise the economy and promote growth; and the enactment of international policies such as the North American Free Trade Agreement (NAFTA) and trade treaties under the World Trade Organization (WTO), designed to facilitate global capital mobility and to buttress the international hegemony of corporate capital (Tomaskovic-Devey and Miller 1983; Navarro 1984; Bodenheimer 1989).

Locally, as well, recapitalisation strategies both legitimise and intensify the role of government as executor of the interests of capital. Beginning in the years following the Second World War, the flight of industrial capital from core urban areas was facilitated by aggressive public-sector investment in projects such as the interstate highway system and home loan programmes to spur further suburban development (Fainstein and Fainstein 1982a). Meanwhile, in the metropolitan regions left behind, the clearing of low- and moderate-income areas under federally sponsored 'urban renewal' programmes provided opportunities for corporate expansion and the creation of new markets for real estate investment, while largely defaulting on their expressed purpose of replacing slums with affordable housing for low-income residents. These residents, increasingly displaced by gentrification, are now being pushed farther towards the cities' peripheral areas. As these trends continue, some analysts believe, the urban poor will eventually be relegated to a peripheral suburban ring, mirroring geographic and spatial relations found in many European cities or in South African cities under apartheid (Fainstein and Fainstein 1982b).

As public policy continues to divert massive resources into private investment and the creation of new markets, increasing numbers of people are thus rendered unable to compete in these new markets for basic services and necessities. Confined in areas drained of resources and human services, they are in jeopardy of becoming, in an economic sense, redundant – discarded 'human capital' with insufficient market value to justify significant public or private expenditures.

Pathogenic pathways: uneven development, public policy and public health

It is among these populations that the deleterious effects of underdevelopment are most directly linked to social, psychological and medical pathologies. Krieger *et al.* (1993: 100) identify four principal pathways through which political, economic and social inequalities may determine patterns of health and disease among at-risk populations:

1 [by] shaping exposure and susceptibility to risk factors, events and processes;
2 by shaping exposure and susceptibility to protective factors, events, and processes;

3   by shaping access to, and type of, health care received; and
4   by shaping health research and health policy.

Data show conclusively how these pathways are operant in exacerbating the risks encountered by residents of communities affected by resource withdrawal and political and economic disenfranchisement – communities that already had few coping resources before the onset of the current crisis. Not only is poverty and economic inequality pathogenic in nature; access to medical care and other necessary human services has declined most seriously in the communities most affected by these pathogenic conditions.

This association between economic underdevelopment, political disempowerment and pathogenesis is especially evident when analysed on the local level. Overcrowding in New York hospitals has been linked to an influx of increasingly sick patients, whose health problems were themselves associated with deterioration of housing stock due to fire damage, following municipal cutbacks in fire protection (Wallace 1990). AIDS, violent crime, tuberculosis and low birthweight are now functional 'index conditions' for 'social disintegration' due to economic and political neglect in poor and minority urban communities (Wallace *et al.* 1997).

The poor face further displacement from the healthcare system as the medical care 'industry', reflecting the overall economic pattern, consolidates increasing amounts of wealth and power among an elite group of corporate providers, reaping unprecedented financial gains through consolidation, integration, and the extraction of higher profits by charging more for services and avoiding uninsured patients (Whiteis and Salmon 1990; Salmon 1994; *Florida Hospital Analysis* 1995; Amsel 1997). Alongside this rampant development in the corporate sector is the inevitable withdrawal of resources from community-based public and not-for-profit providers: disproportionately high closure rates among free-standing public and community hospitals serving poor and minority neighbourhoods have been evident for decades (Sager 1983; McLafferty 1982; Schatzkin 1984; Whiteis 1992). Such closures are expected to increase, perhaps by as many as two to three times the current average rate of approximately fifty per year (McGinley 1995). The result will be increased pressure on the providers that remain: a nationwide 1989 survey found that hospital overcrowding had a 'substantial effect' on quality of care in 65 per cent of the institutions studied. In the most serious cases, patients requiring in-patient care may wait in emergency departments for several days before a bed becomes available (Lynn 1994).

Under these conditions, the two-tiered structure that has long characterised the US medical care system has become increasingly pronounced. A 1994 study of ambulatory care sites in ten cities found that only 44 per cent would provide appointments or authorisation for walk-in visits for Medicaid patients (Medicaid Access Study Group 1994). Children with Medicaid are less likely than other children to receive routine care in physicians' offices, and more likely to lack adequate continuity of care (St Peter *et al.* 1992).

Patients who are black, poor, uninsured or without a regular physician are between 40 per cent and 80 per cent more likely than other patients to delay seeking care (Weissman *et al.* 1991). The care they do receive is often inadequate: nationwide, the uninsured are 29 to 75 per cent less likely than the insured to undergo high-cost procedures; they have shorter lengths of stay for most diagnoses; and they are at a 44 to 124 per cent higher risk of in-patient mortality at time of admission (Hadley *et al.* 1991). Using basic protocols such as history taking, physical examination, and common diagnostic tests and therapies as indices of quality, poor and black Medicare recipients receive lower quality of care than other Medicare recipients (Kahn *et al.* 1994).

These data further illustrate the link among disinvestment and service withdrawal, the concomitant consolidation of wealth and power among the corporate elite, and the pathogenic conditions that threaten the health of poor and minority communities in the USA. Whether on the international, national, regional or local level, whether between the corporate medical care industry and community-based providers, or between downtown corporate headquarters and 'inner-city' neighbourhoods, development and underdevelopment are complementary and contiguous processes.

Implications for social change: challenging the ideology of recapitalisation

Health policy, like other public and social policy in the USA, is debated and enacted largely within the ideological constraints of recapitalisation; it also serves to entrench this ideology further. The passage of the Health Maintenance Organisation Act in 1973, though by no means the only historical case of governmental activism to buttress capital's role in healthcare, provides an important example. Although HMOs did not grow to dominate healthcare as rapidly as their early advocates had hoped (Ellwood and Lundberg 1996), the HMO Act served an important ideological purpose. By placing its *imprimatur* on a profit-driven model of healthcare delivery and financing, government further legitimised corporate enterprise as the driving force in reshaping the US healthcare system (Salmon 1990a).

More recently, the Clinton administration's healthcare 'reform' proposal, based on a model of 'managed competition' developed by economist Alain Enthoven (1993), represented another important stage in the corporate transformation of healthcare. In theory, the programmes would have increased access, primarily through mandating a standard minimum level of universal coverage to be funded by projected cost savings and by taxes imposed on the purchase of more comprehensive plans (Kotelchuk 1994). However, its primary function would have been to harness the power of the state to ensure economic benefit for insurers, and for those providers who could compete successfully in the managed-care 'marketplace' (McKenzie 1994).

Although the proposal failed politically, it furthered the ideological agenda represented by the HMO initiative. In its wake, with the support of many 'mainstream' policy analysts, for-profit corporations and multi-institutional 'not-for profit' firms have succeeded in transforming US medical care into a business very similar to the system envisioned by Clinton's proposal, minus the minimal safeguards for the poor. Membership in HMOs, the dominant form of managed-care organisation, has grown by more than 11 per cent annually since the early 1990s (Anders 1994).

Meanwhile, nearly 20 per cent of all urban Americans and over 43 million Americans nationwide (including 49 per cent of all full-time workers below poverty level) have no health insurance (Levan *et al.* 1998; Kilborn 1999).[2] Public health and wellness concerns have receded from policy discussion except to the extent that they may be commodified and marketed as cost-saving or profit-generating product lines (Salmon 1990b; Whiteis 1997).

As outlined in this chapter, discrepancies such as these between the corporate medical care sector and community-based primary and preventive services reproduce the increasing class disparities, in both wealth and health, that characterise the political economy of the USA. These inequalities are both exacerbated and reflected by recapitalisation policies, such as those that further the withdrawal of resources from poor and minority communities to spur private economic development and profit. Emphasising this link among economic injustice, public health and the commodification and privatisation of public resources can provide an important conceptual framework to challenge the corporatisation of medical care, as well as community disinvestment, unemployment and the privatisation of such public services as education and transportation. The day-to-day stresses that affect low-income urban communities – inadequate housing, poor nutrition, poor public services, inadequate (and abusive) police; the neglect and eventual closure of public schools; the increase of such social pathologies as substance abuse and crime – proliferate alongside declining community health standards and impediments to accessible and affordable care, and have the same causal roots.

Any realistic solution to the public health crises in poor and minority urban communities must thus include attention to economic justice – i.e., a direct challenge to policies that promote capital withdrawal, uneven economic development, and corporatisation – as *an integral health policy issue* alongside such other important considerations as health promotion, prevention, access and affordability of care.

Only by examining and aggressively challenging the ideology of recapitalisation, as well as the policies it sustains – capital accumulation at the expense of community development; corporatisation of medical care, education and other human services at the expense of human need; corporate hegemony at the expense of social justice – can we truly confront the public health crises that threaten the survival of poor and minority urban communities in the USA as well as the ongoing viability of our medical care institutions.

Notes

1   This chapter was first published in *Critical Public Health* (2000) 10: 257–71.
2   Since this article was first published, the proportion and absolute number of uninsured persons in the USA have increased.

References

Abramson, A.J., Tobin, M.S. and VanderGoot, M.R. (1995) 'The changing geography of metropolitan opportunity: the segregation of the poor in US metropolitan areas, 1970 to 1990', *Housing Policy Debate*, 6: 45–72.

Amin, S. (1996) 'On development', in S.A. Chew and R.A. Denemark (eds), *The Underdevelopment of Development*, Thousand Oaks, CA: Sage Publications.

Amsel, L.A. (1997) 'Corporate healthcare', *Tikkun*, 12: 19–25, 76.

Anders, G. (1994) 'HMOs pile up billions in cash, try to decide what to do about it', *Wall Street Journal*, 21: A1, A8.

Bodenheimer, T.S. (1989) 'The fruits of empire rot on the vine: United States health policy in the austerity era', *Social Science and Medicine*, 28: 531–8.

Browne, H. and Sims, B. (1993) *Runaway America: US Jobs and Factories on the Move*, Albuquerque, NM: Resource Press.

Collins, C., Leonard-Wright, B. and Sklar, H. (1999a) *Shifting Fortunes: The Perils of the Growing American Wealth Gap*, Boston, MA: United for a Fair Economy.

Collins, K.S., Hall, A. and Neuhaus, C. (1999b) *US Minority Health: A Chartbook*, New York: Commonwealth Fund.

'Displaced workers face rough road' (1994), *LRA's Economic Notes*, 62(10): 7.

Ellwood, P.M. and Lundberg, G.D. (1996) 'Managed care: a work in progress', *Journal of the American Medical Association*, 276: 1083–6.

Enthoven, A. (1993) 'The history and principles of managed competition', *Health Affairs* (Supplement): 24–48.

Fainstein, N.I. and Fainstein, S.S. (1982a) 'Restoration and struggle: urban policy and social forces', in N.I. Fainstein and S.S. Fainstein (eds), *Urban Policy under Capitalism*, Beverly Hills, CA: Sage Publications.

—— (1982b) 'Restructuring the American city: a comparative perspective', in N.I. Fainstein and S.S. Fainstein (eds), *Urban Policy under Capitalism*, Beverly Hills, CA: Sage Publications.

Fasenfest, D. (1989) 'Race, class, and community development: a comparison of Detroit's Poletown and Chicago's Goose Island', in J. Lembcke and R. Hutchison (eds), *Research in Urban Sociology, Vol. 1*, Greenwich, CT: Jai Press.

Feagin, J.R. and Smith, M.P. (1989) 'Cities and the new international division of labor: an overview', in M.P. Smith and J.R. Feagin (eds), *The Capitalist City*, Cambridge, MA: Basil Blackwell.

Feldman, J.G., Minkoff, H.L., McCalla, S. and Salwen, M. (1992) 'A cohort study on the impact of perinatal drug use on prematurity in an inner-city population', *American Journal of Public Health*, 82: 726–8.

Fischer, D.B. and Boyer, A. (1993) 'State activities for prevention of lead poisoning among children – United States, 1992', *Morbidity and Mortality Weekly Report*, 42: 165–72.

Florida Hospital Analysis (1995), Irving, TX: VHA Inc.

Frank A.G. (1988) 'The development of underdevelopment', in C.K. Wilber (ed.), *The Political Economy of Development and Underdevelopment*, New York: Random House.

—— (1996) 'The underdevelopment of development', in S.A. Chew and R.A. Denemark (eds), *The Underdevelopment of Development*, Thousand Oaks, CA: Sage Publications.

Gordon, D.M. (1984) 'Capitalist development and the history of American cities', in W.K. Tabb and L. Sawers (eds), *Marxism in the Metropolis*, New York: Oxford University Press.

Hadley, J., Steinberg, E.P. and Feder, J. (1991) 'Comparison of uninsured and privately insured patients', *Journal of the American Medical Association*, 265: 374–9.

Hahn, R.A., Eaker, E., Barker, N.D., Teutsch, S.M., Sosniak, W. and Krieger, N. (1995) 'Poverty and death in the United States – 1973 and 1991', *Epidemiology*, 6: 490–7.

Herman, E.S. and Chomsky, N. (1988) *Manufacturing Consent*, New York: Random House.

Ho, M.-S., Glass, R.I., Pinsky, P.F., Young-Okoh, N.C., Sappenfield, W.M., Buehler, J.W., Gunter, N. and Anderson, L.J. (1988) 'Diarrheal deaths in American children: are they preventable?', *Journal of the American Medical Association*, 260: 3281–5.

Howland, M. (1988) *Plant Closings and Worker Displacement: The Regional Issues*, Kalamazoo, MI: W.E. Upjohn Institute for Employment Research.

Jackson, K.T. (1985) *Crabgrass Frontier: The Suburbanization of the United States*, New York: Oxford University Press.

Joint Center for Housing Studies (1995) *The State of the Nation's Housing, 1994*, Cambridge, MA: Harvard University Press.

'The joyless recovery' (1994), *LRA's Economic Notes*, 61(9): 1.

Kahn, K.K., Pearson, M.L., Harrison, E.R., Desmond, K.A., Rogers, W.H., Rubenstein, L.V., Brook, R.H. and Keeler, E.B. (1994) 'Health care for black and poor hospitalized patients', *Journal of the American Medical Association*, 271: 1169–74.

Kaplan, G.A., Pamuk, E.R., Lynch, J.W., Cohen, R.D. and Balfour, J.L. (1996) 'Inequality in income and mortality in the United States: analysis of mortality and potential pathways', *British Medical Journal*, 312: 999–1003.

Kasarda, J.D. (1993) 'Inner-city concentrated poverty and neighbourhood distress: 1970 to 1990', *Housing Policy Debate*, 4: 253–302.

Kennedy, B.P., Kawachi, I. and Prothrow-Stith, D. (1996) 'Income distribution and mortality: cross sectional ecological study of the Robin Hood index in the United States', *British Medical Journal*, 312: 1004–7.

Kilborn, P.T. (1999) 'Uninsured in US span many groups', *New York Times*, 25 February: A1, A14.

Kliegman, R.M. (1992) 'Perpetual poverty: child health and the underclass', *Pediatrics*, 89: 710–13.

Kotelchuk, R. (1994) 'Managed competition', in N.F. McKenzie (ed.), *Beyond Crisis: Confronting Health Care in the United States*, New York: Penguin/Meridian.

Krieger, N., Rowley, D.L., Herman, A.A., Avery, B. and Phillips, M.T. (1993) 'Racism, sexism, and social class: implications for studies of health, disease, and well-being', *American Journal of Preventive Medicine*, 6 (Supplement): 82–122.

Levan, R., Brown, E.R., Lara, L. and Wyn, R. (1998) 'Nearly one-fifth of urban Americans lack health insurance', *Policy Brief*, Los Angeles, CA: Center for Health Policy Research, University of California.

Lynn, S.G. (1994) 'Gridlock in the emergency department', in N.F. McKenzie (ed.), *Beyond Crisis: Confronting Health Care in the United States*, New York: Penguin/Meridian.

MacDorman, M.F. and Atkinson, J.O. (1998) 'Infant mortality statistics from the 1995 period linked to birth/infant death data set', *Monthly Vital Statistics Report*, 46 (Supplement 2): 1–2.

Mason, J. and Proctor, R. (1992) 'Reducing youth violence: the physician's role', *Journal of the American Medical Association*, 267: 22.

McGinley, L. (1995) 'Retooling of Medicare, Medicaid will increase pressure on hospitals', *Wall Street Journal*, 2 October: A1, A7.

McKenzie, N.F. (1994) 'Managed competition and public health', in N.F. McKenzie (ed.), *Beyond Crisis: Confronting Health Care in the United States*, New York: Penguin/Meridian.

McLafferty, S. (1982) 'Neighbourhood characteristics and hospital closure', *Social Science and Medicine*, 16: 1667–74.

Medicaid Access Study Group (1994) 'Access of Medicaid recipients to outpatient care', *New England Journal of Medicine*, 330: 1426–30.

Mishel, L., Bernstein, J. and Schmitt, J. (1999) *The State of Working America, 1998–99*, Ithaca, NY: Cornell University Press.

National Center for Children in Poverty (1999) *Young Children in Poverty: A Statistical Update, June 1999*, New York: National Center for Children in Poverty, Columbia University.

National Center for Health Statistics (1999) *Health, United States, 1998, with Socioeconomic Status and Health Chartbook 1999*, Hyattsville, MD: National Center for Health Statistics.

Navarro, V. (1984) 'The crisis of the international capitalist order and its implications for the welfare state', in J. McKinlay (ed.), *Issues in the Political Economy of Health Care*, New York: Tavistock Publications.

Rich, R. (1983) 'The political economy of public services', in N.I. Fainstein and S.S. Fainstein (eds), *Urban Policy under Capitalism*, Beverly Hills, CA: Sage Publications.

Rowley, D.L. (1995) 'Framing the debate: can prenatal care help to reduce the black–white disparity in infant mortality?', *Journal of the American Medical Women's Association*, 50: 187–93.

Sager, A. (1983) 'Why urban voluntary hospitals close', *Health Services Research*, 18: 450–7.

Salmon, J.W. (1990a) 'The health maintenance organization strategy', in J.W. Salmon (ed.), *The Corporate Transformation of Health Care, Vol. 1: Issues and Directions*, Amityville, NY: Baywood.

—— (1990b) 'Introduction', in J.W. Salmon (ed.), *The Corporate Transformation of Health Care, Vol. 1: Issues and Directions*, Amityville, NY: Baywood.

—— (ed.) (1994) *The Corporate Transformation of Health Care: Perspectives and Implications*, Amityville, NY: Baywood.

Schatzkin, A. (1984) 'The relationship of inpatient racial composition and hospital closure in New York City', *Medical Care*, 22: 379–87.

Schoendorf, K.C., Hogue, C.J., Kleinman, J.C. and Rowley, D. (1992) 'Mortality among infants of blacks as compared with white college-educated parents', *New England Journal of Medicine*, 326: 1522–6.

Sherman, A. (1997) *Rescuing the American Dream: Halting the Economic Freefall of Today's Young Families with Children*, Washington, DC: Children's Defense Fund.

Smith, N. (1990) 'Towards a theory of uneven development II', in N. Smith (ed.), *Uneven Development: Nature, Capital, and the Production of Space*, Cambridge, MA: Basil Blackwell.

Snider, D.E. and Roper, W.L. (1992) 'The new tuberculosis', *New England Journal of Medicine*, 326: 703–5.

St Peter, R.F., Newacheck, P.W. and Halfon, N. (1992) 'Access to care for poor children: separate and unequal?', *Journal of the American Medical Association*, 267: 2760–4.

Texas Employment Commission, Economic Research and Analysis Department (1995) News Release, El Paso: Texas Employment Commission.

Tomaskovic-Devey, D. and Miller, S.M. (1983) 'Recapitalization: the basic urban policy of the 1980s', in N.I. Fainstein and S.S. Fainstein (eds), *Urban Policy under Capitalism*, Beverly Hills, CA: Sage Publications.

Wallace, D. (1990) 'Roots of increased health care inequality in New York', *Social Science and Medicine*, 31: 1219–1277.

Wallace, R., Wallace, D. and Andrews, H. (1997) 'AIDS, tuberculosis, violent crime, and low birthweight in eight US metropolitan areas: public policy, stochastic resonance, and the regional diffusion of inner-city markers', *Environment and Planning A*, 29: 525–55.

Weissman, J.S., Stern, R., Fielding, S.L. and Epstein, A.M. (1991) 'Delayed access to health care: risk factors, reasons, and consequences', *Annals of Internal Medicine*, 114: 325–31.

Whiteis, D.G. (1992) 'Hospital and community characteristics in closures of urban hospitals, 1980–87', *Public Health Reports*, 107: 409–16.

—— (1997) 'Third world medicine in first world cities: capital accumulation, uneven development, and public health', *Social Science and Medicine*, 47: 795–808.

Whiteis, D.G. and Salmon, J.W. (1990) 'The proprietarization of health care and the underdevelopment of the public sector', in J.W. Salmon (ed.), *The Corporate Transformation of Health Care, Vol. 1: Issues and Directions*, Amityville, NY: Baywood.

Wilkinson, R.G. (1992) 'Income distribution and life expectancy', *British Medical Journal*, 304: 165–8.

Wolff, E.N. (1998) 'Recent trends in the size distribution of household wealth', *Journal of Economic Perspectives*, 12: 131–50.

Part II

Making traces: evidence for practice and evaluation

Introduction

Nina Wallerstein

There is no question that health practitioners and researchers value 'evidence' about which interventions improve health outcomes. As health disparities have grown internationally between North and South countries and within industrialised nations, it becomes even more important to focus our energies on what *matters*: what policies, institutional practices, social and community interventions, and behavioural lifestyle actions make a difference to population health.

The key questions, however, are not related to the 'value' of evidence, but instead focus on the 'what' and 'how': *what* constitutes sufficient robustness or 'weight of evidence' to be able to attribute causes to the specific interventions, no matter what level(s) of the socioecologic framework they address; and *how* can we best collect this evidence, or what are the best research and evaluation designs?

The dominant ideology to answer these questions has emerged from the 'evidence-based medicine' literature that privileges the randomised control trial (RCT) as the best mechanism to prove internal validity in efficacy trials, and then testing intervention in effectiveness trials in less controlled community settings (Walker and Jacobs 2002). Inherent in this translational process is the assumption that external validity increases as the settings of the effectiveness trials become more diverse. The Cochrane and Campbell Collaborations and new tools like CONSORT are used in the conduct of systematic literature reviews to identify the best evidence of outcomes and those biases that may compromise study findings (Wormald and Oldfield 1998; White 2001; Bellg *et al.* 2004).

While there is no question that RCTs are best for identifying internal validity and for controlling bias, there are serious limitations to accepting the RCT as the only or even the best evidence for public health or population group interventions which take place in complex social environments, especially in determining external validity (Green and Glasgow 2006). Systematic literature reviews themselves may be limited in their focus on outcome effectiveness, which regards as less important other 'evidence' critical for generalisability: for example, process evaluation, qualitative descriptions of contextual factors, and the quality of the intervention itself (White 2001). Community researchers interested in promoting health improvements as a result of our research face two major challenges: the role of context and the role of the researcher–researched relationship. This introductory chapter will discuss several issues in an attempt to address these challenges:

- The differences between medical and public health/health promotion interventions in dynamic social and community environments.
- External validity and how we can best understand the translation of interventions to multiple settings.
- Empowerment intervention strategies and the role of community-based participatory research and participatory evaluation as parts of the empowerment agenda.

Medical versus community-based public health/health promotion interventions

Medical or pharmaceutical interventions, by their very nature, are discrete treatments, procedures or medications which are tested against an alternative treatment or placebo. Health services research in particular has sought to identify best evidence-supported treatments in efficacy trials that can then be disseminated widely to clinical practice settings. As Chris Bonell (2002) argues, some public health interventions can also fit this model: that is, it is feasible to compare them in community settings. A nutrition education programme within a discrete school setting, for example, may be implemented in multiple intervention schools and tested against control non-intervention schools (or tested against delayed, usual care, or alternative interventions). In this case, the randomised control trial at a population level, or group randomised design, is best applied if the targeted outcomes are at the individual level (Nutbeam 1999), with the goal of holding other factors constant: for instance, assessing intervention effectiveness on the children's nutritional knowledge, attitudes and behaviours.

In the past thirty years, however, public health interventions have shifted dramatically from targeting individual-level changes, especially since the large heart health and tobacco interventions applying behavioural change theory on a community level were largely ineffective (Glanz *et al.* 2003; Murray 2001; COMMIT I 1995; COMMIT II 1995). Several driving forces have been at work:

- The effect of community coalitions, grassroots initiatives, and community-based participatory research which have demanded community-engaged or empowerment models rather than expert-driven community-targeted models (Minkler and Wallerstein 2003; Wallerstein *et al.* 2002; Israel *et al.* 2005; Viswanathan *et al.* 2004).
- The recognition of a comprehensive socioecologic multi-level approach, which integrates individual change targets with goals of organisational, community, economic and policy change (Gebbie *et al.* 2002).
- Critiques of a positivist science which assumes discrete variables that can be controlled and studied objectively (Bonner 2003).

Much has been written about the near impossibility of using RCT methodologies for complex community and social interventions which embrace multi-level community change targets, including community capacity and empowerment, and which usually extend beyond one single programme to evaluate (Goodman 2000; McQueen 2001; Schorr 1997; Kreuter *et al.* 2000). Women's empowerment, for example, may be built into a micro-lending project combined with nutrition, immunisation or family planning educational strategies. Outcomes therefore are only partially related to any one strategy and can be wide-ranging, from changes in individual household decision-making to changes in economic opportunities and policies. With such purposive community-wide interventions, it is not possible to adjust for factors that are simply not known (White 2001).

Policy interventions in particular do not lend themselves to randomisation because of political and ethical considerations. It would, for instance, be impossible randomly to implement needle exchange programmes to prove their effectiveness (Buchanan *et al.* in press). Moreover, the tremendous costs involved have led many to question the value of group-randomised trials because of the small effect sizes, and the difficulty in achieving sufficient community involvement to produce sustainability once the researchers leave (Murray 2001; Thompson *et al.* 2003). Ultimately, expectations for changes in individual health status may be unrealistic in the limited funding periods of RCTs; and actions to transform social determinants and unhealthy conditions may involve even longer-term periods.

Community interventionists, however, have pursued several approaches to address evaluation of complex community interventions: methodological advances within the group-randomised trial, when appropriate; a re-emphasis on process evaluation; and the increasing recognition of alternative evaluation approaches, with quasi-experimental and theory-based design.

Thompson and colleagues (2003) have articulated methodologic advances for community trials, looking at how to maximise power with a small sample size of few randomised communities or using stratification to maximise comparisons. Flay (1986) has recommended testing interventions in phases, from pilot tests, efficacy trials, to effectiveness trials. Statistical methods of multi-level analysis can be used to incorporate the contribution of differences within identified contextual variables. In addition, to mitigate the 'black box' of an RCT (Bonner 2003), process evaluation (assessing dose and fidelity) provides confirmatory evidence to understand how and why the programme is successful; triangulation of evidence gathered by ethnographic study of programme participants, for example, can provide greater understanding of which components of an intervention may matter most.

Quasi-experimental designs comparing communities (Thomson *et al.* 2003) are increasingly used, and theory-based evaluation has emerged as a core strategy for community initiatives to build evidence for social-environmental and policy changes (Bonner 2003; Connell and Kubisch 1998; Fulbright-Anderson *et al.* 1998). A theory of change approach is an interactive evaluation model which enables programmes and community groups to articulate their own assumptions for change, enhance planning, and help them operationalise evaluation indicators. Both the processes and impacts of a community initiative therefore can be 'tested' against assumed pathways for change, and hypotheses can be generated about why the intervention is or is not effective (White 2001).

External validity and translation of interventions to multiple settings

The major challenge for complex social and community public health interventions is how best to understand the role of context in any intervention's effectiveness. One can argue that context may even be equal to or more important than the actual intervention itself. This is the heart of the external validity question: can evidence-based practices and programmes be translated to multiple settings, cultures and contexts, and maintain their comprehensiveness; or does each setting demand cultural and local adaptations? If interventions cannot be transplanted without adaptation, can core components and best practices that have proved to be effective be adopted, yet their implementation be adapted based on the understanding of the 'noise' (the organisational, cultural, personality and policy differences) of each new setting (Hohmann and Shear 2002)? Or can 'effective' interventions be translated to other settings through retaining only the underlying principles and theories, but allowing for flexibility in form (Fixsen *et al.* 2005)?

Green, Glasgow and colleagues argue that the study of external validity has not been sufficiently addressed, given the focus on internal validity in the published literature (Green and Glasgow 2006; Glasgow *et al.* 2006). They cite major failings of the literature in addressing the utility of findings by practitioners and policy-makers. There is, for instance, too little reporting on the feasibility or costs of applying interventions to other settings and insufficient attention to the processes of implementation and dissemination. They argue the need for more practitioner engagement and practice-based evidence, if the field wants evidence-based practice (Green and Ottosen 2004). Participatory planning strategies, which involve practitioners and communities, would assure greater success of implementation, incorporation of theory-driven models, and retention of core conditions of the effective intervention (Green and Glasgow 2006).

Recently, implementation research has emerged as an important addition to the process evaluation literature. Rather than just studying the dose and fidelity of an intervention to uncover why and how it may be effective or not, there is an emerging theory of effectiveness of the implementation, its stages, processes and outcomes (Fixsen *et al.* 2005). In a comprehensive review of the human services and education literature and incorporating learnings from juvenile justice, agriculture, business and medicine, Fixsen and colleagues (2005) articulated core implementation processes. These were: the source of the intervention or best practice to be implemented, its destination, the communication link, feedback elements, and the sphere of influence or context. They also identified three essential implementation outcomes: changes in professional behaviour (with training of staff in the intervention and its implementation proving to be essential); changes in organisational structures and cultures; and changes in relationships to stakeholders and communities. For enhancing translation of findings to diverse settings, they recommend dissemination of information critical to implementation, such as that found in the RE–AIM framework (Glasgow *et al.* 2006; Bull *et al.* 2003): the *reach* of the programme as to participant characteristics; the *efficacy or effectiveness* on the individual level; *adoption* characteristics of the settings; *implementation* findings as to extent of dose and fidelity; and maintenance information. Roth and colleagues (2005) add recommendations to study the facilitating factors and barriers to implementation at multiple levels, from upper echelon and staff practices to organisational cultures of risk-taking and learning. Evans and Killoran (2000) argue for realistic theory of change evaluations (see also Pawson and Tilley 1997), looking at receptive and non-receptive contexts (Pettigrew *et al.* 1992): the political and social relationships and structures; and the mechanisms of change (processes and resources) which may influence outcomes.

Community empowerment and the role of community-based participatory research and participatory evaluation as part of the empowerment agenda

A consistent challenge within the evaluation field has been how to assure the usefulness and use of evidence and evaluation findings by multiple stakeholders. In the last several decades, policy documents encouraging user involvement in the planning and delivery of services have paralleled the call for stakeholder involvement in evaluation (Truman and Raine 2001). More recently, community-based participatory research (CBPR) has emerged within the public health field with a similar agenda (De Koning and Martin 1996; Minkler and Wallerstein 2003; Israel *et al.* 2005; Blumenthal and DiClemente 2004; Viswanathan *et al.* 2004), even including medical researchers advocating consumer involvement (Walker and Jacobs 2002). Levels of participation, however, may vary considerably, from a token co-option to an empowerment collective action agenda (Cornwall 1996; Arnstein 1969).

The key questions for empowerment and CBPR become the role of the 'agency' of consumers and community members in the delivery of services and interventions; and the role of the 'agency' of community members with researchers and within the research agenda. Rather than assuming that interventions can be generalised to other settings, the question becomes: what works best within this cultural setting, within this community, with this group of social actors and influences? Agency means that community engagement or empowerment cannot be done 'to' others, but comes from processes where people act 'with' others and empower themselves and participate directly in the intervention and research processes (Sen 1997; Labonte 1994). Advocates or researchers may catalyse actions or help create spaces for people to learn, but sustainability and empowerment occur only as people gain their own skills and advocate for their own changes.

The premise of empowerment interventions and CBPR practices is of dynamic processes in which participatory processes support continual evaluation and reformulation of strategies and interventions. As empowerment goals and activities purposefully change over time to meet the needs and priorities of the participating stakeholders and settings, the intervention changes and ceases to be the same as a previous intervention, though certain components and evidence-based practices may remain (Rychetnik *et al.* 2002; W.K. Kellogg Foundation 1998). With this model, RCTs can be applied only within similar populations which have been engaged in the creation of their new model.

Empowerment interventions can be characterised both as processes (personal, dialogical and collective political actions), and as outcomes (at multiple interacting psychological, organisational and community levels) relating to social justice and equity (Zimmerman 2000; Wallerstein 2002; Cook 1997; Connell 1995). Once a community is identified as empowered or as producing results, however, maintenance of these conditions cannot be assumed. Empowerment outcomes are not static; they may not be transferable to all issues, or may change over time as political or economic contexts shift. A community may be successful at preventing the installation of a hazardous waste facility, for example, but unsuccessful at increasing funding for local schools the next year. This reinforces the need continually to evaluate changes within institutions, governments and other opportunity structures, to evaluate the targets of change as well as changes in how communities exercise their agency for different goals. Indicators of empowerment at multiple levels are being developed, including through the World Bank (Alsop and Heinsohn 2005; Narayan 2005).

In a recent comprehensive review of the English language literature about the effectiveness of empowerment strategies to improve health, a model of empowerment strategies producing intermediate empowerment outcomes which contribute to health outcomes is articulated (Wallerstein 2006). The review discusses the multiple literatures on women, youth, people living with HIV/AIDS, patients and caregivers, and poor communities which have used triangulation of a wide range of evaluation methodologies to show how empowerment strategies contribute to improved health outcomes. Some of these interventions with subpopulations have used randomised control designs in their evaluations, though the use of comparison studies within the larger complex community and empowerment interventions remains questionable. In one of the few quasi-experimental designs uncovered in this literature review, Eng and colleagues demonstrated that participatory processes at the village level can lead to improved health outcomes, not just in the specific intervention that was promoted, but in subsequent interventions (Eng *et al.* 1990). This study raises an important question: how can we study the added value of participation itself as a contributing factor to improved health?

Within CBPR, much has being written on the added value of local knowledge and interpretation to assess effectiveness of public health and medical interventions. Walker and Jacobs (2002) argue persuasively that despite the apparent scientific value of evidence-based medicine based on systematic literature reviews, medical practitioners often use a highly pluralistic, culturally participative strategy in their treatment approaches. Hall (2001) has argued that culturally supported interventions (those which emerge from indigenous theories and local practices) should be studied independently and integrated with evidence-supported interventions to produce the best interventions for the particular context.

CBPR has also raised serious ethical issues of community-based research, starting from decrying the role of 'helicopter' research, in which researchers fly into a community, extract data, then leave (Buchanan *et al.* in press). CBPR further engages the question of what community consent and community benefit are. Institutional review boards (IRBs) have successfully created structures to protect individuals within a risk–benefit ratio; however, they have not extended their purview to assuring community benefit. As one example of a community-controlled process, the Navajo Nation Institutional Review Board has institutionalised a community approval and benefit process by mandating community engagement, approvals (through chapter resolutions) and plans for community dissemination of findings and benefit before even starting their research.

Introduction to chapters

The readings in this section discuss the issues articulated above and present several recommendations: first, a call for triangulating diverse methods based on the complexity of community interventions; second, a call for reflection about the research process itself, in its effects on a study's findings and on the *utility* of the findings to promote community health improvement; and ultimately, third, a call for community participation and engagement in the research process.

Linda Bauld and Ken Judge present a strong argument for theory-based evaluations for complex health promotion initiatives, especially those based on community development processes. While many health promotion researchers discard the possibility of using randomised control designs, the authors take the refreshing view that the RCT (just like every other methodology) has its place, with strengths and weaknesses, and needs to be considered depending on the context of the programme to be evaluated. With this caveat, however, they make the case for non-experimental evaluation approaches, especially for programmes which have poorly articulated outcomes or documentation of programme delivery. They build on logic-model and theory of change approaches to evaluation in order best to capture the learnings from an extensive body of work from community initiatives which are attempting to tackle intractable social problems (Weiss 1995, 1997; Chen 1990; Wholey 1983). Bauld and Judge provide specific examples of theory of change models from England's Health Action Zones, with excellent illustrations of a range of models, from simple pathways to complex community open systems models. They propose using mixed methods within the theory of change model, and end with a plea not to succumb to the 'tyranny of political business cycles that run the risk of undermining sustainable creativity' in the evaluation process.

Chris Bonell offers an excellent discussion of the importance of researching the 'implementation' process as a core addition to the study of a programme's effectiveness. He presents the challenges faced by the use of a randomised control design for two HIV interventions: a brief counselling intervention in a medical clinic and a longer social intervention within a community agency. The introduction provides an excellent short description of several traditional critiques of RCT – the question of validity of a 'positivist' approach and the feasibility of non-contamination – but then focuses on utility in terms of acceptability to the populations, internal effectiveness, and ultimately its applicability and generalisability (or external validity) to other settings. While many critique RCT applicability from a theoretical stance, Bonell remains open to the benefits of RCT utility, but provides a careful analysis of the challenges of implementation of the research design in two settings, and consequently illustrates the lack of specific utility of the intervention findings in these cases. The challenges included the difficulty in involvement of policy-makers during the different research stages, the potential for lack of efficacy of the brief intervention, the lack of publishing of the process evaluation for the brief intervention which would have supported greater generalisability, and the lack of buy-in and ownership of the staff of the community agency, who had little expertise in the counselling intervention being tested and little interest in RCTs in general. This chapter points particularly to the potential for misuse of intervention results at the community agency when no significance was detected between the group counselling and written materials, and policy-makers decided not to re-fund the counselling programme; subsequent analysis which also incorporated process evaluation showed the effectiveness of both. The complexity of motivations is uncovered at multiple levels, which is instructive for researchers who genuinely care about assessing effectiveness and having their findings used in policy and programme development.

Martin O'Neill and Gareth Williams focus on the process of knowledge creation and policy change within an action research study in South Wales. This is an honest paper, an unfortunate rarity, which provides insights into the challenges and facilitators of community involvement in the research process, including an analysis of community distrust in the initial hiring of a local community coordinator and of community cynicism generated by years of outside researchers conducting 'community consultations' without genuine engagement. The chapter describes the slow development of trust and researcher concern for assuring benefits to the community. As CBPR research moves into greater acceptance and more wide-spread use, it becomes important for all of us to embrace this self-reflective approach towards our work, so that the negative historical and institutional context of many researcher–community relationships, often characterised as 'helicopter' research, is not forgotten. These legacies are still too often current, and remain a challenge as research attempts to become more relevant in community contexts.

Michael Polanyi and colleagues present a call for participatory action research as an ethical stance, in order both fully to understand the context of work conditions and health, and to stimulate commitment and actions to improve work-related health. They present a more structurally based argument for challenging scientist control over the research process, suggesting ways that researcher positionality can limit what is studied, including how exposure and risk are quantified. Arguing against 'positivist' approaches, they advocate for an interconnected understanding of 'wicked' social processes that requires greater praxis and social construction of knowledge between researcher and researched. While not directly addressing the randomised control trial, this chapter recommends using triangulation of mixed methods, critical and appreciative enquiry, and an integration of diverse research traditions. They argue that democratising the research process will ultimately better facilitate worker agency and involvement in actions to improve health.

Conclusion

This introduction has argued for a broad approach to seeking evidence for complex societal and community public health interventions, one that embraces the role of agency of communities in collaboration with evaluators and researchers to enhance appropriateness of interventions and of research methodologies. It parallels several national and international evaluation task forces on evidence that have been convened to make recommendations. A framework for programme evaluation published by the Centers for Disease Control and Prevention (CDC 1999) provides a comprehensive cycle of engaging stakeholders and focusing the evaluation, with four guiding principles to assure evaluation quality: utility, feasibility, ethical standards and accuracy. The World Health Organization's Global Programme on Health Promotion Effectiveness (<http://www.who.int/hpr/ncp/hp. effectiveness.shtml>) has published several reports for researchers and policy-makers, concluding that: evaluation should be participatory, have adequate resources, examine both processes and outcomes, use a mix of methodologies and designs, and foster further development in complex design (WHO 1999; Rootman *et al.* 2001). A Pan-American Health Organisation task force has created a participatory evaluation handbook for healthy municipalities, which contains both a participatory cycle of gathering evidence and recommendations on multi-level outcomes (PAHO 2005).

Ultimately, the search for evidence calls for going beyond the randomised control trial (except in group interventions, when appropriate) to a triangulation of methodologies, using logic models to build theories of change (which could improve comparability across settings), quantitative and qualitative methods, process and outcome evaluations, multi-level targets of change, as well as a study of the implementation process in each context. If the goal of research is to create ethical and effective public health practice, then research methodologies which engage communities and build constituencies have a greater likelihood of changing inequitable social conditions and policies in order to reduce health disparities and promote health.

References

Alsop, R. and Heinsohn, N. (2005) 'Measuring empowerment in practice: structuring analysis and framing indicators', Policy Research Working Paper Series No. 3510, Washington, DC: World Bank.

Arnstein, S.R. (1969) 'A ladder of citizen participation', *Journal of the American Institute of Planners*, 35: 216–24.

Bellg, A.J., Borrelli, B., Resnick, B., Ogedegbe, G., Hecht, J. and Ernst, D. (2004) 'Enhancing treatment fidelity in health behavior change studies: best practices and recommendations from the behavior change consortium', *Health Psychology*, 23: 443–51.

Blumenthal, D.S. and DiClemente, R.J. (2004) *Community-Based Health Research: Issues and Methods*, New York: Springer.

Bonell, C. (2002) 'The utility of randomized controlled trials of social interventions: an examination of two trials of HIV prevention', *Critical Public Health*, 12: 321–34.

Bonner, L. (2003) 'Using theory-based evaluation to build evidence-based health and social care policy and practice', *Critical Public Health*, 13: 77–92.

Buchanan, D., Miller, F. and Wallerstein, N. (in press) 'Ethical issues raised by community based participatory research: balancing rigorous research with community participation in community intervention studies', *Progress in Community Health Partnerships: Research, Education and Practice*.

Bull, S.S., Gillette, C., Glasgow, R.E. and Estabrooks, P. (2003) 'Work site health promotion research: to what extent can we generalize the results and what is needed to translate research to practice?', *Health Education and Behavior*, 30: 537–49.

CDC (1999) 'Framework for programme evaluation in public health', *MMWR–Morbidity and Mortality Weekly Report*, Atlanta, GA: US Department of Health and Human Services.

Chen, H. (1990) *Theory-Driven Evaluation*, Thousand Oaks, CA: Sage Publications.

COMMIT I (1995) 'Community Intervention Trial for Smoking Cessation (COMMIT): I. Cohort results from a four-year community intervention', *American Journal of Public Health*, 85: 183–93.

COMMIT II (1995) 'Community Intervention Trial for Smoking Cessation (COMMIT): II. Changes in adult cigarette smoking prevalence', *American Journal of Public Health*, 85: 193–200.

Connell, J.P. (1995) *New Approaches to Evaluating Community Initiatives: Concepts, Methods, and Contexts*, Washington, DC: Aspen Institute.

Connell, J.P. and Kubisch, A.C. (1998) 'Applying a theory of change approach to the evaluation of comprehensive community initiatives: progress and problems', in K. Fulbright-Anderson, A.C. Kubisch and J.P. Connell (eds), *New Approaches to Evaluating Community Initiatives, Vol. 2: Theory, Measurement, and Analysis*, Washington, DC: Aspen Institute.

Cook, C. (1997) 'Faith-based health needs assessment: implications for empowerment of the faith community', *Journal of Health Care for the Poor and Underserved*, 8: 300–2.

Cornwall, A. (1996) 'Towards participatory practice: participatory rural appraisal and the participatory process', in K. De Koning and M. Martin (eds), *Participatory Research in Health: Issues and Experiences*, London: Zed Books.

De Koning, K. and Martin, M. (1996) *Participatory Research in Health: Issues and Experiences*, London: Zed Books.

Eng, E., Briscoe, J. and Cunningham, A. (1990) 'Participation effect from water projects on EPI', *Social Science and Medicine*, 30: 1349–58.

Evans, D. and Killoran, A. (2000) 'Tackling health inequalities through partnership working: learning from a realistic evaluation', *Critical Public Health*, 10: 125–40.

Fixsen, D.L., Naoom, S.F., Blasé, K.A., Friedman, R.M. and Wallace, F. (2005) *Implementation Research: A Synthesis of the Literature*, Tampa, FL: University of South Florida, Louis de la Parte Florida Mental Health Institute, the National Implementation Research Network.

Flay, B.R. (1986) 'Efficacy and effectiveness trials and other phases of research in the development of health promotion programmes', *Preventive Medicine*, 15: 451–74.

Fulbright-Anderson, K., Kubisch, A.C. and Connell, J.P. (1998) *New Approaches to Evaluating Community Initiatives, Vol 2: Theory, Measurement, and Analysis*, Washington, DC: Aspen Institute.

Gebbie, K., Rosenstock, L. and Hernandez, L.M. (2002) *Educating Public Health Professionals for the 21st Century*, Washington, DC: Institute of Medicine, National Academy of Science.

Glanz, K., Rimer, B.K. and Lewis, F.M. (2003) *Health Behavior and Health Education: Theory, Research, and Practice*, 3rd edn, San Francisco, CA: Jossey-Bass.

Glasgow, R.E., Green, L.W., Klesges, L.M., Abrams, D.B., Fisher, E.B., Goldstein, M.G., Hayman, L.L., Ockene, J.K. and Orleans, C.T. (2006) 'External validity: we need to do more', *Annals of Behavioural Medicine*, 31: 105–8.

Goodman, R.M. (2000) 'Evaluation of community-based health programmes: an alternative perspective', in N. Schneiderman, M.A. Speers, J.M. Silva, H. Tomes and J.H. Gentry (eds), *Integrative Behavioral and Social Sciences with Public Health*, Washington, DC: American Psychological Association Press.

Green, L.W. and Glasgow, R.E. (2006) 'Evaluating the relevance, generalization, and applicability of research: issues in external validation and translation methodology', *Evaluation and the Health Professions*, 29: 1–28.

Green, L.W. and Ottoson, J.M. (2004) 'From efficacy to effectiveness to community and back: evidence-based practice vs. practice-based evidence', *Proceedings from Conference: From Clinical Trials to Community: The Science of Translating Diabetes and Obesity Research*, Bethesda, MD: National Institutes of Diabetes, Digestive and Kidney Diseases, National Institutes of Health.

Hall, G. (2001) 'Psychotherapy research with ethnic minorities: empirical, ethical, and conceptual issues', *Journal of Consulting and Clinical Psychology*, 69: 502–10.

Hohmann, A. and Shear, M. (2002) 'Community-based intervention research: coping with the noise of real life in study design', *American Journal of Psychiatry*, 159: 201–7.

Israel, B., Eng, E., Schulz, A. and Parker, E. (2005) *Methods in Community Based Participatory Research*, San Francisco, CA: Jossey-Bass.

Kreuter, M., Lezin, N.A. and Young, L.A. (2000) 'Evaluating community-based collaborative mechanisms: implications for practitioners', *Health Promotion Practice*, 1: 49–63.

Labonte, R. (1994) 'Health promotion and empowerment: reflections on professional practice', *Health Education Quarterly*, 21: 253–68.

McQueen, D.V. (2001) 'Strengthening the evidence base for health promotion', *Health Promotion International*, 16: 261–8.

Minkler, M. and Wallerstein, N. (2003) *Community Based Participatory Research for Health*, San Francisco, CA: Jossey-Bass.

Murray, D. (2001) 'Efficacy and effectiveness trials in health promotion and disease prevention: design and analysis of group-randomized trials', in N. Schneiderman, M.A. Speers, J.M. Silva, H. Tomes and J.H. Gentry (eds), *Integrating Behavioural and Social Sciences with Public Health*, Washington, DC: American Psychological Association.

Narayan, D. (2005) *Measuring Empowerment: Cross-Disciplinary Perspectives*, Washington, DC: World Bank.

Nutbeam, D. (1999) 'Oakley's case for using randomized controlled trials is misleading', *British Medical Journal*, 318: 944.

PAHO (2005) *Participatory Evaluation of Healthy Municipalities: A Practical Resource Kit for Action*, Washington, DC: Pan-American Health Organization.

Pawson, R. and Tilley, N. (1997) *Realistic Evaluation*, London: Sage.

Pettigrew, A., Ferlie, E. and McKee, L. (1992) *Shaping Strategic Change*, London: Sage.

Rootman, I., Goodstadt, M.H., Hyndman, B., McQueen, D., Potvin, L., Springett, J. and Ziglio, E. (2001) *Evaluation in Health Promotion: Principles and Perspectives*, Copenhagen: World Health Organization Regional Publications.

Roth, D., Panzano, P.C., Crane-Ross, D., Massatti, R., Carstens, C., Seffrin, B. and Chaney-Jones, S. (2005) 'The innovation diffusion and adoption research project (IDARP): moving from the diffusion of research results to promoting the adoption of evidence-based innovations in the Ohio mental health system', in D. Roth and W.J. Lutz (eds), *New Research in Mental Health*, Columbus, OH: Ohio Department of Mental Health.

Rychetnik, L., Frommer, M., Hawe, P. and Shiell, A. (2002) 'Criteria for evaluating evidence on public health interventions', *Journal of Epidemiology and Community Health*, 56: 119–27.

Schorr, L.B. (1997) *Common Purpose: Strengthening Families and Neighborhoods to Rebuild America*, New York: Anchor Books.

Sen, G. (1997) 'Empowerment as an approach to poverty', working paper, Geneva: World Health Organization.

Thompson, B., Coronado, G., Snipes, S. and Puschel, K. (2003) 'Methodologic advances and ongoing challenges in designing community-based health promotion programmes', *Annual Review of Public Health*, 24: 315–40.

Truman, C. and Raine, P. (2001) 'Involving users in evaluation: the social relations of user participation in health research', *Critical Public Health*, 11: 215–29.

Viswanathan, M., Ammerman, A., Eng, E., Gartlehner, G., Lohr, K.N., Griffith, D., Rhodes, S.D., Samuel-Hodge, C., Maty, S., Lux, L., Webb, L., Sutton, S.F., Swinson, T., Jackman, A. and Whitener, L. (2004) *Community-Based Participatory Research: A Summary of the Evidence*, Rockville, MD: Agency for Healthcare Research and Quality, prepared by RTI International – University of North Carolina Evidence-Based Practice Center.

Walker, C. and Jacobs, S. (2002) 'Social structures of science and approaches to outcomes-based medical research', *Critical Public Health*, 12: 309–20.

Wallerstein, N. (2002) 'Empowerment to reduce health disparities', *Scandinavian Journal of Public Health*, 59: 72–7.

—— (2006) *What is the Evidence on Effectiveness of Empowerment to Improve Health? (HEN)*, Copenhagen: World Health Organization Regional Office for Europe.

Wallerstein, N., Polacsek, M. and Maltrud, K. (2002) 'Participatory models for coalitions: the development of systems indicators', *Health Promotion Practice*, 3: 361–73.

Weiss, C. (1995) 'Nothing as practical as good theory: exploring theory-based evaluation for comprehensive communities initiatives for children and families', in J.P. Connell (ed.), *New Approaches to Evaluating Community Initiatives: Concepts, Methods, and Contexts*, Washington, DC: Aspen Institute.

—— (1997) 'Theory-based evaluation: past, present, and future', *New Directions for Evaluation*, 76: 41–55.

White, D.G. (2001) 'Evaluating evidence and making judgements of study quality: loss of evidence and risks of policy and practice decisions', *Critical Public Health*, 11: 4–17.

WHO (1999) *Report on Recommendations for Health Promotion Effectiveness*, Geneva: World Health Organization.

Wholey, J.S. (1983) *Evaluation and Effective Public Management*, Boston, MA: Little, Brown.

W.K. Kellogg Foundation (1998) *Kellogg Foundation Evaluation Handbook*, Battle Creek, MI: W.K. Kellogg Foundation.

Wormald, R. and Oldfield, K. (1998) 'Evidence-based medicine, the Cochrane Collaboration and the CONSORT statement', *British Journal of Ophthalmology*, 82: 597–8.

Zimmerman, M.A. (2000) 'Empowerment theory: psychological, organizational and community levels of analysis', *Handbook of Community Psychology*, New York: Kluwer Academic/Plenum.

5 Strong theory, flexible methods

Evaluating complex community-based initiatives[1]

Linda Bauld and Ken Judge

Introduction

There is a growing recognition that health policies, practices and processes require clear evidence about effectiveness. When resources are scarce and the potential exists for interventions to do harm as well as good, there is a strong ethical case for requiring that new policies should be evidence-based. But in areas such as health promotion there are real questions to be asked about what constitutes an appropriate evidence-base. Traditional approaches to evaluation that emphasise the primacy of experimental approaches are often, although not always, inappropriate for complex, community-based health promotion programmes (Gillies 1999; Speller *et al.* 1997; Green and Tones 1999). We take the pragmatic view that all research methods have their strengths and their weaknesses, and we agree with Chen (1997: 63) that 'a method's usefulness depends on the contextual circumstances surrounding the specific programme to be evaluated'. In our view, mixed methods and the careful triangulation of evidence offer the best way forward in learning about complex health promotion initiatives. From this perspective, theory-driven approaches to evaluation have much to offer. The aim of this paper is to outline the potential benefits of one particular approach to theory-based evaluation that was employed to generate learning about Health Action Zones in England.

Health Action Zones

Health Action Zones (HAZs) were established in 1998 to serve as trailblazers for a concerted effort to modernise the NHS and to tackle health. They were complex, partnership-based entities that set themselves ambitious goals to transform the health and well-being of disadvantaged communities and groups. They were provided with resources, flexibilities and support, but in return they were subject to tough performance management processes. One important requirement was that HAZs were expected to set out clear plans that not only indicated how they would achieve social change in the longer term but demonstrated a capacity to deliver against well-specified targets in the form of 'early wins' to satisfy political expectations. This proved to be difficult to satisfy.

To varying degrees all of the initial HAZ plans were strong on identifying problems and articulating long-term objectives, and to some extent on specifying routinely available statistical indicators that might be used for monitoring progress. On the other hand, they were much worse at filling the gap between problems and goals. Only in very rare cases was it possible at the outset to identify a clear and logical pathway that linked problems, strategies for intervention, milestones or targets with associated timescales and longer-term outcomes or goals.

Many of the HAZs found it difficult to specify precisely how they would intervene to address problems, what consequences they expected to flow from such interventions, and how precisely these related to their strategic goals. As a result, the 'targets' that they included in their plans were not convincing.

Of course, one of the main reasons why HAZs did not develop clear plans in the early stages of their development was that the timetables they were expected to work within were hopelessly unrealistic. But haste was not the only issue and problems of strategic planning were not confined to HAZs. The key difficulty seems to be common to most complex community-based initiatives. Connell and Kubisch (1998: 23) suggest that:

> Experience from a wide range of programmes (in the USA) shows that identifying and agreeing upon long-term outcomes is relatively easy, in part because long-term outcomes are generally so broad as to be uncontroversial . . . Likewise, identifying early activities is relatively straightforward. Intermediate and early outcomes are more difficult to specify because scientific and experiential knowledge about links between early, interim, and long-term outcomes is not well developed in many of the key areas in which [community-based initiatives] operate. Defining interim activities and interim outcomes, and then linking those to longer-term outcomes, appears to be the hardest part of the . . . process.

Theory-based evaluation

What is required is an approach that can help to modify or clarify the design and implementation of initiatives in a way that lends itself to evaluation. This is where theory-driven approaches have a potentially important role to play. As Chen (1990: 22) puts it:

> A social or intervention programme is the purposive and organised effort to intervene in an ongoing social process for the purpose of solving a problem or providing a service. The questions of how to structure the organised efforts appropriately and why the organised efforts lead to the desired outcomes imply that the programme operates under some theory. Although this theory is frequently implicit or unsystematic, it provides general guidance for the formation of the programme and explains how the programme is supposed to work.

The concept of theory-based evaluation has evolved over the past twenty-five years or so in response to the kinds of difficulties outlined above. What has evolved during this time ranges from sophisticated approaches to the evaluation of complex community-based interventions to more pragmatic and practical uses of 'programme logic', 'logical models' and 'logical frameworks' (Funnell 1997). The most comprehensive and persuasive approach to evaluation that follows the logic of theory-based evaluation and seems especially applicable to health promotion initiatives is described as 'theories of change' by the Aspen Institute in the USA (Connell *et al.* 1995; Fulbright-Anderson *et al.* 1998).

The theory of change approach to evaluation

The theory of change approach to evaluation has been developed over a number of years through the work of the Aspen Institute's Roundtable on Comprehensive Community Initiatives for Children and Families (<http://www.aspeninst.org>). It was developed in an effort to find ways of evaluating processes and outcomes in community-based programmes that were not adequately addressed by existing approaches. Comprehensive Community Initiatives (CCIs) aim to: promote positive changes in individual, family and community institutions; develop a variety of mechanisms to improve social, economic and physical circumstances, services and conditions in disadvantaged communities; and place a strong emphasis on community building and neighbourhood empowerment.

These characteristics pose a number of challenges for evaluation because:

- initiatives have multiple, broad goals;
- they are highly complex learning enterprises with multiple strands of activity operating at many different levels;
- objectives are defined and strategies chosen to achieve goals that often change over time;
- many activities and intended outcomes are difficult to measure;
- units of action are complex, open systems in which it is virtually impossible to control all the variables that may influence the conduct and outcome of evaluation.

In order to address some of the complexity of CCIs, a new conceptual framework for evaluation was developed. This 'theory of change' approach is defined as 'a systematic and cumulative study of the links between activities, outcomes and contexts of the initiative' (Connell and Kubisch 1998: 17). The approach aims to gain clarity around the overall vision or theory of change of the initiative, meaning the long-term outcomes and the strategies that are intended to produce them. In generating this theory, steps are taken to link the original problem or context in which the programme began with the activities planned to address the problem and the medium- and longer-term outcomes intended. This framework has much in common with the development in the UK of so-called 'realistic evaluation'

(Pawson and Tilley 1997), with the added element that theory generation is conducted by and with those involved in planning and implementing an initiative.

Connell and Kubisch (1998) provide a number of convincing reasons why this approach to evaluating complex and evolving initiatives is attractive. First, a theory of change can *sharpen the planning and implementation of an initiative.* An emphasis on programme logic or theory during the design phase can increase the probability that stakeholders will clearly specify intended outcomes of an initiative, the activities that need to be implemented in order to achieve them, and the contextual factors that are likely to influence them. Second, with a theory of change approach, *the measurement and data collection elements of the evaluation process will be facilitated.* It requires stakeholders to be as clear as possible about not only the final outcomes and impacts they hope to achieve but the means by which they expect to achieve them. This knowledge is used to focus scarce evaluation resources on what and how to measure these key elements. Finally, and most importantly, articulating a theory of change early in the life of an initiative and gaining agreement about it by all the stakeholders *helps to reduce problems associated with causal attribution of impact.*

Problems associated with attribution, causation and generalisation are common to most health promotion initiatives. A theory of change approach explicitly addresses these issues. It involves the specification of how activities will lead to intermediate and long-term outcomes and an identification of the contextual conditions that may affect them. This helps strengthen the scientific case for attributing subsequent change in outcomes to the activities included in the initiative. Of course, it is important to acknowledge that using the theory of change approach to evaluation cannot eliminate all alternative explanations for a particular outcome. What it can do is provide key stakeholders with evidence grounded in their own experiences that will be convincing to them. At the most general level, the theory of change approach assumes that the more the events predicted by theory actually occur over the lifetime of an initiative, the more confidence evaluators and others should have that the initiative's theory is right.

Along with clear advantages, however, there are naturally difficult aspects to adopting a theory of change approach to evaluation. For example, the approach requires an analytical stance that is different from the responsive and intuitive stance of many practitioners. There is also the challenge of gaining consensus among the many parties involved in implementing community initiatives. This can be a resource-intensive exercise for evaluators. Despite these problems, evidence suggests that skilled evaluators can and should overcome these difficulties and by doing so they enrich both the programme and the lessons to be learned from it (Jacobs 1999).

Theories of change in Health Action Zones

A theory-based approach informed the national evaluation of Health Action Zones in England (Bauld *et al.* 2005; Barnes *et al.* 2005). Figure 5.1 illustrates the approach that was adopted. The starting point is the context within which HAZs operate – the resources available in the communities and the challenges that they face. Once this was established, the key challenge was for HAZs to articulate a logical way of achieving social change and to specify targets for each of their interventions that satisfy two requirements. First, they should be articulated in advance of the expected consequences of actions. Second, these actions and their associated milestones or targets should form part of a logical pathway that leads towards strategic goals or outcomes.

Initial work with HAZs yielded valuable lessons about the type of information needed if any serious attempt was to be made to learn from their activities. Knowledge was required regarding the ways in which different configurations of contexts, strategies, interventions and their associated consequences contribute to improving health for disadvantaged communities. This type of knowledge can only be gained on a continuous basis, through an approach to evaluation that recognises the evolving nature of HAZ plans and activities.

The need for more flexible planning must be matched by adaptive approaches to evaluation if such complex community-based initiatives are to contribute fully to policy learning. The process of monitoring and evaluation began with trying to persuade HAZ stakeholders to develop and articulate the underlying theories of change that guide their plans.

Practical examples from the Health Action Zones

Theories of change in Health Action Zones had to be developed at a number of different levels. All HAZs started with a vision statement of some kind that embraced their primary goals. In each HAZ a set of strategic goals or 'aspirational' targets was closely related to the vision. These objectives were then pursued through a series of work-streams or programmes that comprised a large number of projects. For example, in their original plans the 26 zones reported that between them they had more than 200 programmes or work-streams with in excess of 2,000 individual projects (Judge *et al.* 1999). Each of these activities was expected to generate a range of outcomes in the short, medium and longer term. At each stage in this process –

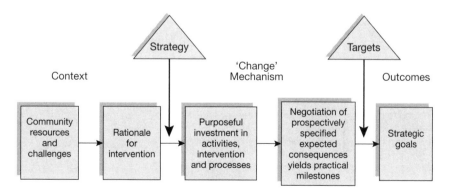

Community Health Improvement Process

Figure 5.1 Realistic evaluation and theories of change

the project, the programme and the overall initiative in each HAZ – it is possible and desirable to develop a theory of change. In practice, it proved easier for the zones to start to develop theories of change for individual projects. A key challenge was to develop convincing and acceptable theory of change models for HAZs as whole systems. The following are simple illustrations of the kind of progress that was made.

Smoking cessation services

Smoking cessation services represent one of the most straightforward areas to illustrate how logic models and a theory of change approach were being developed in HAZs. One of the reasons for this is that evidence-based guidelines exist for smoking cessation interventions, which the Department of Health instructed HAZs to use in developing local services (Raw *et al.* 1998).

Figure 5.2 presents a general overview in logic model form of the approach being adopted by many HAZs. The starting point is the context set out in the White Paper *Smoking Kills* (Department of Health 1998). The rationale for interventions is based on the evidence-base. The expected consequences of these investments are that contacts will be made with smokers for whom cessation rates can, to some extent, be predicted, depending on the form of services that they receive. The number of quitters generated will contribute to achieving reductions in overall smoking prevalence in the longer term.

This kind of logical process can then be taken down to a more practical level, as shown in Figure 5.3. In this example, taken from North Staffordshire, the intervention was nurse-led support for patients in general practice. The expected

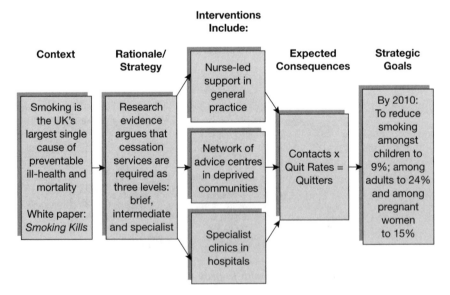

Figure 5.2 Smoking cessation in Health Action Zones

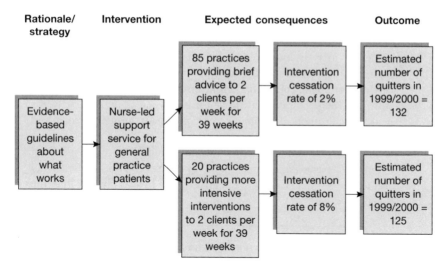

Figure 5.3 Smoking cessation in North Staffordshire HAZ

consequences of the intervention highlight the critical assumptions that specified numbers of practices will be able to recruit modest numbers of patients on a regular basis for a specified time to receive different levels of service. If these assumptions prove to be valid then the evidence-base predicts that a certain number of quitters can be expected.

What is important about these relatively simple examples is that they explicitly draw attention to some critical initial assumptions about the ways in which services will be established and the expected consequences that will result within the context of an overall logical model or theory of change. Moreover, the model clearly shows what data are required to test whether the assumptions are valid.

Capacity for health

Unfortunately, relatively few of the interventions being developed by HAZs were either as straightforward or as clearly linked to evidence-based guidelines as smoking cessation. Many initiatives remained at a relatively early stage of development. But these are exactly the kinds of circumstances in which the theory of change approach has much to commend it. Properly applied, it helps stakeholders to specify programme properties more clearly and so aids processes of implementation and learning.

The next example, taken from the Capacity for Health work-stream in Luton Health Action Zone, illustrates the practical value of the approach.

When we first examined the overall action plan for Luton HAZ, it contained many valuable elements and aspirations. For example, as shown in Box 5.1, there were reasonably clear statements of the approach being adopted and the outcomes that were desired. But at the same time we found it difficult to make logical

---

Box 5.1 Capacity for health in Luton

- General principles: Improved health will come about only if services are more responsive, community participation is enhanced and individuals' capacity for taking control of their health is improved.
- Aim: To increase public ownership, involvement and capacity for healthy living among communities and individuals through personal and community development.
- Outcomes: To reduce inequalities in health by raising rates of community participation, perceptions of control and access to informal and formal social networks in the target areas to levels higher than the (town) average.

---

connections between principles, actions and intended outcomes, a very common problem that we encountered in relation to virtually all HAZ plans at the beginning of the initiative. However, in Luton, as elsewhere, this seemed to be more of a function of people's lack of familiarity with formal planning processes than due to any lack of clarity about what they wanted to do and how they intended to develop new approaches.

In discussions with programme leaders in Luton responsible for developing capacity for health, it rapidly became clear what they were trying to achieve and how they expected to be able to do this. Key assumptions that guided the approach included beliefs about the lack of access to health promoting services and resources, and the need to focus attention on the most disadvantaged communities. These assumptions also included a recognition that although valuable work had already been undertaken, it may not have been as effective as it could have been, and in any event there are significant expectations that have to be met about delivering early successes.

Given these initial assumptions, the programme leaders shared a common view that investing in social capital in general and community participation in particular would yield significant health improvements for disadvantaged people. Three distinct approaches to investing in capacity for health emerged, which entailed:

- Winning hearts and minds – capturing support for community participation activities among all public agencies.
- Empowerment processes – increasing perceptions of control of and access to formal and informal social networks in target areas of Luton.
- Pragmatic opportunities and early wins – investing in a range of specific projects which will build capacity for health in Luton.

Programme leaders articulated two key requirements of the theory of change approach. First, they specified the expected consequences that would result from the initial investments in each of the three areas. Second, for each of these consequences they identified performance indicators that would allow judgements to be made about the extent to which they succeeded. For example, one important expected consequence of the decision to invest in 'empowerment processes' was that neighbourhood action groups (NAGs) and youth actions groups (YAGs) could be established and that these would generate activities that directly address deficits in health-related networks in the most disadvantaged areas. The associated early performance indicators are relatively simple but essential. The targets are expressed in terms of achieving the establishment of NAGs and YAGs in target areas and the accomplishment of specific tasks.

The final step in the logical process of setting out a strategy is to have very explicit *long-term goals*, although discussing these is often the starting point of a planning cycle that then requires creative thinking about how to develop interventions to achieve them. Figure 5.4 shows the strategic goals for the capacity for health programme. What is still missing is a set of clear performance measures so that progress against goals can be evaluated, which were next developed by the capacity for health programme board in Luton.

Conclusion

Complex community-based initiatives (CCIs) like English HAZs were typically established as demonstration programmes to tackle configurations of longstanding social problems. They were initiatives with very ambitious goals that required sustained investments over time if they were to have any chance of achieving social change. Their evaluation represented as much of a challenge as did their design and implementation. If they were to achieve their purposes they had to deliver on the promise of substantial social change (impact) but it was also essential to understand how observed benefits were actually brought about (process). However,

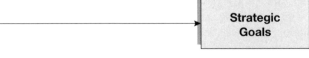

Strategic Goals

- To win support and ownership among public agencies for the importance of and need to invest in community participation;

- and to promote effective investment in community participation in Luton HAZ's target areas

- As a result, to make a contribution to reducing health inequalities in these target areas,

- by increasing perceptions of control, social cohesion and access to formal and informal resources, services and social networks

Figure 5.4 Capacity for health: outcomes

an understanding of cause and effect is remarkably difficult to establish in complex open systems. It is for these kinds of reason that the more imprecise objective of 'learning' often replaces the more common use of the term 'evaluation', which frequently carries with it the unrealistic burden of excessive 'scientific' expectation.

But no matter how creative researchers prove to be, the process of learning about and evaluating CCIs will remain a very challenging business. Our experience of working with HAZs was that there will be more scope for productive action and learning if a theory-based approach to design, implementation and evaluation is adopted at the earliest possible stage (Barnes *et al.* 2005). As Carol Weiss (1995) has persuasively written, there is 'nothing as practical as good theory'.

In following this approach a wide range of methods can be employed to learn about processes and their impact. But there are some essential requirements associated with the theory of change approach. Policy-makers and practitioners must be able to:

- explain their starting assumptions and how they are related to critical aspects of the economic, social and political environments in which they work;
- specify in a plausible, and preferably evidence-based, way why their chosen investments in interventions and process will take them in the direction of the long-term outcomes they are seeking to achieve;
- identify in advance the expected consequences of their actions in ways that lend themselves to being monitored and evaluated;
- commit themselves to a continuous process of learning from the feedback that they obtain;
- and be willing to modify their theories of change and the associated investments in the light of what is observed during the life of an initiative.

If these requirements are satisfied, and if politicians and other stakeholders can restrain their impatience and find ways of escaping from the tyranny of political business cycles that run the risk of undermining sustainable creativity, then we believe that positive learning can be generated from complex community-based health promotion initiatives. Practical learning about such social problems as avoidable inequalities in health is not only complex in scientific terms but it takes time, which seems to be one of the most precious but least appreciated resources required by CCIs. The pressure of the electoral clock and the demands for seemingly instant measures of success may undermine a community's capacity to deliver social change more than any shortage of human and financial resources. We hope that a wider understanding of theory-based approaches to improving the design, implementation and evaluation of complex community-based initiatives may do something to redress the balance. It is important that it should.

Note

1   This is a revised version of a paper originally published by K. Judge and L. Bauld in *Critical Public Health* (2001) 11: 19–38.

References

Aspen Institute (1997) *Voices from the Field: Learning from the Early Work of Comprehensive Community Initiatives*, Washington, DC: Aspen Institute.

Barnes, M., Bauld, L., Benzeval, M., Judge, K., Mackenzie, M. and Sullivan, H. (2005) *Health Action Zones: Partnerships for Health Equity*, London: Routledge.

Bauld, L., Judge, K., Barnes, M., Benzeval, M., Mackenzie, M. and Sullivan, H. (2005) 'Promoting social change: the experience of Health Action Zones in England', *Journal of Social Policy*, 34(3): 427–45.

Chen, H. (1990) *Theory-Driven Evaluation*, Thousand Oaks, CA: Sage Publications.

—— (1997) 'Applying mixed-methods under the framework of theory-based evaluations', *New Directions for Evaluation*, 74: 61–72.

Connell, J.P., Kubisch, A.C., Schorr, L.B. and Weiss, C.H. (1995) *New Approaches to Evaluating Community Initiatives: Concepts, Methods, and Contexts*, Washington, DC: Aspen Institute.

Connell, J.P. and Kubisch, A.C. (1998) 'Applying a theory of change approach to the evaluation of comprehensive community initiatives: progress, prospects, and problems', in K. Fulbright-Anderson *et al.* (eds), *New Approaches to Evaluating Community Initiatives, Vol. 2: Theory, Measurement, and Analysis*, Washington, DC: Aspen Institute.

Department of Health (1998) *Smoking Kills: A White Paper on Tobacco*, London: Stationery Office.

Fulbright-Anderson, K., Kubisch, A.C. and Connell, J.P. (eds) (1998) *New Approaches to Evaluating Community Initiatives, Vol. 2: Theory, Measurement, and Analysis*, Washington, DC: Aspen Institute.

Funnell, S. (1997) 'Programme logic: an adaptable tool for designing and evaluation programs', *Evaluation News and Comment*, July: 5–17.

Gillies, P. (1999) *Evidence Base 2000: Evidence into Practice*, London: Health Education Authority.

Green, J. and Tones, K. (1999) 'Towards a secure evidence-base for health promotion', *Journal of Public Health Medicine*, 21(2): 133–9.

Jacobs, B. (1999) 'Partnerships in Pittsburgh: the evaluation of complex local initiatives', in S. Osbourne (ed.), *Managing Public–Private Partnerships for Public Services: An International Perspective*, London: Routledge.

Judge, K., Barnes, M., Bauld, L., Benzeval, M., Killoran, A., Robinson, R. and Wigglesworth, R. (1999) *Health Action Zones: Learning to Make a Difference*, PSSRU Discussion Paper No. 1546, Canterbury: University of Kent at Canterbury. Available at: <http://www.ukc.ac.uk/pssru/download.html>.

Pawson, R. and Tilley, N. (1997) *Realistic Evaluation*, London: Sage Publications.

Raw, M., McNeill, A. and West, R. (1998) 'Smoking cessation guidelines for health professionals: a guide to effective smoking cessation interventions for the health care system', *Thorax*, 53: S1–S9.

Speller, V., Learmouth, A. and Harrison, D. (1997) 'The search for evidence of effective health promotion', *British Medical Journal*, 315: 361–3.

Weiss, C. (1995) 'Nothing as practical as good theory: exploring theory-based evaluation for comprehensive community initiatives for children and families', in J.P. Connell, A.C. Kubisch, L.B. Schorr and C.H. Weiss (eds), *New Approaches to Evaluating Community Initiatives: Concepts, Methods, and Contexts*, Washington: The Aspen Institute.

6 Developing community and agency engagement in an action research study in South Wales[1]

Martin O'Neill and Gareth Williams

Introduction

Wales has poor health compared with other European countries (National Assembly for Wales 2002). The populations of former coalfields in general have particularly high rates of limiting long-term illness (Joshi *et al.* 2000). The determinants of poor health in parts of Wales are not very different from those found in other post-industrial areas: poverty, inequality, poor housing, educational underachievement, health-damaging ways of life. However, the spatial distribution of the population has produced numerous relatively small, contained areas of social exclusion, close to but dislocated from major sources of economic growth.

Against this background, recent health policy in Wales has been marked by a number of themes. A particularly strong emphasis on the cross-cutting nature of health has emerged, supported by an emphasis on the need for partnership working (National Assembly for Wales 2000; Welsh Assembly Government 2002). There is also growing evidence of a political philosophy that places less emphasis on healthcare deliverables, and more on social determinants, public participation and citizenship:

> The Assembly has developed . . . a number of strategies to counteract social exclusion and to create a *socially inclusive* Wales. It recognises the importance of building and supporting strong *communities* where the values of citizenship and collective action can grow . . . This (Health) Plan builds on wide consultation over the elements that make it up and is part of the process of replacing elite policy making by participative policy development. Our policy here is to build on this commitment and to continue to *enhance the citizen's voice* at the heart of policy.
>
> (National Assembly for Wales 2001: 5; emphasis in the original)

Part of the context for this rediscovery of partnership approaches to health policy with the involvement of citizens is the recognition that modern cultures and societies exhibit a growing mistrust of experts of all kinds, and unwillingness to accept uncritically their advice and recommendations (Williams and Popay 1994). As politics and policy become more concerned with 'evidence', the relationship between 'expert evidence' and political judgements and decisions becomes increasingly complicated. This shift towards a more citizen-based policy-making process, which draws on lay knowledge and popular epidemiology, hints at an emerging recognition of the 'collective intelligence' (Brown and Lauder 2001) or 'civic intelligence' (Schuler 2001) that both challenges a traditional demarcation between different forms of expertise and creates public spaces that provide the basis for new opportunities of democratic renewal. Public participation means inclusion in arguments about knowledge and evidence, as much as it means involvement in discussion and decision-making; and it means, above all, that lay knowledge needs to be taken into account as a form of expertise.

One practical arena in which the possibilities of knowledge-based policy and politics are being expressed is within community-based, participatory action research, where there is a strong emphasis on broad stakeholder involvement and on producing evidence-based recommendations to adjust policies, programmes and projects to maximise health gain and reduce inequality in exposure to health risk.

This chapter considers the issues intrinsic to developing lay participation in a partnership approach by examining a case study of a participatory action research project that sought to tackle the determinants of ill-health in South Wales. The 'Triangle Project' was so called because its focus was on three contrasting post-industrial areas. The project was also triangular in that it sought to focus on three separate dimensions of community health initiatives: communities, agencies and the relationships between the two. The project successfully secured funding from the Sustainable Health Action Research Programme in September 2000. This chapter focuses on one of the three communities in which the project was developed.

Gurnos and Merthyr Tydfil

> The Gurnos estate is not just full of skinheads and yobs, you know. It's also full of their mams, a fair proportion of whom might very well be decent people. And some not, no doubt. Maybe the estate is not so full of their dads.
>
> (Barry 2002: 62)

> Now yer's fuckin pressure for yer, livin on-a Gurnos; yer wunner see oppression? In action, like? Look-a a New fuckin Gurnos, boy, down in Merthyr Tydfil. At's-a real fuckin Wales fer yer, yer twat.
>
> (Griffiths 2001: 84)

Merthyr Tydfil played a pivotal role in the Industrial Revolution as a major site of iron and steel production, a stronghold of political radicalism and the location for 'the most ferocious and bloody event in the history of industrial Britain', the 'Merthyr Rising' of 1831 (Davies 1993: 366; see also Williams 1978). Historically the male population found employment in the foundries or coalmines of the surrounding area. It was for a long time the largest settlement in Wales (Davies 1993). However, as a result of the long decline throughout the twentieth century and the eventual demise of these heavy industries in the 1970s and 1980s, the area, like many others in South Wales (Bennett *et al.* 2000), is now characterised by long-term unemployment, low incomes, poor housing and all the problems typically associated with social exclusion.

The area of Merthyr Tydfil in which our action research took place was generically referred to as 'Gurnos', on the outskirts of the town in the upper reaches of the Taff valley on the northern boundary of the former South Wales coalfield. The Gurnos estate, or estates, was initially constructed during the late 1950s and early 1960s to rehouse the population displaced by the clearance of the industrial slum areas that had grown up around the former iron works during the Industrial Revolution. At this time the area was seen as a symbol of renewal and regeneration, with modern housing offering hot and cold running water and indoor bathrooms and toilets. The estate continued to expand until the late 1970s but the loss of industrial production and rising levels of unemployment in the area were followed by corresponding increases in social problems, such as crime, educational under-achievement and substance dependence.

Currently the estate comprises more than 2,500 council-built properties, of which a significant number are void or difficult to let. The Gurnos estate today is one of the more deprived parts of a deprived area, and is the fourth most deprived electoral ward in Wales, according to the Welsh Index of Multiple Deprivation.

In addition to the formal statistical evidence, the social reality of the area is also informed by a certain reputation and notoriety well beyond the immediate locality. The extracts with which this section began come from two works of mainstream, contemporary English-language fiction. The first was written by a novelist, Des Barry, who was born and brought up on the Gurnos estate. His novel is set in the 1970s. The second is from Niall Griffiths, born in Liverpool of Welsh parents, who has returned to Wales and made it the subject of much of his writing. His novel is a description of the lives of a number of disenfranchised characters living in Wales in the 1990s. The one speaking in the quotation above is from Gurnos, and is arguing in a pub with some Welsh nationalists about the nature of oppression. These are works of fiction, imaginative constructions, sociologically illuminating, but not themselves sociological documents. Nevertheless, in presenting the Gurnos area in the way that they do, these novelists can be seen to be using it as a symbol of contemporary post-industrial South Wales, consciously drawing on, and perhaps reinforcing, the more general notoriety of the area. The sense of inequality and injustice that Niall Griffiths' character expresses is made all the more understandable by the fact that the area is only twenty-four miles from economically buoyant Cardiff, and a short distance from other affluent areas. The important point to take from this is that the residents of the neighbourhoods that make up Gurnos are themselves only too conscious of its reputation. They know how it is regarded, and they also know that this can compound the already harsh difficulties many of them face. It also means that there is a high degree of suspicion and cynicism regarding the attentions of outsiders; and this makes the development of research or development projects led by people from outside the area difficult.

Entering the field

In order to facilitate acceptance in the area, the project team decided to appoint local researchers, employed by the university but from the area, rather than more typical university researchers who would then try to gain access. Appointing a person with strong local networks was one of the early challenges that the project faced. The post of 'local sustainable health coordinator' (more acceptable, we thought at the time, than 'community researcher') was advertised in the local press, indicating that it was a Cardiff University post but with the successful applicant located in a local community facility. No applicants from the estate itself applied. Indeed, the applications that were received came from traditionally qualified people from the relatively more affluent areas of the town. Early interviews with community development workers, who had lived and worked in the area for many years, indicated that although this was a community that was very familiar with the concepts of research and community development, they were accustomed to being passive subjects in these processes. This confusion, uncertainty and wariness about active participation is symptomatic of disengaged communities (Smithies and Webster 1998).

We therefore entered into discussion with local people to identify the barriers preventing members of the community applying for the post. Local people told us that although they had seen the post advertised, the term 'local sustainable health coordinator' meant nothing to them, and although no qualifications were stipulated they felt that, because it was a university post, academic qualifications would be required. At the simplest level, for example, the application forms from the university personnel department asked applicants for their higher educational qualifications and to which professional bodies they belonged. All these questions are loaded with symbolic markers that would indicate to prospective applicants from the estate that they were not the category of person required. On the other side, the personnel department of the university found it difficult to categorise and process a research project wanting to employ local researchers who were not based in the university and did not possess the qualifications traditionally associated with university-based research.

Once appointed, the local researcher, working with the university-based team, was attached to a local community centre at the heart of the area, and began the process of introducing the project to local workers and local residents. It soon became clear that gaining access to the community for research purposes was going to meet resistance. In an area with so many problems, and a reputation of which the residents are very well aware, negotiating the basis for doing research was far from straightforward, even with a local resident working for the project.

Barriers to action research partnerships

Over the years since the locality started to develop a stigma in the late 1960s or early 1970s, the neighbourhood has attracted numerous social scientists, and has provided a rich seam of the fuel that drives research and community development initiatives

(Kynch and Maguire 2000; Mendola-Byatt 2002). However, there are many ways in which the problems of deprivation and exclusion have become more severe. This history of 'policy failure' is very much alive for many residents in the area, and early interviews with community activists and workers revealed that this historical context had precipitated a situation where the local population were, at the very least, sceptical of any further research or regeneration initiatives (Fieldnotes, January 2001), an observation that is supported by studies elsewhere (Mallinson *et al.* 2003).

Although in the past community members may have been willing to cooperate with researchers, in the hope that such activity may provide some of the solutions to the area's problems, years of evidence to the contrary have cultivated, at best, mild cynicism and an unwillingness to waste time on such research. One local resident complained: 'We've had six years of consultation and no benefit' (Fieldnotes, May 2002). Another went to the heart of the relationship between research findings and social change: 'Well, what's happened to all the other reports that have been fed back?' (Fieldnotes, May 2002). Indeed, local people's observations of this process were that those who came into the area to conduct such initiatives were often supported by quite significant funding and after writing their reports they returned to their own communities in the more affluent areas of Wales and beyond. One local agency worker observed that over recent years in excess of four million pounds had been spent on regeneration initiatives on the estate, but still the area suffered higher than average levels of unemployment and poverty (Fieldnotes, March 2001). Although it is difficult to convey in fieldnote data, decades of these experiences of disappointment had generated outright hostility and a feeling that more research was not what was needed. In the early months of the project members of the project team experienced this directly.

If the Triangle Project were to have any possibility of making progress in the context of such deep-rooted fatigue and alienation then one of the key challenges to establishing a partnership approach would be to develop strategies and approaches that provided coalescence of desired outputs and outcomes, not just for the funders and the university but for the people living and working in the area. This is, of course, what action research is supposed to be about, but, in the context of the kind of circumstances we have described, meeting the various expectations for research and action and demonstrating a link between the two was a complex goal. It is probably impossible to attain a situation where multiple agendas can be replaced by one participatory schema towards which all parties can work. However, adopting a reciprocal approach to managing these different agendas has the possibility of a mutually enlightening experience for those concerned. The following section discusses the implications of this for conducting research on health in the area.

From extraction to reciprocation

One of the most complex and challenging issues facing the development of a partnership approach is developing relationships based on genuine mutual trust and respect (Speller 1999). A participative approach involves a complex model of research where the roles of researcher and researched are not so clearly defined as in conventional research, and both are involved in a reciprocal enterprise. Developing greater reciprocity also relates to the products of the process whereby the reports and other outputs that it generates need to be fed back to those who cooperated in their production. To do this, it was necessary for the project team to develop an approach that fostered a willingness in people to engage with the process. This involved first integrating the research process into other community development events, a process that we came to refer to as 'social event methodology'. Second, we attempted to make sure that the findings from the research were fed back into the research process and to local people very quickly, so that some immediate benefit could be seen.

The event that provided the initial focus for this was developed in partnership with the local electricity board in South Wales (SWALEC) to incorporate the sale of discounted low-energy kettles and light bulbs to the local community as part of a healthy living/community consultation event in October 2001. Rather than being a traditional extractive information-gathering exercise, members of the community who took part were provided with something that they found useful. The event was organised in a sports hall on the estate and advertised via the local press and through word of mouth. It was a great success, with people queuing for over an hour beforehand and over 300 people attending and obtaining kettles, light bulbs and information about local services. The research element consisted of a 'research tree', with residents asked to write down on paper, cut into the shape of leaves, the 'best' and 'worst' aspects about living in the neighbourhood, and what single thing would most improve the neighbourhood. Once filled in these leaves were attached to the tree. The use of the research tree, although limited as to the thickness or richness of data it produced, enabled immediate feedback to community members of the issues identified.

Following on from this, a meeting was held of a steering group of local people who had expressed an interest in being involved in the research and consultation process. The group engaged in systematic reflection on the process, and concluded that although the healthy living event was a success, the responses to the event and to the research tree were mainly from middle-aged and older people, especially women. This was seen to be important in interpreting the findings from the research tree; for example, fear of crime and anxiety about groups of children and young people hanging around the estate.

In response to these biases in our 'sampling', additional proactive strategies were used to reach younger people, who were far less inclined to participate voluntarily. The consultation team, in partnership with Valley's Pictures, a local voluntary organisation, established a film club for children between five and eleven years. The estate no longer had a video rental shop, and the club organised free film shows of recently released children's films. These events were very well attended, with up to seventy children attending some sessions. The parents also received them very positively. Not only did it provide some activity for the children, but it involved residents in locally based activities and often provided them with respite from some of their childcare responsibilities. Local volunteers, mainly mothers of the children who attended, came forward to help run the club and were encouraged and supported to take ownership of this initiative to foster sustainability.

Over time, the film club became the forum for a number of research and community development initiatives. For example, some 'fun with smiley faces' was used to find out what the children thought of their locality. The volunteers also provided 'naturally occurring' focus groups to discuss their experiences as young mothers in the neighbourhood. The issue that emerged most strongly from these sessions was the concern women had for the family diet. They were aware of what constitutes a good diet and were concerned about the detrimental effect on their health of their poor diets. In order to address this issue, the Triangle Project is now working collaboratively with the local population and agency representatives such as the local Health Promotion team to identify strategies to overcome the barriers that they face in accessing healthier foods.

In order to extend our 'sampling strategy' still further, the team, together with local community development workers, took the method out into different parts of the housing estates to engage members who otherwise would not get involved. A double-decker bus was hired and decorated in bright colours in order to attract attention. The bus was then parked in various strategic positions on the estate during the day and in the evening, and the researchers and volunteers encouraged community members to give their views via various methodologies, such as community mapping, a graffiti wall and a 'Wish Wizard', a variation on the research tree. Local children were encouraged via a competition to draw pictures and write poems and stories about what they wanted in their area. Over 300 people recorded contact with the bus.

However, these developments in themselves were not without their difficulties. Throughout this process, on a number of occasions, members of the team encountered outright hostility from certain sections of the community who saw these initiatives as an irrelevance. For example, on one occasion a group of local women expressed great displeasure when saying that the money spent on hiring and staffing the bus could be better spent on improving the physical environment of the estate. Their frustration was compounded by their experience of having been consulted for nearly a decade, during which time their concerns had been consistent, and then being consulted again. This revealed to the research team the importance of demonstrating immediate 'pay-offs' if successful engagement were to be developed.

In relation to the developments from the 'kettles' initiative, in the most immediate sense local people have benefited from energy-efficient products that can make a significant difference to people on a low income. The development of the film club not only provides entertainment for the children but acts as a community focus to ameliorate the serious problem of social fragmentation in the area. The healthier-eating initiatives that are emerging from the activities of the film club focus groups are addressing the issues that local people face, and developing an indigenous approach rather than promoting more conventional healthy-eating regimes. Evidence from these consultation and research exercises has been fed back to members of the community, and to the 'power structures' – agencies that are driving forward the local implementation of health improvement plans, community action plans and other local political developments. Nevertheless, the antagonism displayed by certain sections of the community to the 'big bus' consultation demonstrates that, even with a carefully constructed strategy for engagement, parts of the community may still feel excluded.

Conclusion

There are significant difficulties involved in doing partnership-based participatory action research in neighbourhoods that have undergone many years of research, consultation and regeneration. All research is based on multiple agendas and differential power. In attempting to subvert some of the conventional research relationships, participatory action research serves to make interests and power relationships more visible: relationships between the members of the community and local agencies, between local agencies and the researchers, and between the locally based researchers and those in the university, between those working to traditional notions of 'good research' and those trying to build acceptance and trust in the community.

Partnership approaches profess to offer a more democratic knowledge and service-generating process, one that strives to be by the people, of the people and for the people. However, as this case study has highlighted, to achieve effective participation it is not enough simply to invite people to take part in the process. There are many material and symbolic barriers to be overcome and these need to be addressed in imaginative ways. At its most basic, if this knowledge process is going to be available to the people, there is a need to consider and address how such knowledge is to be made accessible to all project partners.

All communities, large and small, are multi-voiced and therefore there is a need to develop multifaceted reciprocal consultation and research strategies that connect with these various voices. For example, artwork, poems and stories produced by community members can provide powerful insight into people's experience, hopes and aspirations while at the same time providing an opportunity to develop their skills, confidence and social capital. From the professionals' perspective, one of the biggest challenges is overcoming the fear of having their expertise challenged and possibly changed, and recognising the opportunities offered by working with the 'civic intelligence' of local residents and *animateurs*.

Acknowledgements

The authors would like to thank other members of the Triangle Project team involved in this work: Neil Caldwell, Jeanne Davies, Pat Gregory, Carolyn Lester and Deanne Rebane. Gratitude is also expressed to the local community and agencies in Gurnos and Galon Uchaf for their help and support. The project was funded by the Welsh Assembly Government under its Sustainable Health Action Research Programme.

Note

1   This chapter is a revised version of a paper originally published in *Critical Public Health* (2004) 14: 37–47.

References

Barry, D. (2002) *A Bloody Good Friday*, London: Cape.

Bennett, K., Beynon, H. and Hudson, R. (2000) *Coalfields Regeneration: The Consequences of Industrial Decline*, Bristol: Joseph Rowntree/Policy Press.

Brown, P. and Lauder, H. (2001) *Capitalism and Social Progress: The Future of Society in a Global Economy*, London: Palgrave.

Davies, J. (1993) *A History of Wales*, Harmondsworth: Penguin.

Griffiths, N. (2001) *Grits*, London: Vintage.

Joshi, H., Wiggins, R.D., Bartley, M. *et al.* (2000) 'Putting health inequalities on the map: does where you live matter, and why?' in H. Graham (ed.), *Understanding Health Inequalities*, Buckingham: Open University Press.

Kynch, J. and Maguire, M. (2000) *Community Involvement in Gurnos and Galon Uchaf Regeneration Strategy*, Cardiff Occasional Papers Series. Available at: <http://www.cf.ac.uk/socsi/publications/workingpapers/wrkgpapers7.pdf>.

Mallinson, S., Popay, J., Elliott, E. and Williams, G.H. (2003) 'Using historical materials in health inequalities research: a pilot study', *Sociology*, 37: 771–80.

Mendola-Byatt, A. (2002) 'Regeneration strategies – a personal to political perspective', in S. Clarke, A. Byatt, M. Hoban and D. Powell (eds), *Community Development in South Wales*, Cardiff: University of Wales Press.

National Assembly for Wales (2000) *Strategic Plan of the National Assembly for Wales*, Cardiff: National Assembly for Wales. Available at: <http://www.betterwales.com>.

—— (2001) *Improving Health in Wales: A Plan for the NHS with its Partners*, Cardiff: National Assembly for Wales.

—— (2002) *Health in Wales: Chief Medical Officer's Report, 2001/2002*, Cardiff: National Assembly for Wales.

Pickin, C., Popay, J., Staley, K., Bruce, N., Jones, C. and Gowman, N. (2002) 'Developing a model to enhance the capacity of statutory organizations to engage with lay communities', *Journal of Health Services Research and Policy*, 1: 34–42.

Sanders, D. and Hendry, L. (1997) *New Perspectives on Disaffection*, London: Cassell.

Schuler, D. (2001) 'Cultivating society's civic intelligence: patterns for a new "world brain"', *Information, Communication and Society*, 4: 157–181.

Senior, M.L. (1996) 'Area variations in self-perceived limiting long-term illness in Britain, 1992: is the Welsh experience exceptional?', *Regional Studies*, 32: 265–80.

Smithies, J. and Webster, G. (1998) *Community Involvement in Health: From Passive Recipients to Active Participants*, Aldershot: Ashgate.

Speller, V. (1999) *Promoting Community Health: Developing the Role of Local Government*, London: Health Education Authority.

Welsh Assembly Government (2002) *Well-being in Wales: A Consultation Document*, Cardiff: Welsh Assembly Government.

Williams, G.A. (1978) *The Merthyr Rising*, London: Croom Helm.

Williams, G.H. and Popay, J. (1994) 'Lay knowledge and the privilege of experience', in J. Gabe, D. Kelleher and G.H. Williams (eds), *Challenging Medicine*, London: Routledge.

7 How useful are trials of public health interventions?

An examination of two trials of HIV prevention[1]

Chris Bonell

Introduction

Randomised controlled trials (RCTs) aim to compare the outcomes of participants in one or more intervention groups with those in a control group who received 'care as usual', which might be nothing (Cochrane 1989). Randomisation is used as the method of allocating participants to intervention and control groups because, if enough participants are involved, the different groups closely resemble one another so that any differences in outcomes are unlikely merely to represent pre-existing differences between groups (Oakley 1990).

The RCT is often regarded as the 'gold standard' of rigorous evaluation of clinical (Cochrane 1989) as well as public health interventions (Oakley *et al.* 1996). However, some criticise the validity of trials, suggesting they are epistemologically 'positivist' and thus invalid for investigating the social processes inherent in most public health interventions (Tones 1997). Others criticise their lack of feasibility, arguing that randomising participants and maintaining a strict separation between intervention and control groups are usually impossible (Kippax and Van den Ven 1998). This paper does not discuss these matters further and assumes that trials of public health interventions are often feasible and generate evidence regarded as valid by many if not all researchers. Instead, it explores utility: whether trials in practice provide useful evidence.

Utility is defined as the ability to inform policy and practice (Walt 1994). To provide useful evidence, trials should generate evidence about interventions which, according to existing knowledge, are good candidates for implementation but for which we do not have definitive evidence about effectiveness (Oakley *et al.* 1996). Clinical interventions are subject to trials only after earlier evaluation of biological effects in laboratories and clinical effects in case studies. Proponents of trials of public health interventions also recommend that evaluation is phased (Oakley *et al.* 1996), with RCTs being done only where there is prior evidence of acceptability and appropriateness in meeting population needs. Such evidence might be derived from formative research, employing mostly qualitative data to examine intervention provision and receipt (Ramos *et al.* 1995), or from evidence of prior successful deployment to meet similar needs elsewhere.

To be useful, trials must also provide planners and implementers with evidence that the intervention might work in their own site. This requires information not only about effectiveness in the study site but about whether this might be repeated if the intervention were undertaken with the population and context with which the planners and implementers are engaged (Peersman *et al.* 1998). The issue of generalisability is arguably more important with regard to public health than clinical interventions because while we might reasonably expect, for example, that a drug for treating migraine will have similar effects in the USA and UK, we would be less certain that a mass-media healthy-eating campaign would have the same effects in each country. Thus, to be useful, trials of public health interventions must also provide evidence about what contextual factors act to promote or impede the feasibility, acceptability and, ultimately, effectiveness of an intervention (Bonell and Imrie 2001). Such evidence might be derived from a 'process evaluation' that explores providers' and participants' views of the intervention.

It is frequently argued that, if research is to be useful, stakeholders should be involved in determining its focus and design. Trials are more likely to focus on the right interventions and deliver the right information if those who would plan and implement the services in question are involved in their development. The trials of HIV prevention on which this paper focuses were conducted using National Health Service (NHS) funding. At the time of the case studies, the NHS was initiating for the first time its own research and development programme (Peckham 1991), managed by the NHS Executive, which had responsibility for overseeing NHS operations. The programme aimed to develop a system for prioritising, undertaking and disseminating research about health services which involved NHS stakeholders at every stage. At this time, one of the key stakeholding groups was NHS commissioners, a group arising from the government's 1989 healthcare reforms (DoH 1989) which introduced NHS 'internal markets' in each local district, with commissioners being responsible for determining priorities and contracting with hospital and community 'trusts' to provide services. Commissioners, alongside other stakeholders, such as academics, clinicians and service users, were invited to sit on the committees convened by the NHS to commission and manage research, and each health authority was asked to participate in research topic priority-setting exercises. Agencies involved in the production or collation of research were to distribute the conclusions of research in an easily digestible manner to health authorities so that commissioners could use it to inform local decisions.

Our research aimed to explore the potential utility and use by the NHS of two RCTs of public health interventions being undertaken, and in particular to examine a number of questions:

1   Did the trials focus on interventions that were regarded as prime candidates for being effective, according to existing evidence?
2   Did the trials aim to collect evidence on the generalisability as well as the effectiveness of the interventions?
3   Were key stakeholders (and especially health authority commissioners) involved in planning the trials?

4   Was the evidence that was produced used in informing health service decisions made by health authority commissioners or others?

Methods

This chapter focuses on two case studies of attempted RCTs of HIV prevention. One of these aimed to evaluate a one-day group-counselling intervention for gay men attending St John's (a pseudonym), an NHS genitourinary medicine (GUM) clinic. The other was a trial of a similar but longer intervention within a voluntary agency, 'Gay Health' (another pseudonym). Doctors, nurses, health advisers, clinical psychologists and health promotion staff worked at St John's. Also attached to the clinic was an academic department undertaking clinical, epidemiological and social science research on sexual health. Gay Health employed a number of staff and involved gay men as volunteers. Some of the latter were professional health researchers.

Fieldwork was undertaken in 1997 and 1998 and examined events occurring in 1996 and 1997, using interviews and documents as data sources. Suitable NHS R & D organisations were identified that were: engaged in HIV prevention; NHS-funded; and aiming to undertake an RCT of HIV prevention with NHS funding. Forty-two interviews in total were conducted. Interviews and examination of documents focused on how evidence was defined, produced and used, and the context within which such activity proceeded. Interviews were audiotaped and transcribed. Transcripts and documents were coded in an iterative process (Lofland and Lofland 1995).

Results

Trial of St John's group-counselling intervention

The St John's clinic and academic department together submitted a proposal to the local NHS Executive regional office for an RCT of group counselling. Within the clinic there existed an informal 'effectiveness movement'. The proposal for the trial was led by two individuals – a medical epidemiologist and the medical director – who were key individuals in this movement. These stressed the particular importance of evaluating the effectiveness of HIV prevention using RCTs. Some clinic staff, particularly nurses and health promoters, were more sceptical about RCTs of HIV prevention. Some staff in the clinic complained that other staff groups had not been sufficiently involved in developing the proposal. One health promotion manager commented:

> They didn't consult at all. They put in this proposal, and then, when they got the money, it was like, 'Ah, what are we going to do? . . . They're health promotion sessions, aren't they? Gosh, so they are! Well, we know about that now – don't we? Do we?' . . . The health advisers were angry, the health promotion people were angry.

The funding committee convened by the NHS Executive office mainly comprised medical academics, with very few commissioners or other managers involved. The St John's proposal was awarded funding and the project ran from 1995 to 1998. The trust housing St John's committed additional funds. This money came out of its allocations from the health authority, which thus indirectly part-funded the trial. The health authority commissioner, though keen to encourage trials of HIV prevention, knew little about the intervention or evaluation. The NHS Executive R & D manager, when asked, said he had not considered the use to which the evidence produced by the trial might be put.

Those who developed the proposal had considered trialling a multi-session group-counselling intervention that was already provided in the clinic and had previously been evaluated using a non-controlled design. However, there was concern that retention would be difficult so the team decided to develop and evaluate a one-day intervention in order to maximise – as they saw it – trial feasibility. A health adviser involved in the study commented: 'We did have to tailor the intervention to some extent and that isn't really what I think should happen with sexual health; we should be finding research . . . that fits in with the intervention.' The reduction in length came despite the conclusion from the earlier non-controlled evaluation that addressing clients' behavioural issues required several sessions of counselling. Several referees appointed to review the bid had also suggested that the intervention was rather brief, when one considered its aims: 'It is questionable whether one single session of intervention . . . would be expected to enable participants to acquire more than superficial understanding of the principles of [the intervention].'

Gay men who gave consent to be involved were randomised either to group counselling or to a control group to be offered standard care (one-to-one consultations with various clinic staff). Evaluators took baseline and outcome measurements of the men's knowledge, attitudes, behaviour and sexually transmitted infections. Another academic department undertook an evaluation of the process of delivery and receiving of the intervention, employing focus groups with trial participants.

The study was successfully completed and written up for a prestigious medical journal. The word limit of this did not allow reporting of the trial's process evaluation, which remains unpublished. Results of the outcome evaluation indicated those in the intervention arm were no less likely to be at risk of HIV infection than those in the control arm. In other words, there was no evidence for effectiveness. This result informed a decision by the clinic's medical director and the trust manager to discontinue the intervention. Some individuals, such as the academic department's director, suggested that the intervention chosen might indeed not have been the best candidate for a trial both because it had not been subject to pre-trial evaluation of its acceptability with clients, and because of its brevity.

Trial of Gay Health group-counselling intervention

In 1996, Gay Health's general manager initiated the development of what was intended to be an RCT of a group-counselling intervention for gay men, occurring over several sessions. A number of sources provided funding, including a national HIV prevention programme, a gay magazine and the local health authority. A research assistant was employed to undertake the evaluation, and two freelance facilitators developed and delivered the intervention. Men who agreed in an initial interview to participate were initially randomised by the research assistant to the group-counselling arm, to a second arm (who would receive an information booklet) or to a no-treatment arm. The research assistant took baseline and two sets of outcome measurements from participants, focusing on knowledge, attitudes and behaviour, as well as conducting a process evaluation. Unlike the majority of the agency's services, volunteers played only a small part in the planning, delivery and evaluation of the service.

Many Gay Health staff and volunteers called for evaluations of effectiveness. One director wrote in the organisation's newsletter that:

> It's all very well demanding more money for gay men's work, but . . . more money doesn't necessarily equal fewer infections. It may just be money down the drain . . . Until recently the success of prevention work has been judged according to the number of people it reached and whether people liked it or thought its message relevant to them . . . All prevention projects, not just Gay Health, need to be looking at their effects on behaviour.

A small minority were proponents of RCTs. Most staff and volunteers were, however, sceptical about the feasibility of using this design to evaluate their services. Commissioners who funded Gay Health were, in contrast, enthusiastic about RCTs and perceived most providers as being unnecessarily resistant to them. One commissioner commented: 'The very mention of the words evaluation, methodology, random, control or trial can reduce the most dedicated HIV prevention worker to a whingeing mass of indifference and excuses.'

Several of those interviewed within Gay Health considered that the manager's main motivation in initiating a trial was to demonstrate to commissioners the unfeasibility of trialling HIV prevention. The assistant manager, for example, commented:

> It's [the manager's] baby . . . I spoke to him beforehand about it, and I was going, 'You can't do this, you can't do this, it just won't work.' But I think . . . he understood what the problems were before. So, knowing what the problems were, but doing it anyway, I can't say that he was doing it on purpose . . . but it wouldn't be a complete surprise.

Gay Health's manager said this was indeed one of his motivations for conducting the trial. Attempting to undertake a trial would enable Gay Health to argue that any criticisms of RCTs it expressed in the future were themselves informed by research. The evaluation was not motivated by a desire to prioritise existing Gay Health services on the basis of effectiveness because, prior to the trial, Gay Health had not delivered group counselling. The intervention was widely regarded, however, to be a good candidate for implementation and evaluation; evidence from an evaluation of a similar intervention in Australia was referred to in support of this.

Commissioners' motivations, according to views expressed in internal correspondence, also did not centre on their desire to know whether Gay Health could effectively deliver group counselling. Commissioners saw other organisations, employing specialised staff, as being better placed than Gay Health to deliver such a service. Commissioners instead regarded the project as a way of developing Gay Health's capacity to produce and use evidence, and as an indication that the organisation was adopting a view of trials closer to the commissioners' own.

Because of problems with participant drop-out, randomisation was eventually abandoned, with participants instead being allocated in order to maintain balance between trial arms. Despite this, the trial continued to be referred to as 'randomised'. Gay Health presented trial results in a poster at a conference in 1998. This poster emphasised the limitations of the trial design:

> [The RCT design] compromises validity by limiting scope for interventions . . . Random allocation fails to acknowledge individual preferences and needs . . . Evidence-based commissioning and health promotion have been dominated in recent years by the elevation of Control Trials as the Gold Standard of evaluations. Despite our best efforts we found it difficult to answer the commissioners' question: just tell me what works?

The poster also reported that no statistically significant differences in outcomes were found between the three arms of the trial and suggested this lack of difference could be explained by the positive effects of the initial interview which all participants received. A report that Gay Health subsequently published suggested the results indicated that both the group counselling and the booklet were effective, since men in both of these groups reported less risk-taking behaviour after receiving these interventions. This report included some information from the process evaluation but this did not focus on contextual factors that might promote or impede implementation of the intervention and so offered little guide to the potential generalisability of the intervention.

No further funding was provided by the local heath authority for the intervention. However, the commissioner who had part-funded the study believed, as did Gay Health managers, that the trial had indicated that both group counselling and the written material were effective. This commissioner suggested that the intervention should not be recommissioned, despite its perceived effectiveness, because other specialist organisations were already providing group counselling. However, Gay Health did continue to provide the intervention for several years, funded by the agency's own reserve funds.

Discussion

Choice of interventions

In the case of St John's, an intervention that appeared, according to existing evidence, to be the prime candidate for being effective was rejected because it was not felt amenable to being trialled. The intervention chosen instead was felt by some to be inappropriate in addressing the needs identified because of its brevity but was chosen because it was easier to trial. Such a decision is explicable because those planning the trial viewed successfully undertaking a trial of HIV prevention (and therefore demonstrating this was feasible) as the prime objective, with producing evidence of use to service planners as only a secondary objective. Demonstrating the feasibility of trials of public health interventions was central to the maintenance and development of occupational and organisational identities for many of those within the clinic and attached academic department's 'effectiveness movement'.

In the case of the voluntary agency trial, the intervention was considered a prime candidate for success by the agency and by commissioners, and evidence was referred to in supporting this view. However, the commissioners did not consider that the agency itself was the appropriate one to deliver such an intervention and actually funded the trial because they thought it would be useful for organisational development. The voluntary agency undertook the study partly motivated by a desire to prove to commissioners that while Gay Health was capable of doing a trial, RCTs were not the most useful or feasible design for evaluating HIV prevention services.

Thus, in both cases the motivation behind trials was complex and not conducive to evaluations that focused on a good candidate intervention being delivered by an appropriate agency.

Process evaluation and generalisability

Both trials that were undertaken did successfully collect information on the process of delivery of the interventions as well as the outcomes achieved, and thereby could produce evidence on the potential generalisability of the interventions. The academics leading the St John's trial sought to conduct a rigorous evaluation and saw a process evaluation as an integral part of this. They involved external evaluators to conduct such an evaluation. However, because of the word limit of the peer-reviewed journal in which the study was published, the academics were not able to include information from the process evaluation. These data were not published elsewhere. This would severely impede the ability of service planners and implementers to use the evaluation to assess whether the intervention was appropriate to generalise to their own populations and settings.

The Gay Health process evaluation was less comprehensive and was not undertake by external evaluators. Although some information from the process evaluation was included in the project report, this did not provide information that could inform decisions about the generalisability of the intervention.

Stakeholder involvement

Both trials were funded mainly by NHS bodies. The GUM trial was funded through the NHS R & D programme; the committee approving funding consisted over-whelmingly of academic doctors and other researchers but few commissioners. The proposal was drafted mainly by academic doctors in the department attached to the clinic and by the clinic's medical director. Other practitioners felt marginalised. A trust manager provided some additional funding to the project in the form of dedicated health adviser time. The local commissioner was not involved in the development of the project.

The voluntary agency trial was part-funded by local commissioners who oversaw the project as part of the overall work of the voluntary agency and were not greatly involved in study design. The project was led by agency managers with minimal involvement of volunteers.

Thus, both trials – despite being funded by the NHS – did not significantly involve NHS commissioners in planning and excluded other stakeholders, such as health promotion staff and volunteers.

Use of evidence

Evidence from the St John's trial was used to inform planning in that the inter-vention was discontinued on the basis of lack of evidence for effectiveness. This decision was made by the clinic's medical director and trust managers rather than by commissioners. Commissioners did not formally fund HIV prevention work in the clinic (since this was regarded as integral to the clinic's work) and so did not make decisions about this.

The voluntary agency referred to evidence from its trial in justifying its decision to continue with the intervention. However, the agency's interpretation of the trial's results – i.e., as indicating the effectiveness of the interventions – was unusual, given the lack of differences in outcome between the three arms of the trial. Commissioners shared this interpretation of the results but nevertheless decided not to fund the intervention further, informed not by the results of the trial but by their view that the agency was not an appropriate one to do such work.

Thus, in neither case did the trials inform commissioning in the way that proponents of the NHS R & D programme might have hoped.

Conclusion

These case studies have demonstrated that, irrespective of whether RCTs can provide valid evidence on the effectiveness of public health interventions, they may be undertaken and/or reported in a manner which hinders utility. While the case-study trials may not be representative of all RCTs of public health interventions, it is likely that other trials are often even less useful, given that these case studies were at least NHS-funded and not solely academic-led.

Machiavellian motives on the part of provider and commissioners underlay the Gay Health trial. These arose in a climate of conflict, and greatly hindered the possibility of useful evaluation. This might suggest that research should be taken out of the hands of local funders and instead be led nationally. However, the St John's trial illustrates important limitations of the NHS R & D programme as it was then managed: the committee funding the trial involved few non-academics; and R & D managers barely considered the potential utility of trial findings. The St John's case also demonstrates the limitations of academic articles for disseminating evidence. Although a comprehensive process evaluation was completed, this was not reported at all in the main journal article and was never published elsewhere. This reflects the negative consequences of journal word-length restrictions and the greater priority given to quantitative rather than qualitative reports in academic research assessment exercises

If RCTs of public health interventions are to provide useful evidence, they must be managed in a way that prevents local tensions from hijacking evaluation priorities and also ensures that all stakeholders' needs and ideas inform the prioritisation of topics and planning of evaluations. Otherwise, the lack of utility of RCTs, rather than any lack of feasibility or validity, might prompt their abandonment.

Note

1   This chapter is a revised version of a paper which first appeared as 'The utility of randomised controlled trials of social interventions: an examination of two trials of HIV prevention', *Critical Public Health* (2002) 12: 321–34.

References

Bonell, C. and Imrie, J. (2001) 'Behavioural interventions to prevent HIV infection: rapid evolution, increasing rigour, moderate success', *British Medical Bulletin*, 58: 155–70.

Cochrane, A. (1989) *Effectiveness and Efficiency: Random Reflections on Health Services*, London: BMJ.

Department of Health (DoH) (1989) *Working for Patients*, London: HMSO.

Kippax, S. and Van den Ven, P. (1998) 'An epidemic of orthodoxy? Design and methodology in the evaluation of the effectiveness of HIV health promotion', *Critical Public Health*, 8: 371–86.

Lofland, J. and Lofland, L.H. (1995) *Analyzing Social Settings: A Guide to Qualitative Observation and Analysis*, Belmont, CA: Wadsworth.

Oakley, A. (1990) 'Who's afraid of the randomized controlled trial?' in H. Roberts (ed.), *Women's Health Counts*, London: Routledge.

Oakley, A., Oliver, S., Peersman, G. and Mauthner, M. (1996) *Review of the Effectiveness of Health Promotion Interventions for Men who Have Sex with Men*, London: EPI Centre.

Peckham, M. (1991) *Research for Health*, London: Department of Health.

Peersman, G., Harden, A. and Oliver, S. (1998) *Effectiveness of Health Promotion Intervention in the Workplace: A Review*, London: Health Education Authority.

Ramos, R., Shain, R. and Johnson, L. (1995) 'Men I mess with don't have anything to do with AIDS: using ethno-theory to understand sexual risk perception', *Sociological Quarterly*, 36: 483–504.

Tones, K. (1997) 'Beyond the randomized controlled trial: a case for "judicial" review', *Health Education Research*, 12: i–iv.

Walt, G. (1994) *Health Policy: An Introduction to Process and Power*, London: Zed Books.

8 Understanding and improving the health of workers in the new economy

A call for a participatory dialogue-based approach to work-health research[1]

Michael Polanyi, Tom McIntosh and Agnieszka Kosny

Introduction

In this chapter, we first describe what we consider to be the prevailing approach to work-health research. Second, we discuss changes to the experience of both work and health or illness in today's globalised economy, and question the capacity of scientist-led, positivist-based research to comprehend and address these experiences. Third, we outline the basis for a more participatory approach to work-health research.

The prevailing approach to work-health research

Mainstream occupational research has several key characteristics. It is driven and controlled by scientists, with minimal engagement of workers themselves; it undertakes to draw cause–effect linkages between quantified risk exposures and measures of ill-health; and it aims to translate this neutral or value-free knowledge into rational actions by workers, employers and governments to reduce exposure to risk.

This approach is built on the tradition of epidemiology, which is interested in the assessment and quantification of risk. Occupational epidemiologists calculate relative risk: how much greater is an exposed individual's chance of developing a disease or an injury compared with a non-exposed individual (Lupton 1995)? This search for objective statistical links between exposure and illness is important. Quantitative studies have been useful in identifying the gender and race distribution of particular social problems (such as poverty), influencing policy development and directing legislative formulation and change (Westmarland 2001). Positivist, quantitative research has the potential to be used as a tool for the emancipation and empowerment of marginalised groups.

However, we question the mainstream approach to work-health research on four grounds. First, we argue that the undemocratic nature of the research process engenders a definition and focus of research that tends to ignore key worker concerns, particularly concerns of marginalised groups. Second, the attempt to establish objective and quantitative relationships between work-related exposures and health-related outcomes limits and distorts our understanding of the complex relationship between work and health. Third, such research fails to stimulate commitment and actions to improve the health of work experiences. Finally, we take the position that such an approach is ethically untenable in the face of growing expectations for democratic participation in social institutions.

Context and experience: limitations of current work-health research

The economies of the industrialised world are being transformed. The widespread introduction of new technology, the massive shift of employment away from manufacturing into the service sector, the rise of participation of women in the labour market, the freeing up of the international flow of capital and goods, and intensive efforts to increase productivity and international competitiveness are leading to fundamental changes in the nature and experience of work.

The increasingly globalised economy requires that firms be lean, dynamic and responsive to market shifts in order to survive, pressuring firms and managers to search for new strategies to remain competitive. Firms are both demanding more from core workers and seeking to reduce costs associated with marginal tasks. This is leading to the intensification of work (working at higher speed, tighter deadlines) (Burchell *et al.* 2002; EFIWLC 2002; Landsbergis 2003), the actualisation of work (Polanyi and Tompa 2002), and increased job insecurity (Betcherman and Lowe 1997; Heery and Salmon 2000; Burchell *et al.* 2002) as well as income insecurity (due to concurrent cuts to the social safety net in English-speaking industrialised countries) (Burke and Shields 1999). Labour market experiences are becoming more transitory, as workers move in and out of jobs more frequently, hold multiple jobs more often, and work in arrangements in which job demands are regularly changing. The nature of work-related illnesses and injuries is also changing. Emerging occupational injuries with non-specific diagnoses, unclear aetiology and prognosis, and an increased psychosocial dimension are becoming more prevalent. These disorders include soft-tissue injuries, environmental and chemical sensitivities, and chronic fatigue. Since pain and disability associated with these conditions are difficult to measure objectively, the legitimacy of these conditions is often questioned. Hence there is a gap between workers' experiences of non-acute occupational injuries and illnesses and the way that these injuries are described and managed by government, medical and academic researchers and practitioners. In this changing context of experiences of work and health, we believe that both the scientist-led model of conducting research and the positivist focus on establishing cause–effect relationships between quantitative variables is no longer epistemologically, method-ologically or ethically appropriate.

Inadequacy of a scientist-led process

Scientist control over the process of research means that the values, interests and beliefs of researchers shape the research enterprise in various ways. Researchers have often chosen to focus on workers who are most accessible or researchable, rather than most in need, and on workplaces and injuries for which funding from companies, unions, government and compensation boards has been available. This has led to a tendency to focus on unionised workers, workers in large companies and workers facing compensatable and clearly defined injuries and illnesses.

The medical control of health research in Canada, and the involvement of compensation boards in funding and providing data for research, has likewise led to a focus on traditional occupational injuries and illnesses rather than emerging, ambiguous illnesses and injuries. The framing of injury and illness by dominant institutions such as workers' compensation boards, which tend to draw sharp distinctions between injury sustained in the public sphere and injury sustained in the private sphere, hinders the exploration of chronic, multi-causal injuries and illnesses, which disproportionately impact on female and immigrant workers and are often not covered under workers' compensation. Several authors (Eakin 1995; Gunderson and Hyatt 2000; Messing 1998; Vosko 2000) note that those employed as domestics, teleworkers, temporary employees, and those working for themselves, in non-profit and small workplaces are often excluded from coverage. Those doing unpaid work (volunteering, housework) and those doing illegal work (sex work and working 'under the table') are also not covered. Women workers and visible minorities predominate in these types of workplace and work situations. As a consequence research into the health hazards of this sort of work is not a priority and the development of policy that protects workers in these jobs is thwarted.

Finally, researchers' implicit definition of 'work' as paid employment outside the home has further influenced and limited the focus of research. Yet work can take a number of different forms and the traditional distinction that work-related policy is only about that activity which takes place in the 'public' sphere is no longer tenable. Work in the home, work caring for children, adults or elders (most often performed by women), volunteer 'work' and even recreational occupation have been ignored even as these forms of work are becoming increasingly common. Features associated with this sort of labour (for example, 'emotional labour') have also been neglected in mainstream occupational health research (Hochschild 1983).

Inadequacy of focus on establishing statistical relationships between variables

The pursuit of statistical relationships between objective exposures and illnesses has influenced the way that both exposure and outcomes have been conceptualised. First, work has traditionally been assumed to be an 'exposure' or a risk, rather than something that gives positive meaning to people's lives. However, studies of workers identify a range of aspects of work that were deemed desirable by different workers: success, fame, money, socialisation, creativity, etc. (Polanyi and Tompa 2004).

Scientific and technical discourses also assume that risk can be measured objectively. However, perceptions and responses to 'risks' and 'hazards' are shaped by personal and political considerations. It is clear from the health and safety literature that the perception and meaning of risk depends on the subjective or lived experiences of those who are 'at risk' (Fox 1999). Work plays different roles in different workers' lives, and the meaning or worth ascribed to work affects the perception and experience of risk, discomfort or injury. For example, depending on the individual and on the characteristics of work, risk can be viewed as a source of excitement, nuisance or danger (Nelkin 1989; Polanyi and Tompa 2004). Moreover, people may derive pleasure from particular activities precisely because they are forbidden or dangerous. In the pursuit of objective relationships between exposure and health outcomes, mainstream research on work and health often reduces gender, race and class into neat, seemingly controllable variables, failing to recognise that these variables are only crude representations of very complex social relations. Messing (1998) argues that in an effort to promote 'objectivity' in data analysis scientists may control for variables such as age, gender and race automatically and this can obscure important associations. For example, if women workers are assigned to particular jobs – like cleaning work – more often, and these jobs expose workers to a particular hazard, controlling for gender prevents the discovery of a connection between gender-specific working conditions and a greater exposure to this hazard. Gender, race and class positions are associated with social and economic locations that often channel individuals into particular industries and working conditions that put them at greater risk of injury and ill-health, a risk obscured by crude adjustment for variables such as gender, race and class.

The pursuit of objective measures of work-related health outcomes is also problematic in the face of emerging complex and ill-defined work-related injuries and illnesses. Many injuries in contemporary workplaces are non-specific, difficult to diagnose objectively, and result from a complex interplay of physical and social factors and processes. They are 'political' in the sense that their legitimacy is contested, and they seem to depend on social, political and economic – as well as medical – factors. Researchers, employers, injured workers, unions and others have very different perspectives and beliefs about these injuries, making policy-making and collaborative responses difficult.

Towards a new approach to work-health research

If the current approach to work-health research is no longer adequate, what should be done to understand and respond better to the complex linkages between work and health? We argue the need for a more participatory approach to work-health research rooted in an ongoing, iterative dialogue between workers, employers, researchers and policy-makers.

Epistemological implications

Conventional, positivist work-health research assumes that researchers external to a social setting can independently understand workplace settings and experiences. As we have already discussed, it is assumed that the social reality of workplaces can be represented and understood as an interaction between measurable variables. This constitutes what the Russian literary theorist Mikhail Bakhtin calls a 'monological' epistemological framework. In monologism, cognition precedes communication; ideas are represented and then transmitted in communication. Systems of thought can be understood and contained in a single consciousness. Bakhtin (1984) wrote that the monological view of knowledge and truth has been mistakenly considered to be the only one. Instead, he suggests: 'It is quite possible to imagine and postulate a unified truth that requires a plurality of consciousness . . . not fitted within the bounds of a single consciousness . . . by its very nature full of event potential and born at a contact among various consciousnesses' (Bakhtin 1984: 81). This is the basis of dialogism, whereby meaning is made in dialogue and with reference to the world. The fundamental units of knowledge are no longer separate 'no-man's thoughts' but an idea that 'is a live event played out at a point of dialogical meeting between two or several consciousnesses . . . the idea wants to be heard, understood and "answered" by other voices from other positions' (Bakhtin 1984: 88). Bakhtin (1986: 69) sought to shift our focus from representational understandings to responsive understanding, arguing that 'all real and integral understanding is actively responsive, and constitutes nothing other than the initial preparatory stage of a response'. There is an emerging critique of the prevailing monological epistemological paradigm from a number of quarters. Indeed, there is a growing sense in philosophical, sociological and organisational behaviour literatures that knowledge-making is a social, interactive process, and that understandings of social issues are reached through processes of open and reflective dialogue.

There has emerged over the past thirty years a growing sense that fundamental social problems are often interconnected, uncertain, ambiguous and conflictual, or in Rittel and Webber's (1973) terminology, 'wicked'. This term distinguishes complex problems from simple problems, which can be bounded, managed or 'tamed'. Problems become wicked, in part, because they exist amid organised complexity – acted upon by multiple yet interrelated pressures. New injuries and illnesses exhibit the characteristics of complex or 'wicked' problems rather than simple problems conducive to technical resolution.

In arguing that almost all policy problems are wicked, Mason and Mitroff (1981) suggest that there is a need to incorporate a wider spectrum of information and actors in order to understand and respond to such problems. They claim that:

> The raw materials for forging solutions to wicked problems is not concentrated in a single head, but rather is widely dispersed among the various parties at stake . . . Every affected party is an expert on some aspect of the problem and its solution.
>
> (Mason and Mitroff 1981: 11–12)

Complex or wicked problems are not conducive to being understood solely by outside researchers, and require the integration of what Evered and Louis (1981) call 'outsider' and 'insider' enquiry. Outsiders (researchers) provide rigour and standardised knowledge, while the involvement of insiders ensures that understandings are relevant and grounded. Both are needed in order to understand organisations in ways that are experientially rooted, praxis oriented and self-reflective.

Methodological implications concerning knowledge transfer

The implicit assumption behind much of population health research is that the provision of researcher-generated information to decision-makers will lead to healthier decisions. Likewise, work-health researchers and policy-makers often assume that workers are rational actors who, given adequate information, can and should avoid unsafe work, and hence the moral culpability for injury falls on the worker who has somehow 'failed' to protect him- or herself (Lupton 1995). There are problems with this assumption. We should have learned by now that research evidence on its own is not sufficient to stimulate social and political change. Even if there is knowledge of potential health impacts, decision-makers and those in power may not want to, or be able to, take action on this information, given the upfront investments required, their own competing interests (e.g., maintaining control over production processes), pressures from groups with vested interests, and lack of institutional capacity. Conventional research transfer practices which focus on a rational and linear conception of disseminating and applying knowledge as though it is a static 'thing' are seriously flawed (NCDDR 1996), being insufficiently focused on interaction between researchers and users of information. Emerging approaches to community development, health promotion and organisational change suggest that action is more likely to result from a focus on capacities rather than deficits (Kretzman and McKnight 1993; Watkins and Mohr 2001). This suggests that understanding better what is 'working' well and is healthy is as important as analysing what is not.

Conventional scientific standards also marginalise values, desires and emotions as biasing or distorting knowledge. However, these are the core human dimensions that can stimulate the enthusiasm and commitment needed for change and have the capacity to unite people, while analysis and critique tend to divide. A major challenge for those who want to encourage reflective utilisation of research is therefore to develop innovative and participatory methods for joint reflection and learning by researchers and users to work towards a mutual understanding of both the research evidence and the social and political constraints of the world of practice.

Ethical implications

The approach to ethics in conventional work-health research is focused on avoiding harm to participants. Yet growing demands for democratic participation in research suggest that this focus is insufficient. Social research does not just impact on research participants; it impacts on the settings and issues more broadly. For example, research can either reinforce or challenge ideologies and belief systems that shape policies, practices and behaviours relating to a group or community. Given that research has implications for groups – often marginalised groups – should the subjects of research not have the right to influence the focus, conduct, interpretation and dissemination of research findings? There are growing pressures for the democratisation of institutions that affect people's lives, as well as a greater emphasis on the right of individuals, groups and communities to speak for themselves. Universities and research organisations have lagged behind in responding to these pressures.

Likewise, there is a strong argument to be made that the needs and desires of research participants should receive at least equal consideration to that which is given to the aims of researchers. Meaningful partnerships between researchers and those researched can 'underscore ethical principles such as self-determination, liberty and equity and reflects an inherent belief in the ability of people to accurately assess their strengths and needs and their right to act upon them' (Minkler 2004: 684). In the realm of work-health research, it is workers who are most directly experiencing the effects of the changing nature of work. Yet, because workers have fewer resources and less power, their voices are often not heard. Increasing the participation of workers in research can work to redress the power imbalances that exist in the health and safety system and perhaps may open up the possibility for practices informed by both researcher knowledge and the experiences, needs and understandings of workers themselves. In sum, meaningful and lasting improvements to working conditions and worker health require deeper and broader participation from workers, decision-makers and researchers utilising a diverse set of theoretical standpoints and methodologies.

Towards a participatory, dialogue-based approach to work-health research

We have put forward above an argument for greater participation of workers in the research process based on the epistemological, methodological and ethical implications of changes to the nature of both work and health. Some preliminary characteristics of a democratic and dialogic approach to research can be suggested: it starts with human experiences and stories; all concerned have the opportunity to participate actively; all arguments are open to examination; the focus is on shared needs, values and desires; the aim is to generate actions based on common ground (Shotter and Gustavsen 1999). Example of approaches falling under these principles include search conferences (Emery and Purser 1996); dialogue conferences (Shotter and Gustavsen 1999), appreciative enquiry (Watkins and Mohr 2001) and learning regions (Shotter and Gustavsen 1999). There is emerging evidence that these approaches lead to a number of common outcomes: shared understanding across difference; new networks and social relationships; a shared vision of the future; a new sense of possibility for change; new enthusiasm and commitment; and action.

There are certainly barriers to engaging in forms of democratic dialogue and enquiry. Entrenched interest groups are leery about cooperating with their foes, which is compounded by professionals' overwork, burnout and a prevailing cynicism that exists on work and health issues. As well, there are structural barriers to be faced by researchers wanting to engage in such enquiry, including current academic reward systems, ethical review systems and financial costs.

There are also challenges associated with increasing collaboration and participation across disciplines. It is important that researchers working together discuss some of the preconceptions and constructions of each other's research disciplines, methodologies and theories. In order for us to use and combine each other's methods, it is necessary that we have some understanding of how they work and for what particular circumstances they are best suited. Although mutual discussion is one way to familiarise ourselves with methods that are not our own, researchers must also take this project on individually. Often when researchers from various disciplines come to work together it is in the context of a funding proposal where time pressures are acute and there is little opportunity for meaningful, in-depth dialogue. Learning about each other's research traditions (at least in part) on our own, will help reduce what Giacomini (2003) has termed 'Exasperation 101' – where researchers continually must explain their canons, theories and methodologies to others within each new transdisciplinary encounter.

There are, then, limitations to more participatory forms of research. There is a danger that collective approaches will gloss over real and important conflicts between various groups, and obfuscate the need to address differences of power. There is difficulty in gaining the participation of certain individuals and groups for the required time, and the capacity of less educated individuals to participate effectively must be taken into account. There is a concern that only easy and non-threatening actions will be taken, and that change on deeper issues will not occur, or will be short-lived. Similarly, there is a fear that such approaches will be watered down to the lowest common denominator, and that the removal of conventional standards of evidence will lead to a free-for-all of arguments without any critical evaluation.

Finally, there is a problem with the 'one-off' nature of much of the research. This is reflective of constraints at various levels. University-based researchers are often constrained by the need to fund 'projects' that have defined beginnings and ends. When these projects involve the sustained engagement of specific communities – be they 'workers', 'First Nations', 'women', etc. – there is a very real prospect of the researcher having to abandon those with whom he/she has engaged as the funding for the project ends. Thus, those who have been mobilised to create change can feel let down and might become cynical or reluctant to engage further with researchers.

Similarly, attempts by policy-makers to engage (rather than merely consult) with citizens on specific issues are faced with the dilemma that such iterative, ongoing dialogues do not fit easily into the traditional policy-making processes and, in practice, are often grafted onto such processes without fundamentally changing the decision-making process within governments (Mendelsohn and McLean 2001). Too often they are designed to 'answer a problem' with which governments are concerned. These one-off engagement exercises can also serve to deflate the enthusiasm and momentum they create if they cannot be sustained over the longer term.

We also should acknowledge the danger of glossing over these real differences (Polanyi 2001). Indeed, these processes do not aim to resolve conflict but instead to create a deeper appreciation of others' experiences and views, which can, we believe, broaden the scope of common ground upon which joint action can be taken. In terms of their impact, it is certainly important for these processes to be carefully evaluated. However, evaluation should be critically applied, and should be broad enough in scope somehow to monitor those hard-to-measure, systemic and institutional 'ripples' that these processes can generate. Indeed, these processes may have the most potential in terms of their ability to engender reflective action over the longer term. Finally, it would be unfair to judge these processes on their ability to deal with the most difficult and intransigent of issues, which other approaches have not been able to address.

Note

1 This is a revised version of a paper originally published in *Critical Public Health* (2005) 15: 103–19.

References

Bakhtin, M.M. (1984) *Problems of Dostoevsky's Poetics*, ed. and trans. C. Emerson, Minneapolis: University of Minnesota Press.

—— (1986) *Speech Genres and Other Late Essays*, trans. V.W. McGee, Austin: University of Texas Press.

Betcherman, G. and Lowe, G.S. (1997) *The Future of Work in Canada: A Synthesis Report*, Ottawa: Canadian Policy Research Network.

Burchell, B., Ladipo, D. *et al.* (2002) *Job Insecurity and Work Intensification*, London: Routledge.

Burke, M. and Shields, J. (1999) *The Job-Poor Recovery: Social Cohesion and the Canadian Labour Market*, Toronto: Ryerson Polytechnic University.

Eakin, J. (1995) 'The health and safety of women in small workplaces', in K. Messing, B. Neis and L. Dumais (eds), *Invisible: Issues in Women's Occupational Health and Safety/ Invisible: La Santé des Travailleuses*, Charlottetown, PEI: Gynergy.

Emery, M. and Purser, R.E. (1996) *The Search Conference: A Powerful Method for Planning Organizational Change and Community Action*, San Francisco, CA: Jossey-Bass.

European Foundation for the Improvement of Work and Living Conditions (EFIWLC) (2002) *Quality of Work and Employment in Europe: Issues and Challenges*, Dublin: EFILWC.

Evered, R. and Louis, M.R. (1981) 'Alternative perspectives in the organizational sciences: inquiry from the inside and inquiry from the outside', *Academy of Management Review*, 6: 385–95.

Fox, N. (1999) 'Post-modern reflections: deconstructing risk, health and work', in N. Daykin and L. Doyal (eds), *Social Perspectives on Work and Health*, London: Macmillan.

Giacomini, M. (2003) 'Interdisciplinarity in health services research: dreams and night-mares, maladies and remedies', *Journal of Health Service Research Policy*, 9: 177–83.

Gunderson, M. and Hyatt, D. (2000) *Workers' Compensation: Foundations for Reform*, Toronto: University of Toronto Press.

Heery, E. and Salmon, J. (2000) *The Insecurity Thesis: The Insecure Workforce*, London: Routledge.

Hochschild, A. (1983) *The Managed Heart: Commercialization of Human Feeling*, Berkeley: University of California Press.

Kretzman, J.P. and McKnight, J.L. (1993) *Building Communities from the inside out: A Path toward Finding and Mobilizing a Community's Assets*, Evanston, IL: Institute for Policy Research, Northwestern University.

Landsbergis, P.A. (2003) 'The changing organization of work and the safety and health of working people: a commentary', *Journal of Occupational and Environmental Medicine*, 45: 61–72.

Lupton, D. (1995) *The Imperative of Health: Public Health and the Regulated Body*, Thousand Oaks, CA: Sage.

Mason, R.O. and Mitroff, I. (1981) *Complexity: The Nature of Real World Problems: Challenging Strategic Planning Assumptions: Theory, Cases and Techniques*, New York: Wiley-Interscience.

Mendelsohn, M. and McLean, J. (2001) 'Getting engaged: strengthening SUFA through citizen engagement', in T. McIntosh (ed.), *Building the Social Union: Perspectives, Directions and Challenges*, Regina: Canadian Plains Research Center.

Messing, K. (1998) *One-Eyed Science: Occupational Health and Women Workers*, Philadelphia, PA: Temple University Press.

Minkler, M. (2004) 'Ethical challenges for the "Outside" researcher in community-based participatory research', *Health Education and Behaviour*, 31: 684–97.

NCDDR (1996) *A Review of the Literature on Dissemination and Knowledge Utilization*, National Center for the Dissemination of Disability Research (NCDDR), July. Available at: <ww.ncddr.org> (accessed 13 April 2005).

Nelkin, D. (1989) 'Communicating technological risk: the social construction of risk perception', *American Review of Public Health*, 10: 95–113.

Polanyi, M.F. (2001) 'Toward common ground and action on repetitive strain injuries: an assessment of a Future Search conference', *Journal of Applied Behavioural Science*, 37: 465–87.

Polanyi, M.F. and Tompa, E. (2002) *Rethinking the Health Implications of Work in the New Global Economy*, Toronto: Comparative Programme on Health and Society, Munk Centre for International Studies, University of Toronto. Available at: <http://www.utoronto.ca/cphs/WORKINGPAPERS/CPHS2001_Michael_Polanyi.pdf>.

—— (2004) 'Rethinking work-health models for a new global economy: analysis of emerging dimensions of work', *Work: A Journal of Prevention, Assessment and Rehabilitation* (special issue on 'Organizations, Organizational Change and Working Life'), 23: 3–18.

Rittel, H. and Webber, M. (1973) 'Dilemmas in a general theory of planning', *Policy Sciences*, 4: 155–69.

Shotter, J. and Gustavsen, B. (1999) *The Role of 'Dialogue Conferences' in the Development of 'Learning Regions'*, Stockholm: Stockholm School of Economics, School of Advanced Studies in Leadership.

Vosko, L.F. (2000) *Temporary Work: The Gendered Rise of a Precarious Employment Relationship*, Toronto: University of Toronto Press.

Watkins, J.M. and Mohr, B.J. (2001) *Appreciative Inquiry: Change at the Speed of Imagination*, San Francisco, CA: Jossey-Bass.

Westmarland, N. (2001) 'The quantitative/qualitative debate and feminist research: a subjective view of objectivity', *Forum Qualitative Sozialforschung/Forum: Qualitative Social Research* [Online journal], 2(1). Available at: <http://www.qualitative-research.net/fqs-texte/1-01/1-01westmarland-e.htm> (accessed 10 April 2003).

Part III

Colonising places: public health and globalisation

Introduction

Ronald Labonté

> We no longer inhabit, if we ever did, a world of discrete national communities.
> [T]he very nature of everyday living – of work and money and beliefs, as well as
> of trade, communications and finance . . . connects us all in multiple ways with
> increasing intensity.
>
> (Held 2004)

An introductory tale

The underlying premise of the readings in this Part is that the health gains or losses
concomitant to humanity's ever-extending patterns of interconnectedness have
never been resolvable simply at the proximal level at which they are noticed as
disease. The history of civilisations has been one of straining against borders and
pushing against what they considered to be the edges of their world (Diamond 1997).
Similarly, disease has invariably followed the pathways of trade, from infectious
plagues in earlier centuries to the socially communicable chronic afflictions of the
twenty-first. There is no more urgent example of this than the present HIV
pandemic in sub-Saharan Africa.

Consider the story of Chileshe, a Zambian woman who, like tens of thousands
of others, is waiting to die from AIDS. The anti-retroviral roll-outs and Global Fund
initiatives have been too late and (still) too little. But that is only the immediate cause
of her impending premature mortality. Chileshe acquired the disease from her now
dead husband, who lost his job in a textile plant and moved to the capital, Lusaka,
where he sold used clothing as a precarious street vendor. Alone and lonely, he
traded money for sex with women desperate to support their own lives, and those
of their children. HIV – known in Africa in a play on its French acronym of SIDA
as '*salaire insuffisant depuis des années*' – is a disease of desperation. And so the pandemic
has surged.

But Chileshe's disease has two causes: one pathological, the other political. Its
political origins lie in the global colonisation of neoliberal policies through the macroeconomic policies imposed by the World Bank and the International Monetary
Fund as conditions for new loans or grants to help Zambia cope with its debt crisis.
In the early 1990s Zambia was required to open its borders to textile imports,

including cheap, second-hand clothing. Its domestic, state-run clothing manufacturers, inefficient in both technology and management by wealthier-nation standards, could not compete, especially when the importers of second-hand clothing had the advantage of no production costs and no import duties. Within eight years, almost all of Zambia's clothing and textile mills closed and 30,000 jobs – including that of Chileshe's husband – disappeared (Labonte *et al.* 2005).

Other facets of structural adjustment also played roles in her disease. Part of the standard adjustment package is privatisation of state industries to raise short-term revenue to continue servicing overseas debts. This privatisation robs a country of the ability for profitable state-run sectors to cross-subsidise social spending in such crucial areas as education and health. Liberalisation of financial markets makes it easier, in turn, for foreign-owned firms to move their profit offshore and avoid having it taxed for public spending or reinvested for domestic growth within the country. This is precisely what happened in Zambia. As well, the assumption that growth would inevitably follow such shock treatment, leading to new forms of employment and taxation to replace the sources lost by unemployment and tariff revenues, proved theoretically sound but empirically false. The net result was a dramatic drop in the monies available to the state to invest in health and education. This was buttressed by other adjustment requirements – a decrease in public spending, a cut in public sector wages and the introduction of cost-recovery (user-fee) programmes in health and other social services. All of this was imposed precisely when the AIDS pandemic was starting to surge.

In varying degrees this story recurred throughout many southern African countries. While the economic outcomes of adjustment remain equivocal (some countries weathered the changes better than others), and the World Bank and IMF argue that things would likely have been worse without these changes, in Africa they were largely negative and, in the case of health impacts, singularly destructive (Breman and Shelton 2001). Roberto de Vogli and Gretchen Birbeck (2005), using a simplified model linking globalisation to health outcomes similar to that in Chapter 10 of this book, identified the five-step multiple pathways by which neoliberal adjustment policies increased HIV vulnerability for sub-Saharan African women and children: currency devaluations, privatisation, financial and trade liberalisation, and implementation of user charges for both health services and education. The first two pathways reduce women's access to basic needs, because of rising prices or reduced opportunities for waged employment. The third increases migration to urban areas, which simultaneously may reduce women's access to basic needs and increase their exposure to risky consensual sex. The fourth pathway (health user fees) reduces both women's and youths' access to HIV-related services, and the fifth (education user fees) increases risk of exposure to risky consensual sex, commercial sex and sexual abuse by reducing access to education.

In effect (and this finding has been supported by the evidence marshalled by de Vogli and Birbeck), African people (particularly women and children) not responsible for the debts that precipitated the adjustment process were (and still are) sacrificing their health to ensure those debts will be repaid.

Globalisation as colonisation

The African AIDS and health governance story has been retold to the point of becoming inadvertently (perhaps only unconsciously) racist. The sequelae of imperial decolonisation and burden of infectious ills (of which HIV is only one of many), followed by tribal allegiances that undermine Western notions of democracy and prematurely coerced integration into the global economy, interspersed by famines and resource wars of horrific brutality, are becoming a disempowering caricature that gives rise to short-term, feel-good, celebrity-driven philanthropies. The richness and potential of the people and the continent, however badly misshapen by the 'white man's burden' of nations carved across traditional lines and boundaries to meet European countries' interests, are largely ignored.

The metaphoric power of the HIV/Africa tragedy, however simplifying, nevertheless attests to one of the principal colonising aspects of globalisation that Larkin (Chapter 9) identifies: the reflexive quality by which 'increasingly we are seen to reference events in relation to the global and through increasing flows of communication we are able to monitor, reflect upon and alter our activities'. We cannot view what happens in Africa without assessing our own roles in its fates, however remote – a point consistent with both the cosmopolitan and especially the relational justice ethics described in the introductory chapter to Part II. Larkin also identifies some of the major globalisation theories: a Western-based post-feudal extension of rationalism and modernity, an unstoppable dynamic embedded in industrialisation and the rise of nation-states, a 'World Systems' logic in which capitalism from its very inception was inherently globalising. These explanatory tropes are explicated by reference not only to the economic inequalities that might arise (as in the case of structural adjustment policies) but in the way in which the global instantiates itself in the local: witness the diffusion of Western medical technologies in India colliding with patriarchal norms, leading to increased abortion of female foetuses in an engendered genocide that others have estimated as 100 million missing women worldwide, and almost 40 million in India alone. (These estimates are based on what a 'normal' distribution of male/female populations should be against what exists; see Sen 2003.) Of particular concern to Larkin in the (still nascent) health studies of globalisation is a tendency to treat the phenomenon as exogenous, an external condition one needs to account for but not critique more thoroughly for its deeply contested and uncertain practices. There is no one globalisation, even if its multiple shapes are constrained by the dominance of deep market integration.

As Chapter 10 concludes, globalisation's 'momentum may be unstoppable, but its shape is not ineluctably determined (the notion that "there is no alternative" is a specious simplification) and its human impacts are readily malleable to human-made policies and regulations'. This chapter builds on Larkin's by describing a simple, syncretic framework for understanding how globalisation affects daily life and health. Labonté and Togerson expand upon Larkin's characterisation of contemporary globalisation as increased reflexivity by regarding this as a hopeful shift from a past paradigm of international health (where one's concern is with the greater burden of disease of the poor in poorer countries) to an emergent one of global health (where the causes and consequences of that burden are located within new forms of global capitalist relations and the past two decades of market-driven reforms). They similarly emphasise the economic aspects of contemporary global-isation, not to the exclusion of other facets but because, they contend, it is the economics of globalisation that shapes its health beneficence or harm. This economic colonisation operates through multiple channels at multiple levels of social organisation captured in their framework. In popular politics (think 'Live 8', white arm bands to 'make poverty history' and the shallowness of new celebrity campaigns such as 'Red', in which overconsumption by the world's more affluent somehow makes a saving statement about global poverty) these disparate channels distil to a simple, though not simplistic, trinity: aid, trade and debt. Since the article on which Chapter 10 is based was published, aid levels and commitments from rich donor countries have increased somewhat, along with efforts to untie this aid from purchases of the donor countries' goods and services, a practice known as 'phantom aid' that is more about subsidising domestic producers in the donor country than meeting people's requirements in the recipient one. But the sums are still insufficient and often distributed on the basis of donors' strategic global interests than the world's development needs. Despite the ballyhooing about increased aid and debt cancellation following the UK-hosted G8 Summit in 2005,[1] all of the new increases came in the form of debt cancellation to just two countries: Iraq and Nigeria (Africa's oil-rich country). There was actually a net decrease in new aid to sub-Saharan Africa (Labonté and Schrecker in press). Similarly scant progress has been made in transforming trade negotiations from the mercantilist arm-twisting of the more powerful nations on behalf of their economic elites to the putative role of such agreements in enhancing global economic welfare for all (which is the foundational goal of the World Trade Organisation).

One of the more neglected areas of enquiry has been the role of debt and financial market liberalisation as global capitalism's colonising force. Larkin puts the debt outflows from developing to developed countries between 1982 and 1990 at around US$72 billion a year, far outstripping reverse transfers in the form of development assistance. In 1993 (as Figure III:1 shows) the combination of aid and foreign direct investment led to a niggardly capital flow from rich to poor countries. Leaving aside whether much of that small cash flow trickled down to the poor within poor countries, what is striking in Figure III:1 is the impact of debt interest payments and profit repatriation in creating a massive redistribution of wealth from poor to rich countries, reaching a staggering US$483 billion in 2005 (United Nations Department of Economic and Social Affairs 2006). (The data used to calculate net financial transfers exclude two important forms: remittances – the money sent home by overseas workers, which now exceeds the value of development assistance – and capital flight. Since these have opposite signs they likely cancel out each other.) Much of this outflow eventually finds its way into US currency reserves, sustaining that country's economy through the greatest debt-financed consumption binge in history. How might one reasonably expect poorer countries to move beyond aid dependence to autonomy in reaching the Millennium Development Goals when so

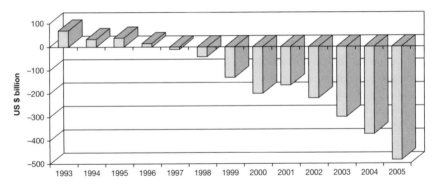

Figure III.1 Net capital flows, rich (OECD) to poor (developing) nations (foreign direct investment + official development assistance – debt servicing costs + profit repatriation)

much of their financial wealth (never mind their resource wealth or, increasingly, their human capital in the form of highly skilled people) migrates to the global centres of capital concentration?

The 1911 *Devil's Dictionary*, in a prescient application of Foucauldian argument, defined debt as 'an ingenious substitute for the chain and whip of the slave-driver'. Almost a century later, a curious account was published in which John Perkins wrote of his experience as an 'economic hit man'. Despite nominally working for a US-based financial institution, Perkins'

> real job . . . was giving loans to other countries – huge loans, much bigger than they could possibly repay . . . [and that would be used to employ] a US company to build . . . services . . . [for] a minority of the wealthiest . . . So we make this big loan most of which comes back to the United States, the country is left with the debt plus lots of interest, and they basically become our servants, our slaves. It's an empire we've built this way, a huge empire.
>
> (Perkins 2005: 15)

How much of Perkins' tale is empirically true is almost beside the point; the effect has been the same, regardless of its *modus operandi*.

What both readings lack, unfortunately, is a sense of possibility – the critical component of a theory of change – and perhaps also of the anger that can spark such possibility. 'That nearly half the world's population should live in the twenty-first century in such poverty that up to a third of their children die before they reach the age of five, at a time of unprecedented wealth among the world's rich,' David Woodward and Andrew Simms (2006: 2) write, 'can only be described as moral outrage.' It is an outrage that has led to an outpouring of global advocacy, much of it initiated from within poor countries and abetted by the research of activist civil society organisations, and a platform of technically feasible and much healthier international or multilateral options. These include fulfilment of commitments to increase aid, an end to lending conditionalities based on neoliberal economic nostrums, deeper debt cancellation, a recognition that much of the developing world's remaining debts are 'odious' and uncollectable under international law, and more emphasis in trade agreements on ensuring policy flexibilities for poorer countries to grow their economies using the same forms of protectionism and technology copying by which today's wealthy nations became so.

If we take seriously the exhortation in Chapter 10 – that we are now facing inherently global health issues – then solutions must also become inherently global rather than merely international or multilateral, however much global solutions might first require agreements among nation-states. Effective systems of wealth redistribution – not as charity, but as rights-based obligation – are one such solution. This entails closing offshore tax havens, in which corporations and the wealthy (including Make Poverty History poster-boy Bono and legendary bad boys the Rolling Stones) increasingly store much of their money.[2] The IMF estimates at least US$8 trillion sits untaxed in such accounts (and hence unavailable for even domestic, much less global, redistribution); the Tax Justice Network estimates it at over US$11 trillion. Based on 5 per cent growth and a nominal OECD tax rate of 40 per cent, a tax on interest earnings alone would bring in US$160–$220 billion annually – roughly double the value of present aid spending. What is further required are simple systems of global tax collection and disbursement. The former (collection) is technically easy if politically formidable, while the latter (disbursement) requires considerable forethought to avoid the inadequacies of current systems of aid distribution and the messy polyphony of disease-siloed global health initiatives. There is some reason for cautious optimism on both counts. The recent tax on airline tickets initiated by France (and now joined by many other countries) hypothecated to the purchase of anti-retroviral drugs for countries that cannot afford them is a small foot in the door through which financial transaction and carbon taxes might follow, and was itself considered inconceivable just a few short years ago.

Colonisation as globalisation

Chapter 9 makes the point that 'contemporary processes of globalisation are constituting themselves within a context already marked by inequalities carried over from the earlier colonial phase'. As Eduardo Galeano wrote of Latin America, 'the soil, its fruits and its mineral-rich depths, the people and their capacity to work and to consume, natural resources and human resources' have 'always been transmuted into European – or later United States – capital' (Galeano 1973: 12). Latin American colonisation by the Portuguese and Spanish set up a structure intended not for internal economic development but to profit the ruling class through export to foreign markets. It left a legacy of inequalities in the continent based on gender, race and wealth that persists to the present day.

A similar legacy constrains the health of indigenous peoples in most parts of the world and has included – until very recently – silencing of, or simply silence on, their traditional forms of knowledge. The special knowledge and 'lifeways' of indigenous peoples, as Lambert and Wenzel argue in Chapter 11, have been largely ignored in public health and health promotion. As if attesting to this, the article by Lambert and Wenzel is the only one specific to indigenous peoples' health to have appeared in *Critical Public Health* in its publication history. While this near silence has somewhat been broken since this article was first published, the voices of *indigena* around the world have still not been given much expression in debates on globalisation (Blaser *et al.* 2004). Yet their link to globalisation is an especially powerful one, since the very definition of 'indigenous' is that of 'colonised' – a locally born population in a land settled by others, largely during Western globalisation's first great wave of exploration, exploitation and conquest between the fourteenth and seventeenth centuries. Thus, even while recognising the plurality of aboriginal tribal identities in North America, Lambert and Wenzel somewhat apologetically conflate these to a more singularly constituted form: that of the colonised.

Readers may sense an idealised romanticism in their chapter, although it is noteworthy for dealing with how indigenous peoples understand health, rather than the more usual recitation of their comparative ills. (Indigenous peoples world-wide do poorer than the descendants of their colonisers on almost every metric of morbidity and mortality, with life-expectancy gaps ranging from 19–21 years in Australia, 8 years in Aotearoa/New Zealand, 5–7 years in Canada and 4–5 years in the United States; Ring and Brown 2003). Certainly, prior to European contact, tribal battles over land and resources were common among many indigenous populations. Some writers (e.g., Wright 2004) have even argued that eventual population pressures might have led to similar forms of environmental alienation as that encountered in today's industrialised capitalist cultures – and indeed did in the civilisations of Mesoamerica – had not European diseases wreaked such devastating depopulation impacts on most indigenous peoples between the sixteenth and eighteenth centuries, with estimates as high as 90 per cent of tribal groups dying of smallpox, measles, plague and influenza. Nevertheless, that a different and more animist *episteme* of knowledge and ecology existed, and still persists, among most indigenous peoples (however diluted by colonisation) is not seriously disputed. Nor is its positive impact on health: cultural revalorisation.

As background to this, colonised indigenous peoples have among the world's highest rates of addiction – to alcohol, tobacco, glue, sugar and other drugs. A report on a 2006 study released by the Australian Commonwealth government cites 'poor nutrition, obesity, smoking, alcohol and drug abuse' as the main causes of high death and illness rates among Australian Aborigines; and 'overcrowded housing, unsafe drinking water and poor sanitary conditions' as the contributing factors. To which the government responded by claiming that the 'idealisation of communal life might be the biggest obstacles to the betterment of Aborigines' – a slap in the face of almost two centuries of evidence of the addictive harm induced by the free market disintegration of such life ('Child death rate three times higher among Aborigines' 2006: 11). Specifically, addictions specialist Bruce Alexander published a compelling essay on the relationship between free markets and addiction, mustering historic Western evidence that alcohol and other forms of substance addiction were little known before the severe 'dislocations' brought about by capitalism's triumph over feudalism (Alexander 2001). Market capitalism requires individual consumers and wage labourers, which in turn requires loosening of the traditional bonds of culture, reciprocity, family and civic obligations and well-defined (if not always empowering) social roles. Into this normative gap or moral vacuum creeps what French sociologist Emile Durkheim labelled 'anomie' to describe the escalating rates of suicide that accompanied capitalism's dislocating rise in nineteenth-century Europe. Durkheim's solution back then was to urge creation of new collective associations that would imprint new moral orders and social roles, or what we now euphemise and theorise as building social capital (on which see Chapter 2). Alexander posits that the erosion of those collective associations in the new dislocations of late twentieth-century global capitalism – from trade unions to churches to public schools or other non-consumer-based public gathering places – leads an increasing number of people to seek meaning through 'substitute lifestyles', of which compulsive morbid behaviour ranks high.

How this pertains to cultural revalorisation is that strong communal identities play a role in the decommodification of the consumer-life, a fact recognised by early colonists forbidding the ritual sharing of gifts and material goods that characterised many indigenous cultures but threatened market capitalism. As if attesting to both Durkheim's and Alexander's insights, a Canadian study found that, as First Nations reserves revitalised cultural practices (from increased authority over the programmes on reserves to traditional ceremonies and language renewal), their excessively high suicide rates dropped in gradient fashion to at, or below, the non-aboriginal Canadian average (Chandler and Lalonde 1998). While precise data on addiction rates are not available, given their close relationship to suicide, we can assume that they also dropped.

Globalisation perpetuates indigenous peoples' colonisation but, as Larkin cautions in her contribution, it is a site of both struggle and possibility. Not only does economic power supplant 'guns, germs and steel' for indigenous groups; it wears a dialectically spinning Janus face. Stephen Kunitz (2000), in a penetrating essay, notes that economically wealthy countries, as they become so, move to a benign or less malign policy relationship with their indigenous populations: hence the various land rights and treaty settlements experienced in North America and Oceania in recent decades. He worries that weak or failed states (which, under conditions of globalisation, may remain stuck in this condition) will be unable to do a similar *volte face*. On the other hand, it may force, with sufficient local indigenous activism, a globally weak but domestically more democratic state. In a two-fisted way, globalisation homogenises consumer culture while also increasing awareness of cultural diversity. It displaces people 'in the way of development', as Mario Blaser and colleagues (Blaser *et al.* 2004) title their text on this topic, even while it constitutes a *global* indigenous identity in which the local power struggles of one group become both strategy and inspiration to another. This creates political tensions within many indigenous communities. Their economic empowerment, in turn, often lies in the unhealthy periphery of the mainstream: gambling and tobacco sales have been the major sources of tribal income for many North American First Nations, largely owing to arcane treaty exemptions that free them from government taxation and regulation and despite this leading to higher rates of problem gambling and tobacco use among their own members.

As well, and almost by definition, indigenous peoples are less removed from the physicality of their environments. This became recognised both as 'globalised' fact (in the United Nations' Agenda 21 on sustainable development, as one example; see United Nations 1992), and as an important survival strategy: 'The focus [of Agenda 21] on the environment is important for Indigenous peoples in part because it provides a narrative anchor by which their concerns for survival can be articulated with non-Indigenous peoples' concerns for survival' (Blaser *et al.* 2004: 10). Western-style resource extraction, however, often follows land claims settlements that are partly prompted by the needs of non-indigenous resource industries for clarity on legal title; whether such extraction is managed in more ecologically sustainable ways than past European practices remains a future imperfect.

Constraining the flows of people

Perhaps what remains most compelling and critical in Lambert and Wenzel's contribution is its insistence on, however Western-influenced, differing indigenous epistemologies. These differences require creation of what some have described as an 'ethical space' for respectful engagement between indigenous and non-indigenous peoples. This necessity is broader and more urgent given that an important and enduring aspect of globalisation has been the movement of people across borders.

Much of the critique of contemporary globalisation has been its liberalisation in the flow of capital of goods while increasingly curtailing the flow of people, at least from poor to rich countries (most migration remains within the same continent and over half of émigrés shift from one developing country to another). Exceptions to the poor–rich flow are made for highly skilled workers (particularly health workers), a phenomenon described as 'brain drain', in which the human capital of poorer countries is deliberately mined ('give us your brightest and your best') along with its natural capital, or flows of its own voluntary pursuit of opportunity, following the increasing accumulation of capital by elite groups in high-income countries and the media-beckoning illusion of wealth and opportunity in Europe, North America or Oceania (Labonté *et al.* 2006). Exceptions are also made for special lesser-skilled labourers, such as farmworkers, construction workers and other seasonal employees, though such groups are routinely denied the benefits of citizenship in their host countries and frequently subsist in conditions akin to nineteenth-century slavery. But the heightened alerts about terrorism, which many view sceptically as creation of a post-communist 'other' to justify the militarism and state retrenchment policies of the USA and other Anglo-American liberal market nations (the UK, Australia and Canada, at time of writing), has led to a new era of protectionism with respect to people flows. So, too, has the carving out of the middle classes in many high-income countries due to a perceived loss of their jobs to less costly and more easily exploited migrant workers. The irony, however, is that most of these economic losses arise from transnational companies outsourcing their production to lower-cost workers in low- and middle-income countries (or at least threatening to do so, to obtain wage concessions) and not to these workers pushing themselves across borders to steal jobs, as in the media-fed imagery.

A growing and more invidious rationale for raising the drawbridge on new migrants is that, once they enter high-income countries, they start to consume like high-income country residents, something the planetary resources cannot sustain (Abernethy 2006). This concern has led some environmentalists and 'steady-state' economists (including such notables as Herman Daly) to call for a curb on migration in the name of achieving ecological sustainability. The counter-argument is that the problem is not with migration, but with the excess consumption of and, via global market integration, appropriation of ecological resources from around the world by citizens of wealthier nations (Neumayer 2006). Ethically, and empirically, the raising of border barriers for ecological reasons is a red herring; albeit the impact of excess consumption and population growth on environmental resources is not. The barely beneath-the-surface problem for those interested in a critical approach to public health is the rise in xenophobia and intolerance that might come in its wake. People across cultures and countries seem to grasp that inequalities in access to resources are unfair and amenable to state correction (see Part I). The analysis of economic inequality is less tinged with emotive or prejudicial undertones. Racism, however, is ineluctably irrational and much harder to address.

Notwithstanding these recent and rising barriers, people still are on the move, including from low- to high-income countries. And they change not only countries but cultures. With this shift we encounter health- (and equity- or empowerment-) related issues of cultural conflict, similar to the concerns expressed in Chapter 11. A few points are worth stating at the outset: cultures are dynamic and routinely absorb elements of other cultures with which they come in contact. Even in the instance of the (important and health-enhancing) recreation of indigenous culture noted earlier, several Amerindian tribes have revitalised the ritual use of sweat lodges, a form of indigenous sauna but with strong spiritual as well as health connotations, despite such use having never been part of their particular tribal culture prior to European colonisation. Also (another point emanating from Chapter 11), many cultures that may be patriarchal and gender-disempowering on the surface (or at least from the Western feminist 'view from the tent' – an expression once used to describe the gross misinterpretation of other cultures' behaviours viewed by early anthropologists from the safety of their tents and entirely through the prism of Western intellectual constructs) often have gender-empowering aspects in their social organisation beneath the surface. The emancipatory health approach to such issues is never an easy one to ascertain, though with globalisation's compression of time, space and cognition, it is one that requires every practitioner's or policy-maker's attention.

Confronting globalisation's racist by-product

It is also a topic with which Pascale Allotey and her colleagues, Lenore Manderson and Sonia Grover, grapple. At the time they crafted their contribution (2001), 'female genital cutting' (a less harshly judgemental way of stating the more commonly used term, 'female genital mutilation', or FGM/C as it is now referenced) was one of the most difficult intercultural health issues confronting practitioners. The authors accept the well-intended motives of the international movement to restrict or ban this practice, noting that several countries in which FGM/C is a cultural practice have fallen in line with 'global' thinking on the issue. (That these countries have done so also indicates the empowering and health-promoting possibility of multilateral institutions in their various rights-based declarations or legal covenants in shaping policy discourse and practice.) They question, however, the somewhat tenuous health grounds on which the practice might be considered a health risk; there may be increased risks of neonatal or maternal mortality due to complications during delivery, but even FGM/C's recent and much touted elevated risk for HIV lacks solid clinical evidence even though its plausibility is strong. Instead, the authors consider FGM/C on gender rights or empowerment grounds, on which their case study of the Australian state of Victoria discloses a discomforting double-standard that, for the affected migrant women they interviewed and for the authors themselves, smacked of institutional racism.

First, there are the pronounced differences between what health professionals might expect from and how affected women experience surgical reversal of infibulations. While some of this could be dismissed as affected women's inter-nalisation or normalisation of something objectively unhealthy or disempowering, such exogenous conclusions are risky to generalise. (That these differences could only be uncovered through the use of qualitative methods and 'giving voice' to the women themselves attests to the importance of multiple methods in the armamen-tarium of critical public health research.) Second, and more at issue: why should FGM/C as practised on certain (black) women from certain cultural backgrounds be perceived with horror – and legislation applied accordingly – while labial surgeries, clitoral jewellery or even tattooing by young white women of the dominant culture undertaken for virtually the same reasons (identity, belonging) is given short shrift? Indeed, the trend towards such cultural adornment noted by Allotey and her colleagues in the late 1990s has, if anything, greatly accelerated, likely outstripping the 1–2 per cent annual increase in FGM estimated by the World Health Organisation. A website devoted to labial surgery – in which normal physical variations are pathologised 'misshapenness and irregularities' – even refers to its procedures as 'Female Genital Surgery'; that is, female genital cutting with an anaesthetised name. The 'dramatic increase' in this procedure is

> largely being driven by societal evolution regarding sexual habits, wants, and expectations . . . [A]s women in everyday life are now demanding more options when it comes to another openly accepted, self-esteem, minor surgical

procedure. Most women seek sculpting of the labia, or vaginal beautification to achieve a better look for themselves, and their sexual partner.

(Vaginal Cosmetic Surgery 2006)

This question may be less a double standard (at least in the sense of applying different standards to different groups) than the differential application of the same standard to different groups. And that is the definitional basis of racism. It is also a question that will not go away in our hegemonically articulated '9/11' world. In 2006, senior UK Labour MP Jack Straw stirred his country's uncomfortably stewing race/religion pot by expressing his discomfort when in the presence of women in the Islamic *niqab*, the veil and accompanying robes that cover all but a woman's eyes. The media debate vacillated between those (including many Muslim women) arguing that the *niqab* was less a religious symbol than a means of gender oppression and those questioning whether the same discomfort might be felt in the company of Catholic nuns in traditional garb, certainly still a common sight in many parts of Europe. Debates such as these are healthy, particularly when they incorporate differences expressed from within as well as across cultures. What can become toxic, however, is the lack of reflexivity on the part of dominant cultural groups over what embedded assumptions gird their response. To my own shock, I recall some years ago walking down a New York street in a poor neighbourhood when a young black man in rather tatty clothing approached asking me something that I couldn't hear well. I shrugged that I had no spare change (which was true). He (rightfully) angrily replied in a louder voice that he was looking for directions to a particular street.

But Allotey *et al.*'s caution extends beyond the personal internalisation of stereotypes: as it concludes, a central issue lies with public policies or laws that, however well meaning in intent, can marginalise ethnic minority groups. This probing across multiple dimensions of exclusion and inequitable differentiation, even if it does not always yield clear answers or what may seem later to be the better one, is another quality that distinguishes a critical from mainstream public health approach. This probing can often be personally disquieting and dystopian, leading to 'paralysis by analysis' – the pessimism of the intellect that for the Italian radical Antonio Gramsci could be countered only by an optimism of the will.

Notes

1   The G8 comprises eight of the world's wealthiest and most powerful countries: Canada, France, Germany, Italy, Japan, Russia, the UK and the USA. These countries account for about half the world's economic activity, hold effective vetoes at the World Bank and the IMF, and dominate trade negotiations at the World Trade Organization.

2   In both instances, these performers have their royalties paid to accounts in the Netherlands, which charges 10 per cent or less tax on such earnings (Murphy 2006). The Rolling Stones reportedly paid a paltry 1.6 per cent in taxes on some US$450 million in royalties earned over the past twenty years (*Globe and Mail*, 16 December 2006: R6). That the Netherlands offers such tax sheltering, as do other European countries and British and American protectorates, should disabuse us of the image of shady-dealing tropical islands and see it as another example of the logic of globalising capitalism itself.

References

Abernethy, V.D. (2006) 'Immigration reduction offers chance for softer landing', *Ecological Economics*, 59: 226–30.

Alexander, B. (2001) *The Roots of Addiction in Free Market Society*, Ottawa: Canadian Centre for Policy Alternatives.

Blaser, M., Feit, H.A. and McRae, G. (2004) 'Indigenous peoples and development processes: new terrains of struggle', in M. Blaser, H.A. Feit and G. McRae (eds), *In the Way of Development: Indigenous Peoples, Life Projects and Globalization*, New York: Zed Books.

Breman, A. and Shelton, C. (2001) *Structural Adjustment and Health: A Literature Review of the Debate, its Role-players and Presented Empirical Evidence* (Rep. No. WG6: 6), WHO: Commission on Macroeconomics and Health.

Chandler, M. and Lalonde, C. (1998) 'Cultural continuity as a hedge against suicide in Canada's First Nations', *Transcultural Psychiatry*, 35: 191–219.

'Child death rate three times higher among Aborigines' (2006) *Guardian Weekly*, 30 June–6 July: 11.

de Vogli, R. and Birbeck, G.L. (2005) 'Potential impact of adjustment policies on vulnerability of women and children to HIV/AIDS in sub-Saharan Africa', *Journal of Health Population and Nutrition*, 23: 105–20.

Diamond, J. (1997) *Guns, Germs and Steel: The Fates of Human Societies*, New York: W.W. Norton.

Galeano, E. (1973) *Open Veins of Latin America: Five Centuries of the Pillage of a Continent*, New York: Monthly Review Press.

Held, D. (2004) 'Globalisation: the dangers and the answers', *Open Democracy* (online). Available at: <http://www.opendemocracy.net/globalization-vision_reflections/article_1918.jsp>.

Kunitz, S.J. (2000) 'Public health then and now: globalization, states and the health of indigenous peoples', *American Journal of Public Health*, 90: 1531–9

Labonté, R., Packer, C. and Klassen, N. (2006) 'Managing health professional migration from sub-Saharan Africa to Canada: a stakeholder inquiry into policy options', *Human Resources for Health*, 4: 22.

Labonté, R. and Schrecker, T. (in press) 'Foreign policy matters: the case of the G8 and population health, *Bulletin of the World Health Organization*.

Labonte, R., Schrecker, T. and Sen Gupta, A. (2005) *Health for Some: Death, Disease and Disparity in a Globalized Era*, Toronto: Centre for Social Justice.

Murphy, R. (2006) *Tax and Corporate Accountability*, Tax Justice Network, UK (online). Available at: <http://www.taxresearch.org.uk/Blog/2006/08/20/100/>.

Neumayer, E. (2006) 'The environment: one more reason to keep immigrants out?', *Ecological Economics*, 59: 204–7.

Perkins, J. (2005) 'Interview with John Perkins, author *Confessions of an Economic Hit Man* (Berret and Koehler, 2005)', *CCPA Monitor*, 1 June: 15.

Ring, I. and Brown, N. (2003) 'The health status of indigenous peoples and others', *British Medical Journal*, 327: 404–5.

Sen, A. (2003) 'Missing women revisited', *British Medical Journal*, 327: 1297–8.

United Nations (1992) *Agenda 21: Report of the United Nations Conference on Environment and Development*, New York: Division for Sustainable Development, United Nations Department of Economic and Social Affairs. Available at: <http://www.un.org/esa/sustdev/documents/agenda21/english/agenda21toc.htm> (accessed 9 December 2003).

United Nations Department of Economic and Social Affairs (2006) *World Economic Situation and Prospects 2006*, New York: United Nations.

Vaginal Cosmetic Surgery (2006) (online). Available at: <www.labiaplastysurgeon.com>.

Woodward, D. and Simms, A. (2006) *Growth is Failing the Poor: The Unbalanced Distribution of the Benefits and Costs of Global Economic Growth* (Rep. No. 20), New York: United Nations Department of Economic and Social Affairs.

Wright, R. (2004) *A Short History of Progress*, Toronto: House of Anansi Press.

9 Globalisation and health[1]

Maureen Larkin

Introduction

Influenced by broader trends in social science literature in the 1990s, health and healthcare research has begun to acknowledge a global dimension to health. Some of this research notes the expansion of American 'for profit' healthcare plans into the developing countries (*British Medical Journal* 1996), or convergence towards the bureaucratisation and rationalisation of healthcare systems around the globe (Turner 1995). Here, the concept is deployed to describe what is seen as a growing internalisation of medical knowledge, technology and healthcare systems. Other studies have identified links between the growth of tobacco consumption and the export of Western lifestyles around the globe (Potter 1997), and the growth in global liberalisation of trade and markets with knock-on effects for health linked to restructuring of labour markets and uncertain employment prospects (Walt 1998). Potential threats to health are also being identified in relation to global changes in the physical environment, such as ozone depletion and skin cancers or global warming and alterations in vector habitats and disease patterns (Bentham 1994; McMichael and Haines 1997).

What is common with much of this research is that while acknowledging a growth in the scale and complexity of health issues associated with 'the global', the term itself and its implied characteristics are not critically examined. Instead, the existence of a global dimension to health is unwittingly constructed as some external and uniform process that will inevitably have consequences for health. What is not addressed is the complex and contested nature of these processes and, in particular, the uncertain ways in which they may come to insert themselves into local cultures and social relations. The active, transforming processes that work to shape how global influences are expressed is not acknowledged; instead, the social context and local social relations are constructed as passive recipients of external forces.

There is thus a need to problematise the global, a need that is also evident in contemporary attempts to understand and redefine the uncertain roles of the WHO and other UN bodies within the international health policy arena. It has been suggested that emerging global health problems call for a refocusing of the afore-mentioned organisations' priorities and greater collaboration and vision in providing stronger international leadership (Walt 1998). Useful though these insights may perhaps be in terms of the survival interests of bodies such as the WHO, a more critical analysis would need to consider the variety of ways in which global tendencies have been working to reshape the context within which international organisations operate, and which, in itself, has created new problems and uncertainties for procuring health which may not be amenable to reworked, traditional, bureaucratic forms of intervention. An example here is the ways in which policies and funding for health at an international level have become caught up in global economic policies and the workings of the market, as well as the variety of new agencies and interests which are active in seeking to shape agendas for health.

Making sense of these dynamics requires more in-depth understanding of how global processes operate and how they are mediated through a variety of international agencies and coalitions of interest. To aid in this, this chapter provides a fuller discussion of globalisation theories, and attempts, selectively, to assess how some of the insights gained from these may be utilised towards an understanding of health in developing countries.

Globalisation: themes and issues

Theorisations of the global have a tendency towards excessive abstraction. For this reason it is all too easy to form the impression that globalisation is some sort of uniform phenomenon which everywhere transforms local particularities into global realities. In this respect, a regional focus such as that on the 'developing' world can be helpful in identifying some of the central themes contained in the theories, as well as their usefulness within particular contexts.

Globalisation is a concept which gained currency in academic studies during the 1980s and expanded rapidly in the 1990s (Robertson 1992). Although it is possible to identify a shared concern among theories to understand contemporary processes of change, a variety of different theories of globalisation has developed with conflicting interpretations of its origins, nature and dynamics. For example, some theorists see globalisation as a process stretching back to the decline of feudalism in Europe (Robertson 1992). Others, such as Anthony Giddens (1990), link the process to the development of modern societies and the rise of capitalism and the nation-state. On the other hand, writers in the Marxist tradition, including World Systems theorists such as Immanuel Wallerstein, have emphasised the globalising imperative of capitalism from its inception (Wallerstein 1980; see also Amin 1980).

Disputes about origins notwithstanding, there would appear to be considerable agreement about some of the ways in which globalising tendencies manifest themselves in contemporary times. Globalisation is understood as a multifaceted and speeded-up process of change, which transcends and interconnects people and places across national boundaries. This interconnectedness is achieved through processes relating in the main to trade, financial, technological and communication flows and expanding cultures of consumerism, as well as the growth of international regulatory bodies and agencies (McGrew 1992). These processes are seen to be drawing more and more regions and peoples of the world into a web of shared interdependencies and, according to more recent theories, into a shared conscious-ness of this world as a whole (Waters 1995). In this sense the process of globalisation is understood as essentially reflexive; increasingly we are seen to reference events in relation to the global and through increasing flows of communication we are able to monitor, reflect upon and alter our activities (Waters 1995).

For most writers it would seem to be this reflexive quality which differentiates the modern form of globalisation from its disputed earlier stages. 'Globalization as a concept refers both to the compression of the world and the intensification of consciousness of the world as a whole' (Robertson 1992: 8). This links to other central concepts which are widely used (though in different forms) to understand the global experience, such as 'time–space distanciation' or the way in which travel and telecommunications have disrupted the time–space equation and enabled transactions and social relations to transcend the limitations of local contexts. In this sense, Giddens writes about the 'disembedding of social relations', or 'the lifting out of social relations from social contexts of interaction and their restructuring across indefinite spans of time–space' (Giddens 1990: 21). This suggests that globalisation and how it works cannot simply be read off as some uniform phenomenon but need to be interpreted in terms of the complex and uncertain ways in which globalisation constitutes itself within local contexts and social relations. These themes will be readdressed as my explorations proceed.

Globalisation and inequalities: the poorer regions of the world

That globalisation is not a uniform process is self-evident when we consider the poorer regions of the world in relation to developed countries. While more and more peoples and regions of the world appear to be caught within globalisation's reach, what seems to mark the process is its uneven nature (Kiely and Marfleet 1998). At a global level, whatever flows or indicators are used, whether world GNP, financial, investment or communication flows, what stands out are the massive and growing inequalities between developed and poorer regions of the world, such as sub-Saharan Africa, South Asia and parts of Latin America and the Middle East. This is reflected in the admittedly crude statistic which shows that 22.9 per cent of the world's population is estimated to be living in the industrial countries, but they have over 80 per cent of global GNP (United Nations Development Programme 1992). And in relation to health, huge disparities between developed and developing countries persist, where infant mortality rates of six per thousand in the former compare with an average of two hundred per thousand for low-income countries (World Health Organization 1995).

This is underpinned by the uneven distribution of global investment flows, which (as the research indicates) tends to be highly concentrated within developed regions of the world and among the more successful of the developing countries, such as those in Southeast Asia, and especially China (Hoogvelt 1997; Hirst and Thompson 1996). World trade is equally concentrated in the developed world. with actual shares of most developing regions showing a decline since the 1950s. And though much is made of global communications networks and flows, around 80 per cent of the world's population still lacks access to the most basic forms of communication technology (Kiely and Marfleet 1998). This is not to argue that the poorer regions are outside the reach of globalisation, or that all populations in developed countries are equally integrated into the process, but it is to draw attention to the uneven nature of globalisation and how this works through inequalities already laid down between developed and underdeveloped regions. The longstanding and widening disparities in health chances between developed and poorer countries are a telling example of this (Gray 1993).

In other words, contemporary processes of globalisation are constituting themselves within a context already marked by inequalities carried over from the earlier colonial phase, and it is relative to these patterns of inequality that people and states in the poorer countries must currently engage with globalisation. The importance of these unequal relations can be seen in the ways in which communities and states in the poorer regions have become caught up in Western-driven development agendas which appear to be out of their control and have had serious negative consequences for health. The literature on globalisation recognises that globalising tendencies can have implications for the nation-state, and ongoing debates centre on if and to what extent national and regional autonomies are being eroded by these processes (McGrew 1992).

As activities surrounding production and exchange increasingly transcend national boundaries and as new and related problems, such as environmental threats, unemployment and migration, pose new threats, so the nation-state is seen as either severely constrained or incapable of generating effective policies to meet these challenges (McGrew 1992). While there are a variety of positions on this issue in relation to the Western world, the argument can be seen to have a particular saliency for already weakened national states in the poorer regions of the world. Here, even some of the poorest countries in sub-Saharan Africa have been forced into global markets through the imposition of Western-driven neoliberal development strategies and the necessity of debt service to the West. It is estimated, for example, that over the period 1982 to 1990, debtor countries in the South remitted to their creditors in the North average monthly payments totalling over US$6 billion in interest payments alone (George 1992). (As the introductory chapter to this part makes clear, these net transfers of wealth from poor to rich countries have risen consistently over time and virtually exploded in the first half-decade of the new millennium.) While not all the problems of the poorer countries can be understood in terms of globalisation, there is no doubt that globalising processes, particularly in the form of Western-driven development strategies, have worked to weaken the role of local states considerably and to exacerbate their already disadvantaged position. The scope and detail of combined World Bank/IMF interventions alone have been held by some to match, if not exceed, the direct administration of former colonial governments (Hoogvelt 1997).

Structural adjustment policies and health

This stands out mostly clearly in relationship to structural adjustment policies (SAPs), which were put in place from the 1980s onwards at varying intervals in different countries throughout the so-called developing regions. Put briefly, these policies involved a package of measures allegedly designed to solve the 'debt crisis', whereby new loans were made conditional upon the liberalisation of trade, deregulation of labour markets, the removal of tariffs, price controls and subsidies and the privatisation of public assets (Loewenson 1993). The imposition of SAPs had the effect of forcing already weak economies into the global market place where their struggle for survival has worked to create highly adverse contexts for health. The increase in poverty is a major cause for concern. For example, in the mid-1990s it was estimated that in some of the poorest countries in sub-Saharan Africa, life expectancy would have decreased by the year 2000 (and indeed, it did), by which time the rate for some forty-five countries was estimated at under sixty years (World Health Organization 1996). (Much, though not all, of this decline can be attributed to the HIV pandemic. The introductory chapter to Part III recounts the link between SAPs and the rise of AIDS in sub-Saharan Africa.) Some of the ways in which SAPs have contributed to deteriorating health status are:

- the growth of poverty as labour markets were deregulated, unemployment increased and incomes fell;
- the undermining of food security as subsidies were withdrawn and prices rose; and
- shortage of essential medical and drug supplies and personnel as state expenditure was cut and user charges were imposed (Asthana 1994).

Research from the 1980s for affected regions show increased incidence of infectious diseases and raised infant and maternal mortality rates (Cornia *et al.* 1987).

There are a variety of other less researched ways in which the unequal insertion of poorer countries into world markets can be seen to have implications for health. As the necessity to export increases, there is pressure on countries to create favourable investment environments for industry and agriculture. This means lax safety standards and regulations governing work and the environment. There is currently increasing concern about the high rates of industrial accidents and overuse and misuse of pesticides in developing countries (Cooper Weil *et al.* 1990; World Bank 1996; Dinham 1993).

Under such circumstances, policies for health, whether of an international or national variety, are under considerable strain and intimately linked into the unfolding of the globalising processes. It is notable, for example, how in the 1980s the WHO's primary-care policies became caught up in and attenuated by market-driven ideologies and the preferences and interests of donor aid agencies. As health budgets came under pressure, so technical, cost-effective and targeted measures came to replace the WHO's original comprehensive strategies (Werner 1995). Indeed, in the 1980s, the role of the WHO itself as an international health policy-maker came to be overshadowed by the growing fund-holding power of the World Bank, whose loans for health quadrupled in that decade (World Bank, 1994). In this sense, it is increasingly difficult to separate policies for health from global strategies for development.

Global–local mediations

I now want to consider another central theme in the discourse of globalisation and to suggest ways in which it might be used to deepen an appreciation of the relationship between globalisation and health. As indicated earlier, the operation of global processes is not something that can be read off as unproblematic since it seems to work in often contradictory and unpredictable ways. As Giddens (1990: 64) argues, 'Local transformation is as much a part of globalization as the lateral extension of social connections across time and space.' Crucially, then, globalisation needs to be understood in terms of how it is mediated by local cultures and social relations. This does not, however, mean the simple transformation of the local and the global but rather, as Hall *et al.* (1992) argue, it is more a matter of understanding the new articulations between the global and the local. These interactions can work variously to strengthen old identities (as in the rise of nationalisms) or to create new ones, as cultures mix and flow across national boundaries.

Some of the complexities and implications of this process for health in developing countries can be illustrated in relationship to the global dissemination of Western medical technologies and how they are mediated by local cultures and power relations. For example, in places with strong patriarchal cultures of son preference, such as parts of India and China, the techniques of ultrasound and amniocentesis are widely used to secure families' preference for male children. Sex-determination testing and the abortion of female foetuses are reported to be both widespread and lucrative (Smyke 1991; Koblinsky *et al.* 1993). Feeding into this, in the case of India, is the culture of dowry payments, made all the more demanding and expensive within a growing culture of consumerism. The importance of local meanings and cultures and the complex ways in which they can combine and transform global influences can also provide useful insights into what is seen as a growing problem of drug resistance, particularly in developing countries (Kanji *et al.* 1992). In a variety of direct and indirect ways, this problem is linked to wider issues concerning difficulties in procuring appropriate drug supplies and in regulating markets, prescribing practices and usage (Chetley 1990). A handful of giant pharmaceutical transnational companies (TNCs) monopolise world trade in drugs and much research has understandably centred on the obstacles this presents for controlling the drugs market and attempting to develop rational drugs policies in developing countries (Kanji *et al.* 1992; Chetley 1990). Less attention has been given to the cultures within which users buy and consume drugs and the complex rationalities involved, which may have little to do with orthodox scientific concerns for safety and efficacy (Kanji *et al.* 1992).

The contemporary global context makes understanding these cultural meanings all the more challenging as global–local interactions work to transform meanings into what may be understood as hybrid forms.[2] Western medicines insert themselves into and are appropriated within local contexts with very different health beliefs and therapeutic cultures to those of Western biomedical culture. This can have implications for drug prescribing and drug use as different health beliefs and therapeutic practices combine in complex and uncertain ways to determine drug consumption. For example, Bledsoe (Bledsoe and Goubaud 1985) have shown among some ethnic groups in Africa how traditional cultural beliefs about disease causation, rooted in pre-modern health systems, come to be attributed to Western medicine. Thus, red tablets are sought out for blood disorders, reflecting the principle of fighting fire with fire (Geest 1988). Tablets and pills are also often dispensed individually, in numbers which have significance within local therapeutic cultures (see Wolfers in Geest 1988). The increasing overlap between the traditional and the modern is also powerfully shaped by emerging cultures of consumerism and a growing commodification of all forms of health products. Within such hybridised and commercialised contexts, attempts to regulate drug supplies become highly problematic.

Globalisation, oppositions and resistance

Finally, any attempt to develop analytical insights based on globalisation theories need to be sensitive to its contingent and dialectical nature; in particular, the contradictory dynamics contained within it (Giddens 1990). Globalisation tends to promote homogenisation and centralisation, inclusion and exclusion. Simultaneously, it also engenders decentralising tendencies, including oppositions and resistances, as local communities and transnational coalitions seek to challenge and regain control over what are experienced as impersonal forces (Rosenau 1989; Brecher and Costello 1994). It needs to be noted that there are a variety of different ways in which resistances and oppositions might be interpreted and which cut across modern/postmodern and postcolonial discourses (Williams and Chrisman 1993). These differences might be important for understanding the nature of particular forms of opposition and their potential for politicisation and empowerment. But what is of more saliency for this discussion is the way in which these oppositional tendencies cut across and interlink with a variety of different constituencies and pose new challenges for understanding or attempting to influence policies for health. This is notable from the late 1970s onwards, when, in our case, health and development and their related oppositions became increasingly pronounced and interlinked. What is evident in this period is that, as health became increasingly caught up in the development process through the machinations of debt servicing, restructuring and the dual role of the World Bank in development and health, so a variety of oppositional interests and groups arose to challenge these policies. At local and transnational levels, these interests are expressed through the activities of NGOs, environmental, anti-poverty and indigenous peoples' groups, as well as women, health and consumer groups. While some of the larger movements have gained considerable international recognition, such as the movement of landless people in Brazil, specific movements around health are less well documented.

The struggles of Health Action International against the pharmaceutical TNCs and related action around baby foods are two of the few high-profile exceptions (Chetley 1990). (These struggles, respectively, pertain to the role of extended patent protection in limiting access to essential drugs, and to ongoing violations by baby food producers of the UNICEF/WHO Code of Marketing of Breast-milk Substitutes.)

Considerable mobilisations and activities, especially around women's health issues, however, are a distinct feature of the politics of the 1980s and 1990s across Latin America, Asia and Africa (Safa 1990; Doyal 1995; Correa 1994). While women and women's groups do not speak with one voice and there are a variety of different issues around which women are active, health as a central concern for all women is often an integral dimension of wider concerns for meeting basic needs, such as housing, food and water within local communities (Correa 1994; Stein 1997). Local groups, in turn, are often linked into many wider regional and international women's networks, such as the Latin American Women's Movement and, in the case of reproductive health, the Women's Global Network for Reproductive Rights.

These larger international networks have been particularly vocal in bringing women's health concerns to the attention of international audiences through mobilisation and participation in world conferences. Here, reproductive health issues have been a key theme around which women's groups have been active. However, such movements for change are not without their difficulties and are not easy to assess in terms of their effectiveness in challenging the constraints of a global order and its constellation of commercial and ideological interests. Single-issue based as many of these groups are, their ability to challenge the given power structure is heavily dependent upon their ability to form effective alliances across a wide spectrum of interests and to maintain effective global–local links. In the struggle for recognition and funding, the dangers of subversion and co-option by more powerful interests are ever-present. The alliances formed between women and population and family-planning groups as agendas and budgets have come under threat create a sense of unease and pose difficult questions as to whose interests such mobilisations ultimately secure. For example, does sharing a common rhetoric of women's empowerment and reproductive rights mean that former demographic-driven policies will now be replaced by women-centred ones? Or is it merely a discursive transformation designed to co-opt women's interests to a wider global agenda of neoliberal forms of development?

Conclusion

Globalisation as theory and process poses new challenges for understanding and securing the health of populations in the late twentieth century. As a process, globalisation is more than a simple stretching of health issues, health problems and institutions around the world. What this tentative exploration of the area has demonstrated is that, if the term is to be used critically, the study of health must engage with the complex dynamics involved in this process and how these might be altering not only the wider socioeconomic context but the cultural meanings and practices through which individuals and groups engage in seeking to shape health chances.

The uneven nature of globalisation and how it works through unequal patterns already laid down have been demonstrated through a consideration of North–South inequalities and specifically the impact of Western-driven development strategies on developing countries. A more lengthy analysis of this unevenness would need to explore how this works itself through at a local level, creating advantage as well as disadvantage for different social groups. What is clear, however, is that the dominance of Western-driven interests and their ability to dictate terms and conditions of entry for developing countries into global markets creates serious obstacles for national governments and communities in attempting to control or provide for even the most basic prerequisites for health.

At the same time, as Western knowledge, technologies and ideologies are disseminated around the world, there is a need for a more critical appreciation of how these are mediated and transformed by local cultures and the wider socio-economic context. Whether this be in the case of some of the examples used above, such as reproductive technologies and Western pharmaceuticals, or the myriad other ways in which Western cultural products and practices are inserted into developing countries, failure to problematise the complicated interactions which are set in train is not only poor research. It can also implicate the researcher (or public health practitioner) in the perpetuation of a culture of despair as to the inevitability of globalisation, thus further disempowering already marginalised communities.

Finally, if policies for health are seriously to engage with the globalisation of health problems, then the way in which the international context has changed needs to be addressed. In particular, what needs to be acknowledged is the way in which globalisation has created an international constellation of commercial, technical and political interests that are active within the international policy-making arena and share what has rapidly become a global ideology of the free market. The uneasy roles of the WHO and other United Nations bodies within the health and development fields, and how their aims are often compromised, cannot be understood in isolation from these interests.

Similarly, the variety of coalitions of activists and groups and the resistances and oppositions displayed at both local and international levels constitute an integral part of how health issues and health problems are, and are likely to be, constituted within the new globalised context. How, and to what extent, effective coalitions can be achieved, given the variety of often contradictory interests involved, remains an open question. In a world of intense competition for funding, the dangers of co-option cannot be ruled out. However, as researchers and/or health activists, we cannot uncritically assume that the way forward for health can, or should be, guided solely by the deliberations of technical and professional experts. Globalisation has, paradoxically, opened up new sites of resistance in health as elsewhere, bringing new challenges and uncertainties for understanding future directions. These cannot be ignored or read off as some simple outcome of the hidden hand of globalisation.

Notes

1 This is a revised version of an article originally published in *Critical Public Health* (1999) 9: 335–45.
2 For an interesting discussion on hybridity and representations of the body in postcolonial contexts, see Caroline Allen (1998) 'Health promotion, fitness and bodies in a postcolonial context: the case of Trinidad', *Critical Public Health*, 8: 73–92.

References

Amin, S. (1980) *Class and Nation*, New York: Monthly Review Press.
Asthana, S. (1994) 'Community participation in health and development', in D. Phillips and Y. Verhasselt (eds), *Health and Development*, London: Routledge.
Bentham, G. (1994) 'Global environmental change and health', in D. Phillips and Y. Verhasselt (eds), *Health and Development*, London: Routledge.
Bledsoe, H.C. and Goubaud, F.M. (1985) 'The reinterpretation of Western pharmaceuticals among the Mende of Sierra Leone', *Social Science and Medicine*, 21: 275–82.
Brecher, J. and Costello, T. (1994) *Global Village: Global Pillage*, Boston, MA: South End Press.
British Medical Journal (1996) 'Editorial', *British Medical Journal*, 313: 28.
Chetley, A. (1990) *A Healthy Business: World Health and the Pharmaceutical Industry*, London: Zed Books.
Cooper Weil, D., Alicbusan, A., Wilson, J., Reich, M. and Bradley, D. (1990) *The Impact of Development Policies on Health: A Review of the Literature*, Geneva: WHO.
Cornia, G., Jolly, R. and Stewart, F. (1987) *Adjustment with a Human Face, Volume I: Protecting the Vulnerable and Promoting Growth*, Oxford: Oxford University Press.
Correa, S. (1994) *Population and Reproductive Rights: Feminist Perspectives from the South*, London: Zed Books.
Dinham, B. (1993) *The Pesticide Hazard*, London: Zed Books.
Doyal, L. (1995) *What Makes Women Sick*, London: Macmillan.
Geest, S. (1988) *The Context of Medicine in Developing Countries*, Dordrecht: Kluwer Academic.
George, S. (1992) *The Debt Boomerang: How Third World Debt Harms Us All*, London: Pluto Press/TMI.
Giddens, A. (1990) *The Consequences of Modernity*, Cambridge: Polity Press.
Gray, A. (1993) *World Health and Disease*, Milton Keynes: Open University Press.
Hall, S., Held, D. and McGrew, A. (1992) *Modernity and Its Futures*, Milton Keynes/Cambridge: Open University/Polity Press.
Hirst, P. and Thompson, G. (1996) *Globalization in Question*, Cambridge: Polity Press.
Hoogvelt, A. (1997) *Globalization and the Postcolonial World*, Basingstoke: Macmillan.
Kanji, N., Hardon, A., Harnmeijer, J.W., Mamdani, M and Walt, G. (1992) *Drugs Policy in Developing Countries*, London: Zed Books.
Kiely, R. and Marfleet, P. (1998) *Globalization and the Third World*, London: Routledge.
Koblinsky, M., Timyan, J. and Gay, J. (1993) *The Health of Women: A Global Perspective*, Boulder, CO: Westview Press.
Loewenson, R. (1993) 'Structural adjustment and health policy in Africa', *International Journal of Health Services*, 23: 717–30.
McGrew, A. (1992) 'A Global Society?', in S. Hall, D. Held and A. McGrew, *Modernity and Its Futures*, Milton Keynes/Cambridge: Open University/Polity Press.
McMichael, J. and Haines, A. (1997) 'Global climate change: the potential effects on health', *British Medical Journal*, 315: 805–9

Potter, I. (1997) 'Looking back and looking ahead: health promotion: a global challenge', *Health Promotion International*, 12: 273–8.

Robertson, R. (1992) *Globalization: Social Theory and Global Culture*, London: Sage.

Rosenau, J. (1989) *Turbulence in World Politics*, Brighton: Harvester Wheatsheaf.

Safa, H.I. (1990) 'Women's social movements in Latin America', *Gender and Society*, 4: 354–69.

Smyke, P. (1991) *Women and Health*, London: Zed Press.

Stein, J. (1997) *Empowerment and Women's Health*, London: Zed Books.

Turner, B. (1995) *Medical Power and Social Knowledge*, London: Sage.

United Nations Development Programme (1992) *Human Development Report*, Oxford: Oxford University Press.

Wallerstein, I. (1980) *The Modern World System III*, New York: Academic Press.

Walt, J. (1998) 'Globalization of international health', *Lancet*, 251: 434–7.

Waters, M. (1995) *Globalization*, London: Routledge.

Werner, D. (1995) 'Who killed primary healthcare?', *New Internationalist*, 272 (October). Available at: <http://www.healthwrights.org/articles/who_killed.htm>.

Williams, P. and Chrisman, L. (1993) *Colonial Discourse and Post Colonial Theory: A Reader*, Brighton: Harvester Wheatsheaf.

World Bank (1994) *World Development Report 1993: 'Investing in Health'*, Oxford: World Bank/ Oxford University Press.

—— (1996) *World Development Report 1995: 'Workers in an Integrating World'*, Oxford: World Bank/Oxford University Press.

World Health Organization (1995) *The World Health Report: Bridging the Gaps*, Geneva: WHO.

—— (1996) *Poverty Report 1995*, Geneva: WHO.

10 Interrogating globalisation, health and development

Towards a comprehensive framework for research, policy and political action[1]

Ronald Labonté and Renée Torgerson

Introduction

Understanding how globalisation affects health is not easy; the concept itself is multifaceted, and the breadth and depth of the pathways by which it influences health almost defy study of causal relations. Any explanation for how globalisation affects health becomes an evidence-based argument, in which evidence necessarily derives from multiple studies examining differing aspects of globalisation for their impact on theoretical or empirically established causal chains. The evidence is built up link by link; the problematic becomes one of organising the evidence into a coherent story.

In this chapter we provide an analytical framework for developing such a story, and proffer its usefulness as a heuristic device for organising both past and future research and policy studies. We view the processes through a critical lens by dismantling the dominant discourse around globalisation: that the rising tide of market-driven economic integration raises all ships. While our findings are not sanguine to this conclusion, more evidence is needed around the intersections between globalisation and 'real life' experiences. This includes understanding the policies and programmes which mitigate negative outcomes.

Defining globalisation

Globalisation describes a constellation of processes by which nations, businesses and people are becoming more connected and interdependent via increased economic integration and communication exchange, cultural diffusion (especially of Western culture) and travel. Our particular emphasis is in economic integration as the ultimate driver of the other processes. In this respect we differ from others (e.g., Lee 2002) who consider globalisation more broadly as a function of technology, culture and economics leading to a compression of time (everything is faster), space (geographic boundaries begin to blur) and cognition (awareness of the world as a whole). This is undoubtedly true, but as others have argued, 'economic globalisation has been the driving force behind the overall process of globalisation over the last two decades' (Woodward *et al.* 2001: 876).

Globalisation is not a new phenomenon; the history of humankind – or at least of Western civilisations – has been one of continuous pushing against borders, exploring, trading, expanding, conquering and assimilating, generally driven by an economic pursuit of resources or wealth (Diamond 1997). So the period of rapidly increased integration of global markets that began in the 1980s continues a longer historical trajectory, but it also differs in significant ways: the speed and scale of capital flows, the existence of enforceable trade and investment liberalization agreements and the size of transnational corporations, many of which are economically larger than most of the world's countries. These new global phenomena carry (some) health benefits and (many) health risks that demand critical appraisal, an undertaking that is still in its infancy (Drager and Beaglehole 2001).

The first critical step: from international to global health

Until recently, researchers, development agencies and non-governmental organisations (NGOs) mobilised around 'international health' issues: the greater burden of disease faced by poor groups in poor countries. International health remained essentially an extension of national health, the 'global' component being the rich world's modest efforts to aid in the development of countries that were lagging behind. Four world events changed the landscapes of these international relations irrevocably.

First was the 1970s recession in the industrialised world, compounded by the 'oil crisis' and domestic monetary policies that dramatically increased interest rates. This led many developing countries to default on international loans, and reshaped the International Monetary Fund (IMF) and World Bank into 'watchdog[s] for developing countries, to keep them on a policy track that would help them repay most of their debts and to open their markets for international investors' (Junne 2001: 206). The policy track of 'structural adjustment' embodied the neoliberal economic orthodoxy and conservative politics of the wealthier countries that dominate decisions in both institutions. Second, the fall of the Berlin Wall established the United States as the world's only superpower and created a normative vacuum for alternative models of development that could no longer experiment with 'third way' blends of state centralism and market capitalism. The birth of the World Trade Organisation (WTO) in 1995, with its first set of agreements tilted steeply in favour of transnational corporations based in wealthier nations, followed only a few years later. Third, the 1992 United Nations Conference on Environment and Development (United Nations 1992) fostered a global environmental consciousness with special emphasis on the developing world's need for both economic growth and environmental protection. Fourth, though harder to date, is the ongoing diffusion of information and communications technologies (ICTs) that has transformed the nature of global capitalism, while also increasing the speed and scale with which civil society can analyse and mobilise responses to its economic abuses.

This new landscape demands a shift in how global health is conceptualised. An international concern with poorer countries' greater burden of disease needs to give way to a more critical recognition that both the determinants and consequences of their excess disease are inextricably linked to processes of globalisation; that is, we are now confronting 'inherently global health issues' ranging from climate change and loss of ocean fisheries to financial instability and trade in health-damaging products (Labonte and Spiegel 2003).

Questioning globalisation's dominant discourse

Debates over globalisation tend to be polarised. Proponents claim that it represents the logical triumph of liberal capitalism, a humanising victory that should be propelled more quickly through rapid liberalisation and global market integration. Opponents counter that it represents less a humanising victory than one of corporate and elite group interests based largely in a few high-income countries. More nuanced perspectives argue that globalisation is neither good nor bad. Its momentum may be unstoppable (though that remains a moot point), but its shape is not ineluctably determined and its human impacts are readily malleable to human-made policies and regulations. We take the latter position – there are both positive and negative consequences of these human-made policies. What is needed at this juncture is a critical methodology infused with praxis. One cannot simply understand how globalisation affects population health; the goal is the development and evaluation of policies and actions which enhance population health in an era of continuing structural adjustment and neoliberal agendas.

Contrasting discourses similarly accompany discussion of the health impacts of globalisation. The diffusion of new knowledge and technology through trade and investment, it is argued, can aid in disease surveillance, treatment and prevention (Lee 2001). ICTs can enable more rapid scientific discovery, create virtual communities of support, increase knowledge about human rights and strengthen diaspora communities. The dominant health pro-globalisation discourse, however, rests principally on the rationale put forward by pro-liberalisation economists and trade ministers. Liberalisation (the removal of border barriers, such as tariffs, on the flow of goods and capital), proponents claim, increases trade. This increases economic growth, which decreases poverty; and any decline in poverty is good for people's health (Dollar 2001; Dollar and Kraay 2000). Growth also provides revenue for investments in healthcare, education, women's empowerment programmes and so on. Improved health, particularly among the world's poorer countries, also increases economic growth (Savedoff and Schultz 2000; WHO 2001) and so the pro-globalisation, pro-health circle virtuously closes upon itself.

This virtuous circle, however, has some vicious consequences. These include the more rapid spread of infectious diseases, some of which are becoming resistant to treatment; and the increased adoption of unhealthy 'Western' lifestyles by ever-larger numbers of people (Lee 2001), 'globalising' new pandemics of tobacco-related diseases, obesity and diabetes. The diffusion of new health technologies to developing countries usually benefits the wealthy, often at the expense of already underfunded and fraying public healthcare systems for the poor. And there are important gender relational and power implications. Trade openness might increase women's share of paid employment, an important element of gender empowerment (UNDP 1999; Chinkin 2000; Harcourt 2000; Sen 1999). Such work, however, is frequently in export processing zones that often pay below market wages, have poor health and safety standards and suppress union organisation (Durano 2002; ICFTU 2003) and given the lack of public support for childcare in most countries, women in these conditions have few options where that is concerned. There is also evidence of an emerging global 'hierarchy of care', in which women from developing nations are employed as domestic workers in wealthy countries, sending prized foreign currency back home to their families. Some of this is used to employ poorer rural women in their home countries to look after the children they have left behind. These rural women, in turn, leave their eldest daughter (often still quite young and ill-educated) to work full time caring for the family in the village (Hochschild 2000). More fundamentally, trade and financial liberalisation does not inevitably lead to increased trade or economic growth (Rodrik 1999; Rodriguez and Rodrik 2000). When it does, such growth does not inevitably reduce health-damaging poverty, and almost always (though not inevitably) leads to health-damaging inequality (Cornia 2001; Weisbrot *et al.* 2001; UNDP 2000). Much depends upon pre-existing social, economic and environmental conditions within countries; and upon specific national programmes and policies that enhance the capacities of citizens, such as health, education and social welfare programmes (UNDP 1999, 2000). Yet such programmes and policies are often cut back radically as part of structural adjustment, whether undertaken at the behest of international financial institutions or independently by governments seeking to attract investors with low taxes and an expanding pool of low-cost labour.

Of devils and the details: a framework for critically assessing globalisation's impacts on health

Sufficient evidence now exists to support a profound scepticism about the dominant 'story' that links globalisation, growth, development and health. Two recent reviews comparing economic, health and social development indicators in the 'pre-globalisation' era (roughly 1960 to 1980) with those following structural adjustment and trade liberalisation indicate that the net beneficiaries were the wealthy countries (Weisbrot *et al.* 2001; Milanovic 2003), what Milanovic calls the WENAO (Western Europe, North America and Oceania). Milanovic concludes, 'maintaining that globalisation as we know it is the way to go and that, if [its] . . . policies have not borne fruit so far, they will surely do so in the future, is to replace empiricism with ideology' (Milanovic 2003: 683).

The more specific impacts of globalisation on health, however, are more difficult to trace. They cannot be inferred from one or two independent variables, such as trade liberalisation or levels of inward foreign direct investment (FDI); there are simply too many historical and contingent confounders. The range of health outcome measures (the dependent variables) is vast and the reliability of the historic data in many countries is poor. An especially important point is that national-level comparisons provide little useful information about how health gains or risks are distributed subnationally or by different population groups. Locally oriented research, especially when it gives much needed voice to marginalised groups, can partly address this problem.

Our own approach to this complexity was to undertake a reasonably comprehensive review of analytical frameworks to create a 'map' of the linkages between globalisation and health (Labonte and Torgerson 2003). We defined 'frameworks' as graphic, visual representations of concepts, contexts and pathways that link globalisation to health, whether these pathways are defined in terms of arithmetical

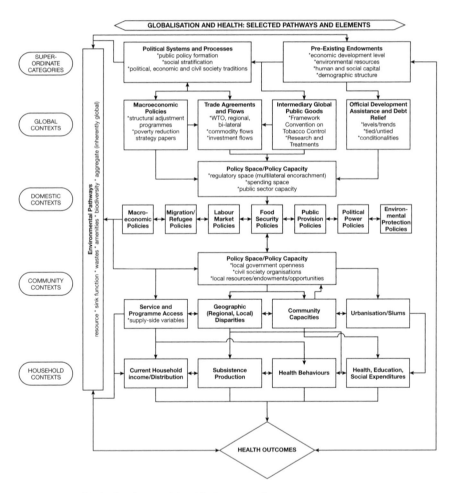

Figure 10.1 Globalisation and health framework

Note: Health systems, and other public infrastructures essential to better health outcomes, are subsumed under the categories of 'Public Provision Policies' and 'Services and Programme Access'.

relationships or qualitative descriptions of causal relations. Most frameworks we found were partial, reflecting the disciplinary or sectoral interests of their creators. Few frameworks incorporated people as social actors able to influence public policies, social norms or macroeconomic contexts. Interestingly, those that identified community organisations or civil society groups as mediators between globalisation and its impacts were non-governmental organisations. The frequent absence of social actors relates to another common omission: analysis of social power relations, by class, gender or ethno-racial background. Such analysis, we argue, is basic to a critical approach to understanding health determinants.

While the many analytical frameworks we encountered generated *partial* answers to *some* questions about globalisation and health, the absence of more comprehensive frameworks makes it difficult to identify the full range of both positive and negative effects. We present below our own composite framework, which incorporates elements that we found from our review to be theoretically and/or empirically 'rich' (substantiated). It is organised as a simple hierarchy. What follows is a brief discussion of the framework's different levels, and their implications for assessing globalisation's impacts on health.

Superordinate categories

Governments' decisions to contribute to, negotiate or abide by globalisation's key economic drivers, and their capacities to mitigate any health-damaging impacts, are conditioned by their national histories. We identify two categories of elements (many are still too broadly stated to be considered variables) that reflect this: pre-existing endowments and political systems and processes.

Pre-existing endowments

Crude measures of pre-existing economic endowments include *per capita* income or wealth, currency reserves and other monetary measures.[2] Natural resources also constitute a pre-existing endowment. Countries facing deficits in water, arable land, fibre (forests), energy and other natural resources will experience the impacts of globalisation more harshly than those with a surfeit of natural capital. Human capital (traditional knowledge, new knowledge, education attainment, individual and collective skills or abilities) and social capital (social networks predicated on trust and reciprocity) are other pre-existing endowments.

Political systems and processes

Political institutions and processes similarly shape the range of possible policy responses. In a case study of post-apartheid South Africa, McIntyre and Gilson (2001) argue that the influence of global contexts on domestic (national) policy space and capacity has been mediated by acceptance of discrimination (on the basis of race, ethnicity or gender), definition of public need and attitudes towards privatisation, determination of public policy (degree of civil society participation), level of unionisation and accountability of public administration. Some of these influences (notably the second, third and fourth) have been found in other cross-national studies (Global Social Policy Forum 2001; Gough 2001), particularly those contrasting the social and labour market impacts of global market integration between different forms of rich world capitalism (i.e., the Nordic social democratic, European corporatist and Anglo-American liberal models; see Esping-Anderson 1990).[3]

The extent of prior social status systems within countries, whether stratified by gender, class, caste, ethnic or wealth-based criteria, is also an important prior condition influencing how macroeconomic policies are selected and implemented, and ultimately shape health outcomes (Diderichsen *et al.* 2001). Countries with unequal power distribution are more likely to support global macroeconomic policies that retain elite group privileges than are those with a broad middle class, gender equity and strong civil society groups and labour unions.

Global policy and economic contexts

A focus of much of our work to date concerns the health impacts of four key elements of the global context, each of which is primarily under control of the rich, industrialised countries and the holders of transnational enforceable property rights: domestic macroeconomic policies, trade agreements (global, regional or bilateral), official development assistance and debt relief. To this list can be added the movement of peoples (over 175 million people lived outside their country of birth in 2000) and the flow of remittances to developing countries (some US$80 billion in 2002, more than double the amount in 1990, and an important source of foreign currency for many poorer countries) (Kapur and McHale 2003).[4]

Macroeconomic policies

The most commonly examined macroeconomic policies are those embodied in the conditionalities imposed by the IMF and World Bank on indebted countries in return for loans, grants or debt relief, collectively known as structural adjustment programmes, or SAPs (Mohan *et al.* 2000). Funds were made available only if the debtor country agreed to a relatively standard package of macroeconomic policies, including reduced subsidies for basic items of consumption, the reduction or elimination of tariffs and controls on capital flows, privatisation of state-owned productive assets, currency devaluations to increase the competitiveness of exports, and domestic austerity measures such as reduced government spending on education and health and the introduction of cost recovery through user fees (Milward 2000). SAPs are associated with the erosion of labour market institutions (full employment policies, decreased minimum wage and reduction in public sector employment), shifts in taxation policies (less progressive) and reduced public spending (e.g., on education, health and environmental protection) (Cornia and Court 2001).

While SAPs have disappeared in name, many of their macroeconomic elements are still found in the conditionalities associated with the Heavily Indebted Poor

Countries (HIPC) initiative launched in 1996 to provide partial debt relief for some of the world's most desperate countries. A key element of eligibility for HIPC is the preparation of a national Poverty Reduction Strategy Paper (PRSP) as the basis for domestic social and economic policy. Key PRSP elements include commitments to poverty reduction, broad public participation and local government ownership. However, the lenders who assess PRSPs operate on the presumption that poverty reduction is best achieved through neoliberal prescriptions for privatisation, deregulation and rapid integration into the global economy. PRSPs sometimes require more rapid liberalisation than that mandated under World Trade Organisation agreements, which is likely to exacerbate existing inequalities (SAPRIN 2002; UNDP 2001; Brock and McGee 2004); and they have failed to ensure increased funding for health and education, or to consider health as an outcome, rather than simply a means, of development (WHO 2001).

Trade agreements, flows and institutions

Trade liberalisation is a subset of macroeconomic policy. The aim of contemporary trade agreements is to facilitate the reorganisation of production or commodity chains across national borders in order to maximise profitability. Considerable disagreement surrounds the question of whether trade liberalisation *per se* will improve or worsen health and health-determining social contexts (Cornia 2001; Cornia and Court 2001; Dollar 2001; Kirkpatrick and Lee 1999; Labonte 2001). Trade liberalisation by definition reduces tariffs. This can shrink the amount of revenue governments have to spend on health, education and environmental protection. Tariff reduction has been particularly hard on developing countries, which used to get much of their revenue from tariffs. Few countries experiencing sharp post-liberalisation declines in tariffs have been able to generate other forms of compensatory taxation (Hilary 2001). This severely reduces their 'spending capacity' – the amount available for key health-promoting investments such as public healthcare, education, water/sanitation and gender empowerment programmes, or to enforce occupational, environmental or labour rights and standards.[5]

Trade policy may have perverse effects on health in two further ways. First, meaningful improvements in market access for the products of the world's poorest countries could result in dramatic increases in income and, therefore, in opportunities to improve health. A recent Oxfam report notes that: 'If developing countries increased their share of world exports by just five per cent, this would generate $350bn – seven times as much as they receive in aid' (Watkins 2002). Despite the free-trade rhetoric of the industrialised countries, and their demands that developing world markets be opened up to imports, they protect their own domestic markets in various ways, ranging from high tariffs on products of special importance to developing countries to trade-distorting subsidies to agricultural producers. Indeed, the industrialised world can be seen as giving with one hand (in the form of limited debt relief and development assistance) and taking away much more aggressively (in the form of trade protection and agricultural subsidies) with the other. The collapse of the WTO trade talks in Cancun in September 2003 can be read as a simultaneous success and failure in this regard. The success is the increased strength of organised developing countries; the failure lies in the apparent commitment of wealthier countries, particularly the USA and those in the EU, to focus now on bilateral and regional trade agreements where economic might can overwhelm a more diluted developing world opposition.

Second, an additional and increasingly scrutinised aspect of trade agreements involves the loss of domestic 'regulatory space' (Rao 1999; Labonte 2001; see Table 10.1). This loss can have positive health consequences if it prevents governments from providing subsidies to domestic companies that lead to resource depletion or environmentally destructive activities (for example, in agriculture or fisheries). But its impact is negative when, for example, 'the ability of governments to enact and implement appropriate environmental regulations is undermined by the provisions of trade and investment agreements' (OECD 2001). Most of the environmental frameworks reviewed in our study, using empirically based modelling experiments or case studies, concluded that increased global trade will create negative environmental externalities through accelerated resource depletion, trade-related energy consumption and greenhouse gas emissions (Labonte and Torgerson 2003), the health implications of which are profound.

Domestic regulatory space is further, if indirectly, encroached by the costs of implementing WTO agreements, which are estimated as far exceeding the total development budgets of the least developed countries (Finger and Schuler 2001); and by the level of public sector employment, which is often severely curtailed as a consequence of austerity measures undertaken in response to pressure from lenders (Cornia and Court 2001; Milward 2000).

Official development assistance

Official development assistance (ODA) is rarely considered in globalisation frameworks, perhaps because of the stagnation and subsequent decline of ODA spending by most industrialised countries during the 1980s and 1990s. (The recent attention given to the Millennium Development Goals (MDGs), and the importance of massively increased levels of development assistance to achieve them, is beginning to focus more media and public attention on ODA.) Only a few European countries ever achieved the internationally agreed target of 0.7 per cent of GDP for official development assistance (see Figure 10.2). Several donor countries have since pledged to reach this target by 2015, although not the USA, Japan or Canada (UN Millennium Project 2005: 252).

Although ODA remains an essential element in many national government budgets among the world's least developed countries, a number of problems (aside from its insufficient value) must be considered. Targeting of countries for assistance is inconsistent, making it difficult for countries to plan sustainable infrastructures and programme expenditures. Much of the aid is tied (requiring purchases from the donor country) or in the form of technical cooperation (requiring employment of donor country nationals). Reflecting an overall pattern of government expenditure in many developing countries, much aid, especially in health and education, does

Table 10.1 WTO agreements and health-damaging loss of domestic regulatory space

Agreement	Health impacts from loss of domestic regulatory space
Agreement on Trade-Related Intellectual Property Rights	Extends patent protection rights, limiting governments' abilities to provide essential medicines at affordable costs. Higher cost of drugs with extended patent protection drains money useful for primary healthcare. Case example: access to anti-retroviral drugs.
Agreement on Sanitary and Phytosanitary Measures	Requires scientific risk assessments even when foreign goods are treated no differently from domestic goods (i.e., even when there is no discrimination between a domestic and a foreign supplier of the good). Such assessments are costly, and are imperfect in assessing the many potential health risks associated with environmental and manufactured products. Case example: the successful challenge to the European Union's ban on the use of artificial hormones in raising beef.
Technical Barriers to Trade Agreement	Requires that any regulatory barrier to the free flow of goods be 'least trade restrictive as possible'. Many trade disputes over domestic health and safety regulations have invoked this agreement. The only WTO dispute where the health exception, allowing countries to abrogate from trade agreement rules for purposes of protecting human, animal and environmental health, was in favour of France's ban on the import of Canadian asbestos products. This occurred under appeal, and followed widespread negative reaction to the initial WTO ruling in favour of Canada.
Agreement on Trade-Related Investment Measures	Limits countries' abilities to direct investment where it would do most good for domestic economic development and employment equity, both of which are important to improving population health.
Agreement on Government Procurement	Limits governments' abilities to give priority to domestic firms bidding on its contracts, or to require purchases of goods from local companies, both of which can promote employment opportunities and regional equity, which in turn have strong links to better population health. This is currently an 'optional' agreement to which few developing countries have 'signed on'.
Agreement on Agriculture	Continuing export and producer subsidies by the USA, EU, Japan and Canada depress world prices and cost developing countries lost revenue which could be used to fund health, education and other health-promoting services. Subsidised food imports from wealthy countries undermine domestic growers' livelihoods. Market barriers to food products from developing countries persist and deny poorer countries trade-related earnings.

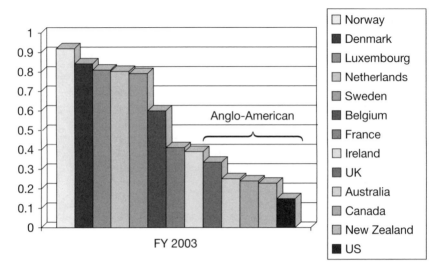

Figure 10.2 Development assistance as a percentage of Gross National Income
Source: OECD/DAC Annual Report 2004

not go to 'basic' services benefiting the least well off, but to technically advanced services benefiting a smaller number of the privileged (World Bank 2000). Finally, high debt and ODA insufficiency are conjoined twins. The problem is that development dollars that are not already tied go indirectly but no less certainly as debt repayments into the pockets of First World bankers, investors, government marketing boards, the IMF and other creditors – many of whom could be held at least partly responsible for these debts in the first place (Stiglitz 2003). In 1995, for all developing countries, debt service costs amounted to 3.6 times the value of ODA receipts. By 2000, the ratio had risen to over 7:1 (Pettifor and Greenhill 2002).

Domestic public policy contexts

A longer and more robust history exists of mapping pathways that link national (as distinct from global) policies to health outcomes, particularly in high-income countries. There is a premise that public policies determine the ultimate allocation of opportunities and resources within a political jurisdiction. We describe these as domestic rather than national policies, since most countries have a complex layering of policy-making rights from national to community levels. The ones identified in our framework are those with the strongest relationship to health outcomes.

Community contexts

Elements from higher-order categorisations recur within community contexts. First, there is the issue of how national resources are allocated to geographic areas, and the nature of local-level endowments capable of generating the means of livelihood and savings within communities. Second, there are aspects of local government itself (i.e., openness) and of civil society strength, both of which can enhance citizen participation in policy, programme and resource decisions. But this participation, in turn, and particularly for poorer groups, is often confined by a deficit in certain 'capacities' identified by the international and community development practice literature (e.g., leadership, resource mobilisation, assessment and analysis skills, organisational skills); hence an emphasis here on strategies that build such community capacities (Labonte and Laverack 2001). Key vehicles for this purpose reside in various publicly provided services; and here disparities in regional or community outcomes reflect responses to a macroeconomic policy context that is determined at national and international levels. Not only might there be geographic or regional disparity; many poorer countries have significantly unequal allocations of public programming and service resources within the same geographic community. A critical juncture between globalisation processes and community contexts is the impact of economic restructuring (via SAPs and free trade agreements) on accelerated urbanisation, creating massive 'slums' in poor countries with sanitation, crowding and poverty problems rivalling the worst of the European urban slums during the early period of nineteenth-century industrialisation (World Resources Institute 1996).

Household contexts

All of the analytical frameworks we reviewed that incorporated a household level describe and analyse gender roles – a perspective whose importance was noted earlier. McCulloch *et al.* 2001: 69) argue that the effects of poverty fall 'disproportionately on women, children and the elderly'. They discuss this in terms of 'gender power within the household', and how trade-related lowered family wage and a rise of female labour, without compensational help with household duties, may decrease women's welfare and compromise any increased household power their income-earning potential might have accrued for them. Greater female control of household income, in turn, is associated with better health and educational outcomes for children.

Health outcomes

Finally, our concern is with greater equity (fairness) in health within and between nations. Difficulties in selection and quality of data have already been mentioned; nevertheless, a useful shortlist of outcomes, particularly for developing countries, is provided by the health targets associated with the first seven of the Millennium Development Goals (Table 10.2), especially since these are the continued focus of progress reviews (e.g., UN Millennium Project 2005). Some caution is still in order because the MDGs are stated in aggregate terms. Improvements in health status and in the determinants of health sufficient to meet the MDG targets when measured at the national level only may not reflect improvements in the situation of the poorest

Table 10.2 The first seven Millennium Development Goals

Goal 1:	Eradicate extreme poverty and hunger
Target 1:	Halve, between 1990 and 2015, the proportion of people whose income is less than one dollar a day.
Target 2:	Halve, between 1990 and 2015, the proportion of people who suffer from hunger.
Goal 2:	Achieve universal primary education
Target 3:	Ensure that, by 2015, children everywhere, boys and girls alike, will be able to complete a full course of primary education.
Goal 3:	Promote gender equality and empower women
Target 4:	Eliminate gender disparity in primary and secondary education preferably by 2005 and to all levels of education no later than 2015.
Goal 4:	Reduce child mortality
Target 5:	Reduce by two-thirds, between 1990 and 2015, the under-five mortality rate.
Goal 5:	Improve maternal health
Target 6:	Reduce by three-quarters, between 1990 and 2015, the maternal mortality ratio.
Goal 6:	Combat HIV/AIDS, malaria and other diseases
Target 7:	Have halted by 2015, and begun to reverse, the spread of HIV/AIDS.
Target 8:	Have halted by 2015, and begun to reverse, the incidence of malaria and other major diseases.
Goal 7:	Ensure environmental sustainability
Target 9:	Integrate the principles of sustainable development into country policies and programmes and reverse the loss of environmental resources.
Target 10:	Halve, by 2015, the proportion of people without sustainable access to safe drinking water.
Target 11:	By 2020, to have achieved a significant improvement in the lives of at least 100 million slum dwellers.

Source: Devarajan *et al.* (2002: 34–5)

or least healthy (Gwatkin 2002). A country could conceivably reach the MDG targets by increasing health inequalities between high- and low-income groups within its borders. Careful monitoring of the incidence of such improvements using national-level equity stratifiers is needed.

Conclusion: towards an empowering methodology

The utility of any analytical framework in population health research depends on its ability to identify (or allow identification of) causal relations in ways that support and inform policy interventions, on scales ranging from the community to the transnational. This brings us to the important issue of *how* globalisation/health research itself might adopt the three tenets of a *critical population health* perspective that informed our own framework study: health is seen as embedded in social relations of power and historically inscribed contexts; research questions to 'unpack' the policy- and programme-relevant aspects of health determinants are shaped by the interests of those who face the greatest burden of disease; and, where applicable, research methods aim to be empowering and health-enhancing in their own right (Labonte *et al.* 2005). This issue is particularly acute when the research questions concern power differentials between the world's wealthiest and poorest citizens. Several broadly stated principles for conducting global health research have recently been proposed (Labonte and Spiegel 2001):

- Give priority to research on inherently global health issues that will reduce the burden of disease.
- Give priority to research on the burden of disease that includes study of inherently global health determinants.
- Within both, give priority to research that represents Southern-defined concerns or questions.
- Within such research, give priority to proposals that will increase equity in health outcomes between groups within nations.
- Within such research, give priority to proposals that have solid civil society engagement.
- Within such research, give priority to proposals that will increase equity in knowledge capacities between the North and South.

Our own efforts to act on these principles include new research work on the 'brain drain' of health professionals from southern African countries to Canada, the UK and Australia. The impetus for this research came from research/civil society networks in southern Africa, which are examining how globalisation processes (from trade agreements to macroeconomic policies to aid/debt trends) affect the supply of health workers in already under-resourced nations. It has an explicit advocacy plan and time frame; indeed, it is the advocacy plan's need for the research that is driving the collaboration.

Underpinning these principles is a more fundamental question, and one that for the moment remains unresolved: Can responses really be 'evidence-based', or will they be shaped by the interests of the world's rich minority. The challenge this poses for critical population health research is the degree to which researchers are committed to the political nature of the project in which they engage. Paraphrasing Marx's famous thesis on Feuerbach, researchers have only studied the world; the point, however, is to change it.

Acknowledgements

Some of the work reported herein was undertaken with support from the Globalisation, Trade and Health Group, World Health Organization, and the Institute of Population and Public Health, Canadian Institutes of Health Research. All opinions expressed in this paper are those of the authors. Thanks to Ted Schrecker, Senior Policy Researcher, Institute of Population Health, University of Ottawa, for contributions to this chapter.

Notes

1 This is a revised version of a paper first published in *Critical Public Health* (2005) 15: 157–79.
2 We emphasise that our use of the term 'pre-existing' refers only to how a country's current endowments affect its ability to respond to future challenges. In fact, most 'pre-existing' endowments are reflections of past historical processes; the current endowments of many developing countries are directly traceable to their colonial past.
3 The loss of domestic regulatory capacity and space that this chapter documents as consequent to contemporary globalisation has tempted some to announce the death of the nation-state as an important political actor. This is not the case. First, nations have created and agreed to the new global economic rules that subsequently diminished their own policy flexibility. Once created, these rules become a path-dependent force making it difficult, although not impossible, to alter the rules in the future. Moreover, considerable variation in domestic policies has persisted over the past two decades of global market integration. The Nordic countries continue to have high-tax, high-welfare, low-poverty capitalist regimes that also perform better, economically, than do most of the Anglo-American low-tax, low-welfare, high-poverty capitalist regimes. More at issue, and the reason why ongoing study of globalisation's health impacts is important, are the effects of new global economic rules on developing countries to achieve the type of welfare capitalism still enduring in much of Northern Europe.
4 Intermediary global public goods (IGPGs) is another element in our list of globalisation processes. IGPGs refer to the agencies and regulatory structures for 'global public goods', or GPGs. The GPG concept is a new expansion of the classical economic construct of public goods. At issue for a critical population health approach is that the GPG concept is beset by definitional disputes. Some claim that free trade agreements are GPGs on the assumption that they promote economic growth, which, by definition, is a public good. Others argue that such agreements are global public 'bads' by virtue of the inequities in wealth distribution they exacerbate and the environmental pollution and resource depletion that usually accompany rapid growth. Detailing the debates over GPGs is beyond the scope of this chapter; for further discussion, see Blouin *et al.* (2004), Kaul *et al.* (1999) and Woodward and Smith (2003).
5 Cornia (2001) and Cornia and Court (2001), among others, argue that liberalisation in capital markets has had far more negative health effects than liberalisation of trade in goods, including the increased vulnerability of national economies to capital flight and currency collapse. In each country affected by such currency collapses, the result has been increased poverty and inequality, and decreased health and social spending (O'Brien 2002).

References

Blouin, C., Foster, J. and Labonte, R. (2004) 'Canada's foreign policy and health: towards policy coherence', in M. Sanger and S. Sinclair (eds), *Putting Canada First: Canadian Health Care Reform in a Globalizing World*, Ottawa: Canadian Centre for Policy Alternatives.

Brock, K. and McGee, R. (2004) *Mapping Trade Policy: Understanding the Challenges of Civil Society Participation*, Working Paper 225, Brighton: Institute for Development Studies.

Chinkin, C. (2000) *Gender and Globalization: UN Chronicle 37* (no. 2). Available at: <http://www.un.org/Pubs/chronicle/2000/issue2/0200p69.htm> (accessed 21 January 2003).

Commission on Macroeconomics and Health (CMH) (2001) *Macroeconomics and Health: Investing in Health for Economic Development*, Geneva: WHO. Available at: <http://www3.who.int/whosis/cmh/cmh_report/report.cfm?path=cmh,cmh_reportandlanguage=english> (accessed 27 May 2003).

Cornia, G. (2001) 'Globalization and health: results and options', *Bulletin of the World Health Organization*, 79: 834–41.

Cornia, A.C. and Court, J. (2001) *Inequality, Growth and Poverty in an Era of Liberalization and Globalization*, Policy Brief No. 4, UN University, WIDER.

Devarajan, S., Miller, M. and Swanson, E. (2002) *Goals for Development: History, Prospects and Costs*, Washington, DC: World Bank. Available at: <http://econ.worldbank.org/files/13269_wps2819.pdf> (30 accessed May 2002).

Diamond, J. (1997) *Guns, Germs and Steel*, London: Random House.

Diderichsen, F., Evans, T. and Whitehead, M. (2001) 'The social disparities in health', in T. Evans, F. Whitehead, F. Diderichsen, A. Bhuiya and M. Wirth (eds), *Challenging Inequalities in Health: From Ethics to Action*, Oxford: Oxford University Press.

Dollar, D. (2001) 'Is globalization good for your health?', *Bulletin of the World Health Organization*, 79: 827–33.

Dollar, D. and Kraay, A. (2000) *Growth is Good for the Poor*, Washington: World Bank. Available at: <http://www.worldbank.org/research> accessed 22 January 2002).

Drager, N. and Beaglehole, R. (2001) 'Editorial: globalization: changing the public health landscape', *Bulletin of the World Health Organization*, 79: 803.

Durano, M. (2002) *Foreign Direct Investment and its Impact on Gender Relations*, Women in Development Europe (WIDE). Available at: <http://www.eurosur.org/wide/Globalisation/IS_Durano.htm>.

Esping-Anderson, G. (1990) *The Three Worlds of Welfare Capitalism*, Princeton, NJ: Princeton University Press.

Finger, J.M. and Schuler, P. (2001) 'Implementation of Uruguay Round commitments: the development challenge', in B. Hoekman and W. Martin (eds), *Developing Countries and the WTO: A Pro-active Agenda*, Oxford: Blackwell.

Global Social Policy Forum (2001) 'A North–South dialogue on the prospects for a socially progressive globalization', *Global Social Policy*, 1: 147–62.

Gough, I. (2001) 'Globalization and regional welfare regimes: the East Asian case', *Global Social Policy*, 1: 163–90.

Gwatkin, D.R. (2002) *Who Would Gain Most from Efforts to Reach the Millennium Development Goals for Health? An Inquiry into the Possibility of Progress that Fails to Reach the Poor*, HNP Discussion Paper, Washington, DC: World Bank.

Harcourt, W. (2000) *Communicable Diseases, Gender and Equity in Health*. Available at: <http://www.hsph.harvard.edu/Organizations/healthnet/Hupapers/gender/hartigan.html> (accessed 16 January 2003).

Hilary, J. (2001) *The Wrong Model: GATS, Trade Liberalisation and Children's Right to Health*, London: Save the Children.

Hochschild, A.R. (2000) 'Global care chains and emotional surplus value', in W. Hutton and A. Giddens (eds), *Global Capitalism*, New York: New Press.

International Confederation of Free Trade Unions (ICFTU) (2003) *Export Processing Zones – Symbols of Exploitation and a Development Dead-end*, Brussels: ICFTU.

Junne, G. (2001) 'International organizations in a period of globalization: new (problems of) legitimacy', in J. M. Coicaud and V. Heiskanen (eds), *The Legitimacy of International Organizations*, Tokyo: United Nations University Press.

Kapur, D. and McHale, J. (2003) 'Migration's new payoff', *Foreign Policy*, November–December: 49–57.

Kaul, I., Grunberg, I. and Stern, M. (1999) 'Introduction', in I. Kaul, I. Grunberg and M. Stern (eds), *Global Public Goods: International Cooperation in the 21st Century*, New York: UNDP/Oxford University Press.

Kirkpatrick, C. and Lee, N. (1999) WTO *New Round: Sustainability Impact Assessment Study, Phase Two Report – Executive Summary*, Manchester: Institute for Development Policy and Management and Environmental Impact Assessment Centre, University of Manchester. Available at: <http://www.europa.eu.int/comm/trade/pdf/repwto.pdf> (accessed 22 January 2002).

Labonte, R. (2001) *Health, Globalization and Sustainable Development*, a draft discussion paper prepared for the World Health Organization meeting 'Making Health Central to Sustainable Development', Oslo, Norway, 29 November–1 December. Available at: <www.spheru.ca> (accessed 30 January 2002).

Labonte, R. and Laverack, G. (2001) 'Capacity building and health promotion: for whom? And for what purpose?', *Critical Public Health*, 11: 111–27.

Labonte, R., Polanyi, M., Muhajarine, N., McIntosh, T. and Williams, A. (2005) 'Beyond the divides: towards critical population health research', *Critical Public Health*, 15: 5–17.

Labonte, R. and Spiegel, J. (2001) *Setting Global Health Priorities for Funding Canadian Researchers*, discussion paper prepared for the Institute on Population and Public Health, Canadian Institutes of Health Research. Available at: <www.spheru.ca> and <www.globalhealth.liu.bc.ca> (accessed 30 January 2002).

—— (2003) 'Setting global health research priorities', *British Medical Journal*, 326: 722–3.

Labonte, R. and Torgerson, R. (2003) *Frameworks for Analyzing the Links between Globalization and Health*, Geneva: World Health Organization.

Lee, K. (2001) 'Globalization: a new agenda for health?', in M. McKee, P. Garner and R. Scott (eds), *International Co-operation in Health*, Oxford: Oxford University Press.

—— (ed.) (2002) *Health Impacts of Globalization: Towards Global Governance*, London: Palgrave Macmillan.

McCulloch, N., Winter, L. and Ciera, X. (2001) *Trade Liberalization and Poverty: A Handbook*, London: Centre for Economic Policy Research. Available at: <http://www.ids.ac.uk/ids/global/pdfs/tlpov.pdf> (accessed 14 February 2002).

McIntyre, D. and Gilson, L. (2001) 'Social Africa: addressing the legacy of apartheid', in T. Evans, M. Whitehead, A. Diderichsen, A. Bhuiya and M. Wirth (eds), *Challenging Inequalities in Health: From Ethics to Action*, Oxford: Oxford University Press.

Milanovic, B. (2003) 'The two faces of globalization: against globalization as we know it', *World Development*, 31: 667–83.

Milward, B. (2000) 'What is structural adjustment', in G. Mohan, E. Brown, B. Milward and A.B. Zack-Williams (eds), *Structural Adjustment: Theory, Practice and Impacts*, London and New York: Routledge.

Mohan, G., Brown, E., Milward, B. and Zack-Williams, A.B. (2000) *Structural Adjustment: Theory, Practice and Impacts*, London and New York: Routledge.

O'Brien, R. (2002) 'Organizational politics, multilateral economic organizations and social policy', *Global Social Policy*, 2: 141–62.

OECD (2001) *Environment Outlook Report*, Paris: OECD.

—— (2005) 'Development co-operation: 2004 report', *DAC Journal*, 6(1) [whole issue].

Pettifor, A. and Greenhill, R. (2002) *Debt Relief and the Millennium Development Goals: Human Development Report Office*, Occasional paper – background paper for HDR 2003, United Nations Development Programme, December, New York: UNDP.

Rao, J.M. (1999) 'Defining global public goods', in I. Kaul, I. Grunberg and M. Stern (eds), *Global Public Goods: International Cooperation in the 21st Century*, New York: UNDP/Oxford University Press.

Rodriguez, F. and Rodrik, D. (2000) *Trade Policy and Economic Growth: A Skeptic's Guide to the Cross-National Evidence*, University of Maryland and Harvard University. Available at: <http://ksghome.harvard.edu/~drodrik/skeptil299.pdf>.

Rodrik, D. (1999) *The New Global Economy and Developing Countries: Making Openness Work*, Cambridge, MA: Harvard University Press.

Savedoff, W. and Schultz, T.P. (eds) (2000) *Wealth from Health: Linking Social Investments to Earnings in Latin America*, Washington, DC: Inter-American Development Bank.

Sen, A. (1999) *Development as Freedom*, New York: Knopf.

Stiglitz, J. (2003) *Globalization and its Discontents*, New York: W.W. Norton.

Structural Adjustment Participatory Review International Network (SAPRIN) (2002) *The Policy Roots of Economic Crisis and Poverty: A Multi-Country Participatory Assessment of Structural Adjustment*, Washington, DC: SAPRIN. Available at: <http://www.saprin.org/SAPRI_ Findings.pdf> (accessed 27 May 2003).

United Nations (1992) *Agenda 21: Report of the United Nations Conference on Environment and Development*, New York: Division for Sustainable Development, United Nations Department of Economic and Social Affairs. Available at: <http://www.un.org/esa/ sustdev/documents/agenda21/english/agenda21toc.htm> (accessed 9 December 2003).

United Nations Development Programme (UNDP) (1999) *Human Development Report 1999*, New York: Oxford University Press.

—— (2000) *Human Development Report 2000: Human Rights and Human Development*, New York: Oxford University Press.

—— (2001) 'UNDP review of the Poverty Reduction Strategy Paper (PRSP)', reproduced as pp. 201–16 in IMF and World Bank (2002) *External Comments and Contributions on the Joint Bank/Fund Staff Review of the PRSP Approach, Volume I: Bilateral Agencies and Multilateral Institutions*, Washington, DC: IMF. Available at: <http://www.imf.org/external/np/ prspgen/review/2002/comm/v1.pdf> (accessed 25 January 2003).

—— (2003) *Human Development Report 2003: Millennium Development Goals: A Compact among Nations to End Human Poverty*, New York: Oxford University Press.

UN Millennium Project (2005) *Investing in Development: A Practical Plan to Achieve the Millennium Development Goals*, London: Earthscan.

Watkins, K. (2002) *Rigged Rules and Double Standards: Trade, Globalisation, and the Fight against Poverty*, Washington, DC: Oxfam International. Available at: <http://www. maketradefair.com/stylesheet.asp?file=03042002121618andcat=2andsubcat=6andsel ect=1> (accessed 12 January 2003).

Weisbrot, M., Baker, D., Kraev, E. and Chen, J. (2001) *The Scorecard on Globalization 1980–2000: Twenty Years of Diminished Progress*, Centre for Economic and Policy Research. Available at: <http://www.cepr.net/globalization/scorecard_on_ globalization.htm> (accessed 29 September 2002).

Woodward, D., Drager, N., Beaglehole, R. and Lipson, D. (2001) 'Globalization and health: a framework for analysis and action', *Bulletin of the World Health Organization*, 79: 875–81.

Woodward, D. and Smith, R. (2003) 'Global public goods and health: concepts and issues', in: R. Smith, R. Beaglehole, D. Woodward and N. Drager (eds), *Global Public Goods for Health: Health Economic and Public Health Perspectives*, Oxford: Oxford University Press.

World Bank (2000) *World Development Report 2000/2001: Attacking Poverty*, New York: Oxford University Press.

—— (2002) *World Development Indicators*, Washington, DC: World Bank.

World Health Organization (WHO) (2001) *Health in PRSPs: WHO Submission to World Bank/IMF Review of PRSPs*. Available at: <http://www.worldbank.org./poverty/ strategies/review/index.htm> (accessed 25 January 2002).

World Resources Institute (1996) *World Resources 1996–97: The Urban Environment*, New York: Oxford University Press.

11 Medicine keepers

Issues in indigenous health[1]

Lori Lambert (Abenaki / Mi'kmaq) and Eberhard Wenzel

> To me, health is being spiritual, keeping in a good mind. Keeping myself away
> from the 'Evil One', keeping spiritual, keeping strong.
>
> Salish cultural leader

> Western medicine is so linear and not very conducive to healing [for me]. There
> is no connection to the spiritual aspect of healing [in Western medicine].
>
> Cree cultural leader

Today, all over the planet, indigenous peoples are in trouble. From the Sami
in Scandinavia, to the Amazonian tribes of the South American rainforest, to
North American First Nations and Australian Aboriginals, traditional lands and
lifeways are being altered in the name of economic development by non-traditional
enterprises such as logging, damming, mining and various other development
projects (Young 1995). Families of indigenous peoples are being disrupted, brought
to settlement, made to move from traditional homelands, from the ashes of their
grandfathers, from their traditional hunting grounds, from their aboriginal fishing
territories. These activities are carried out without consensual agreements of the
indigenous peoples and the projects are affecting social, mental, physical and
emotional health (Colomeda 1996; Indian Health Service 1997; Kelm 1998; Kuletz
1998; Sandefur *et al.* 1996; Waldram *et al.* 1995; Young 1994).

Diseases such as Minamata, lung cancer, breast cancer, congenital anomalies,
lead poisoning, obesity, diabetes and heart disease can all be traced to collisions of
culture in indigenous communities (Colomeda 1996; Cook 1998; Eichstaedt 1994;
Grinde and Johansen 1995, Joe and Young 1994; Kunitz 1996; Ramenofsky 1987;
Reid and Trompf 1991; Robinson 1996; Saggers and Gray 1998; Shephard and
Rode 1996; Spector 1996). When indigenous peoples speak about restoring health,
they talk about restoring the land in the same breath. For indigenous peoples,
health is linked to the health of the land, health of the culture, and spiritual health
(Colomeda 1999).

Although the World Health Organization (WHO) has defined the concept of
health for all populations as being physical, mental, social and spiritual well-being
(WHO 1946), the meaning of health and its application in everyday life is dependent

on the culture and worldview of the population being served. It is easy to agree on generalities; it is more complicated to agree on the cultural and social meanings of health practices in a world that is still diverse in almost every aspect, despite economic and cultural globalisation. As far as North America is concerned, this relates to the large cultural diversity among American Indians (Hodgkenson 1990) which makes it almost impossible to write about indigenous peoples, as they are by no means one distinctive population group. The same is true in Australia, which is home to more than 300 different tribes with different cultures and languages (Horton 1994). To speak of indigenous Australians is misleading. We are aware of this problem, but within the frame of this chapter we are not able to differentiate every issue where differentiation is necessary.

Indigenous peoples

Who are the world's indigenous peoples? In 1977, the Second General Assembly of the World Council of Indigenous Peoples (WCIP) passed a resolution declaring that only indigenous peoples could define indigenous peoples. The formal political definition developed by WCIP is:

> Indigenous Peoples shall be peoples living in countries, which have populations, composed of different ethnic or racial groups who are descendants of the earliest populations which survive in the area, and who do not, as a group, control the national government of the countries within which they live.
>
> (World Council of Indigenous Peoples 1977)

When indigenous peoples from different cultures meet one another for the first time they are overwhelmed by the fact that they share the same basic culture in spite of overt difference. What makes them different from the dominant society is the relationship to the land and how the land helps them to maintain good health. For indigenous peoples, knowledge of the land depends on contracts with the invisible spirit world, which plays its own crucial part in ensuring health, reproduction of society, culture and the environment. Non-indigenous environmentalists deal exclusively with the relationship of human beings and 'nature'. Indigenous peoples have a different way of conceptualising this. Knowledge is both spiritual and conceptual and human beings are not separated from what non-indigenous peoples view as the 'natural world' (Gray 1991).

> Traditional people of Indian nations have interpreted the two roads that face the light skinned race as the road to technology and the road to spirituality. We feel that the road to technology . . . has led modern society to a damaged and seared earth. Could it be that the road to technology represents a rush to destruction, and that the road to spirituality represents the slower path that the traditional native people have traveled and are now seeking again? The earth is not scorched on this trail. The grass is still growing there.
>
> (Mamiwinini 1991)

Indigenous peoples have an ancient and deep respect for the land, embodied in the spiritual concept of the earth as Sacred Mother. Art, cultural ceremonies and indigenous life all reflect this. American Indians believe that the grasses are Mother Earth's hair. When they burn sweet grass in ceremonies the smoke carries the prayers to the Creator, much like the candles and the incense in other religious ceremonies.

Indigenous health

Before contact with Europeans, the health problems that indigenous peoples experienced were not of the magnitude that we see today. For indigenous peoples, the colonisation by Europeans has presented a conflict in cultural values, beliefs and practices, or a collision of cultures until the present day (Colomeda 1999). All indigenous peoples know that health or well-being is directly related to the land on which we live. When we lose our land, when we lose the connection to our land, our well-being is threatened in real terms (Goudie 1997). The technical term 'environment' does not reflect the deep spiritual quality of the human connection to land. Rather, it conceals it, thereby opening the door for reason and rationality to treat the environment as just another commodity (Wenzel 1997), in which land is there to be used since 'Wilderness = Land of no use' (Bass 1996). Land has become a commodity to be consumed by the individual (corporation) for individual needs and purposes.

One of the clear distinctions between industrialised and indigenous cultures is the individualisation of human life. Industrialised societies need mobile and competitive individuals to travel where work is offered. They need individuals who are available for work at any point in time irrespective of their family and kinship relations. In fact, the individual is a product of industrialisation. Only the individual disconnected from land, kinship and culture can function properly in societies, which honour the self-made man and woman as the icon and myth of industrialised societies (Romanyshyn and Whalen 1987).

On the other hand, the concept of community and connectedness is extremely strong in indigenous cultures (Long and Dickason 1999; Stephenson 1995). The solutions indigenous peoples seek for their future do not lie in an individualistic form of thinking. When people in their communities are ill, others bring food and medicines and pray for them. Rarely is this done in non-indigenous communities. The members of the community help form the worldview of all that live in the related community. Worldview consists of the principles that we acquire to make sense of the world around us. It is an especially valid point when we speak of sacred animals or spirit animals and their role in health. Worldview directs everyday practice in every culture. Differences in worldview cause differences in practice in all sectors of everyday life.

For indigenous peoples, good health includes practising cultural ceremonies, speaking the language, applying the wisdom of the elders, learning the songs, beliefs, healing practices and values that have been handed down in the community from generation to generation (Lyon 1998; Vogel 1970). The culture of many indigenous peoples stems from an oral and behavioural tradition. Westerners use the word 'theory'. For indigenous peoples, this may mean 'the way our ancestors thought about things':

> This impersonal academic tradition is a far cry from the highly ritualized bestowal of knowledge upon a neophyte by the custodians of ancient wisdom. The end product of the two traditions results in a very different reading of the environment and a different perception of what, in the West, is identified as science and technology, and in Aboriginal culture is celebrated as ancient wisdom and traditional skills. This is not to say that Aboriginal people did not or cannot think about the environment in a scientific or rational way. They can and do.
>
> (Gostin and Chong 1998: 148)

Indigenous health is built upon their oral and behavioural traditions, especially the meanings given to balance between mind, body, spirit, culture and earth. When these elements are in balance, we may enjoy good health. On the other hand, if we consider Western medicine today, it is clear that its major characteristic is not balance but pre-eminence. Such pre-eminence is not merely that of prestige, but also that of 'expert authority' and power (Freidson 1970). Western medicine claims that its paradigm of scientific conduct is the only one that merits acknowledgement by everyone living on Mother Earth.

Yet the indigenous peoples of the Americas knew many cures for illnesses long before medicine in Europe became a science (e.g., Lacey 1993). The Mi'kmaq of eastern Canada knew about curing goitres by eating harvested sea kelp. The iodine in the kelp kept them free from the condition. The Hurons taught the French explorer Jacques Cartier how to cure scurvy in the 1500s by boiling the vitamin C-rich needles from an evergreen tree. In the 1700s James Lind of the Scottish Navy learned about the Indians' cure from reading an account of Cartier and the Hurons, and then claimed the cure for himself (Weatherford 1988). Indian peoples in northern California and Oregon used a medicine called 'the sacred bark' to evacuate the bowels in cases of constipation. The Spanish mixed the bark with sugar and chocolate. Today, the same ingredients are found in ExLax (Weatherford 1988), a popular product of the pharmaceutical industry in the USA and elsewhere. Curare originally came from the rainforests of the indigenous peoples living in the Amazon Basin. It was painted on the tips of arrows used to kill prey in the canopy of the rainforest. Later, it was used by Western medicine to cure the symptoms of lockjaw. Today, it is used to relax the body before surgery so that the endotracheal tube can be inserted into the windpipe (Weatherford 1988).

> Indian healers developed many drugs to treat the problems of women. They used the trillium erectum to ease the pain of childbirth, which led the pioneers to rename the plant the 'birthroot' . . . In addition, Indian people developed many salves and ointments: among them are witch hazel, wintergreen and Vaseline. Indian healers sewed facial lacerations by using bone needles

threaded with human hair. They set bones in eel skins and plasters made of downy feathers, gum and resin. They gave enemas with rubber hoses and invented the bulb syringe to clean out ear canals.

(Weatherford 1988: 181)

Issues in indigenous health

Today, American Indian people [as well as most indigenous nations] are faced with a number of health related problems. Many of the old ways of diagnosing and treating illnesses have not survived the migration and the changing ways of life of the people . . . skills have been lost . . . modern healthcare facilities are not always available . . . social and economic factors are suspected contributors.

(Spector 1996: 243)

However, 'Native North Americans have demonstrated a remarkable tenacity in the face of adversity inflicted on them from the time of contact' (Young 1994: 216).

Indigenous peoples examine health and well-being from a comprehensive perspective. Key players in this perspective are the elders. They are 'keepers of the wisdom' who help educate tribal members, and remember their history and cultural practices. Traditional wisdom and knowledge of the land and how the land supports the community have been essential foundations of indigenous health and well-being. Elders have always played a critical role in maintaining the health of indigenous nations. They are living libraries, repositories of the oral traditions for their nations. They remember the old ways, old ceremonies, songs to sing for gathering the plants, medicines to use that will cure their people. In the face of environmental degradation and excessive agricultural use of the land, this foundation has been shaken to its core (Eichstaedt 1994; Grinde and Johansen 1995; Kuletz 1998).

We will refer to some key issues of indigenous health in the following paragraphs, but we wish to make clear that our presentation does not go into details of the relations between those issues and the broader worldview of indigenous peoples, particularly in North America and Australia.

The earth as mother: land

One side respected the land; one side exploited the land. One side was basically peaceful and benign; the other was essentially sadistic and autocratic. One sought harmony; the other was driven by aggression and competitiveness.

(Elder 1998: 2)

The land is everything to indigenous peoples. To frame it in biological and environmental terms is abhorrent when we speak of the land. It is a living, breathing entity. To indigenous peoples, land is not just physical and biological environment. It is the ash of their ancestors who fought to keep the land from becoming destroyed by others, the ancestors on whose shoulders we stand in this generation, whose land we must preserve for the next seven generations. The land generously gives plants, animals and a life that contributes to good health (Burden 1998).

> There used to be so many clams on the beach you only had to kick the sand to find them. You could dig them up with your toes. Now they're scarce . . . When I was a girl the sand was pearly white. Now it's covered with that green algae, from pollution, they say. The pesticides, herbicides, and fertilizers run down from the potato fields. Still it is beautiful. It is where the Creator intended us to live.
>
> (Wall and Arden 1990)

Mining, damming, roads, infrastructure planning – all are activities of industrialised societies which exploit land for the benefit of people governed by economies and profit-making.

> The most important concern is our world we live in. People all over this world are ruining the world. Even in the United States, things such as testing bombs are a wound that will never heal. A world that will never grow plants again. This world that we live in must be protected. Where will our children, grandchildren and great grandchildren live if this world is ruined?
>
> (Personal communication: Herman Toolie, Savoonga, Alaska)

In the pre-colonial days of Australia, before the coming of Europeans, penal colonies and the massacre of indigenous peoples, small groups of Aboriginal people moved across the red, parched land in search of water. These were scientific people who, through their observations and deductive reasoning, could predict rainfall by watching the patterns in the sky. By observing weather cycles and climate changes, the people understood the locations of plants and their use as foods or medicines. Depending on the amounts of rainfall, the people knew where animals would be grazing. In their seasonal activities, small groups of men hunted kangaroos and emus, while the women harvested food such as grasses, seeds, fruits, small reptiles, lizards and mammals.

Traditional foods: nutrition

'Many chronic diseases such as diabetes, hypertension, obesity, cardiovascular diseases are the result of rapid changes in lifestyle, particularly in dietary habits and physical activity levels' (Young 1994: 216).

With the loss of the land, or the restricted access to the land, indigenous peoples have lost the foundations of their traditional nutritional practice. In addition, environmental degradation has contaminated many traditional food sources, particularly cultural plants, and game to the extent that their consumption is dangerous to human health:

> Studies of traditional Aboriginal foodstuffs suggest an Indigenous diet high in protein, complex carbohydrates, fibre, vitamins and minerals and low in simple

carbohydrates (sugar) and saturated fats. Aboriginal people have adapted successfully over many millennia to this diet, which met their nutritional requirements. Changes in nutrient intakes as a result of the appropriation by settlers of rich and productive lands, and the concentration of large groups of Aboriginal people in permanent camps are implicated in the subsequent rise in the disorders usually associated with affluence, namely heart disease, diabetes and obesity.

(Horton 1994: 459–60)

A similar history of European culture collision impacted the indigenous peoples of North America. As a result, they have fared no better than the Aborigines of Australia. For the Indian people of North America the coming of the Europeans altered and changed for ever the nomadic hunting lifestyle or farming lifestyle of the indigenous peoples of the Turtle Continent. In addition, Indian removal policies of the nineteenth century and implementation of the reservation system created generations of dependants. No longer free to lead a nomadic life or engage in the hunt for traditional foods and wild game, the people became dependent on store-bought foods and government handouts of flour, bacon, beans and sugar. The combination of increased carbohydrates from flour, bacon and sugar, inactivity and decline in hunting wild game as protein led to obesity, cardiovascular problems and diabetes. These problems continue to impact the health of Native North American peoples:

The situation with obesity is particularly striking. As recently as the 1940s caloric and nutrition deficiency was a real threat in many communities; today, obesity is widespread . . . Many chronic diseases are associated with obesity such as ischemic heart disease, hypertension, diabetes, gall bladder disease, and certain cancers.

(Young 1994: 139)

The way our people learn: education

The concept of education for indigenous peoples varies markedly from that of Westernised Europeans (Cajete 1994; Groome 1998). While Western education is based on linear modes of analysis and synthesis, education in indigenous cultures is more circular and focused on observation, waiting and analysis of situations. For example, hunters observe the minute signs of the land and they know when caribou or fish will migrate; women observe the development of children and know when to implement certain strategies for child development. Storytelling constitutes a major strategy for learning among indigenous peoples. The extended family plays a critical role in education of the indigenous person. Aunts, grandmothers and female cousins teach young girls the skills they will need to be a contributing member of the group; uncles, grandfathers and other males teach the boys the skills they will need to be successful.

Research with American Indians has demonstrated that they learn best in groups and when the learning can be linked to previous knowledge and to life's work. The constructivist theory of education is a viewpoint in learning theory that holds that learners actively construct their own ways of thinking as a result of interacting with the learning experience (Molenda 1991). In the constructivist model, Indian students extrapolate from the subject that which is meaningful to their own lives and life's experience. In other words, they will 'make meaning' of their learning.

In the modern world of academic education put forth in state and public schools, acknowledgement of and teaching to indigenous learning styles and strategies can mean the difference between success and failure for the indigenous child, and for their teacher. Additionally, indigenous children are not made to 'perform' for the family group without practising and feeling confident: indigenous peoples do not make their children perform 'on the spot'. In a classroom situation, the wise teacher of indigenous children must be made aware of these cultural aspects of education (Cajete 1994).

Indigenous education may be more differentiated because it does not rely on a formal educational system to which parents and the community as a whole delegate the education of children and adolescents. Education is practised as a communal task, the responsibility of which lies with every member of the community.

Consequently, regarding health education, indigenous communities prefer approaches which encompass the whole community rather than aiming at certain 'target groups'. The Western model of analytical segregation of communities for the purpose of health education and health promotion can hardly gain support from indigenous peoples as they feel that this approach may result in 'blaming the victim' models of community organisation.

Women's business: power and medicine

> The Native American woman is not a drudge or squaw or princess, she is merely a woman defined by the roles she assumes within her culture. She is a link between the ancestors and the next seven generations. She is vulnerable, poor, and confused as to who she is because of the marginalization of her people.
>
> (Meyer 1993: 242)

Despite widely different environments and social systems, the rearing of little girls remained remarkably similar in many indigenous cultures. Indigenous parents are permissive and the bond between little girls and their mothers is strong. The overwhelming pressures of the dominant culture have produced social problems found in the non-Indian world: rape, incest, alcoholism, lack of self-esteem and loss of identity as an Indian woman.

In the past, in all tribes, women were valued for their skills. They brought forth the future nation and contributed as much as 80 per cent of the labour needed to produce the family food supply. Not only were activities such as gardening, gathering and preparing plants done by women, but butchering, storing and cooking the meat brought in by the men. Women were treasured for their roles as healers, midwives and crafters. They are the sustainers of the people (Colomeda 1996).

Traditionally, in indigenous cultures women have their own power. Some call it Moon Power, and it is a power owned only by women. In the old days, hunters were forbidden to be in the same room as a menstruating woman because female power at this time was so great. In many cultures, it was taboo for a menstruating woman to touch the weapons of hunters. Often the women were isolated in a special building until they completed their cycle. Before the arrival of the Jesuits into North America, many Indian women had their own societies and were leaders of their tribes. The Jesuits changed that way of life to be more congruent with the agrarian European model. However, in many indigenous cultures, the business of women's health, childbirth and child development activities continue to be the pursuance of women (Colomeda 1996).

Conclusion

When cultural contexts and values are not taken into account in health and develop-ment programmes, their usefulness is questionable. To locate culture within the heart of health education, promotion and providers is cultural empowerment in the best sense of the phrase (Cajete 1994; Cornelius 1999; Hill 1996). Cultural empowerment in health takes into account how health knowledge, beliefs and practice are produced and interpreted at many levels, including individual, family and community (Duran and Duran 1998; Fredericks and Schanche Hodge 1998; Koertvelyessy 1996).

> The process of empowering individuals in health education programming is often based on the assumption that individuals, primarily because of their limited economic resources, are powerless. Eurocentrists often consider silence, which makes most Westerners uncomfortable, to indicate voicelessness and weakness, failing to recognize that knowledge borne of Western economic praxis carries questionable values and biases that marginalize traditional and local knowledge.
>
> (Airhihenbuwa 1995: 27)

The local has never been only local, as our ancestors have known. It has always been embedded in much larger contexts, which needed to be respected in order to be able to live in the places for a certain period of time. Nowadays, the local is even more connected to its global neighbours via physical lines of communication, trade and tourism.

Politically and mentally, we have to understand that our very own lifeways are dependent on the lifeways of all humans dispersed on every part of the planet. No one is independent, no one is superior, and no one has more rights than others (Bretherton 1996). Mother Earth never thought of different rights for different people and species. The fundamental reality is that only equality between all of us will help to maintain material living conditions on earth in a sustainable way. Everything else contributes to annihilation (Escobar 1995).

Note

1   This chapter was first published as Colomeda, L.A. and Wenzel, E. (2000) 'Medicine keepers: issues in indigenous health', *Critical Public Health*, 10: 241–56.

References

Airhihenbuwa, C.O. (1995) *Health and Culture: Beyond the Western Paradigm*, Thousand Oaks, CA: Sage.

Bartlett, B. (1998) *Constructs of Community*, unpublished manuscript.

Bass, R. (1996) *The Book of Yaak*, Boston, MA/New York: Houghton Mifflin.

Bretherton, C. (1996) 'Universal human rights: bringing people into global politics?', in C. Bretherton and G. Ponton (eds), *Global Politics: An Introduction*, Oxford: Blackwell.

Burden, J. (1998) 'Health: an holistic approach', in C. Bourke, E. Bourke and B. Edwards (eds), *Aboriginal Australia: An Introductory Reader in Aboriginal Studies*, St Lucia: University of Queensland Press.

Cajete, G. (1994) *Look to the Mountain: An Ecology of Indigenous Education*, Durango, CO: Kivaki Press.

Colomeda, L. (1996) *Through the Northern Looking Glass: Breast Cancer Stories Told by Northern Native Women*, New York: National League for Nursing.

Colomeda, L. (1999) *Keepers of the Central Fire: Issues in Eecology for Indigenous Peoples*, New York: Jones and Bartlett/National League for Nursing.

Cook, N.D. (1998) *Born to Die: Disease and New World Conquest, 1492–1650*, Cambridge/New York: Cambridge University Press.

Cornelius, C. (1999) *Iroquois Corn in a Culture-Based Curriculum: A Framework for Respectfully Teaching about Cultures*, Albany, NY: SUNY Press.

Duran, B.M. and Duran, E.F. (1998) 'Assessment, program planning, and evaluation in Indian Country', in R.M. Huff and M.V. Kline (eds), *Promoting Health in Multicultural Populations: A Handbook for Practitioners*, Thousand Oaks, CA: Sage.

Eichstaedt, P. (1994) *If You Poison Us: Uranium and American Indians*, Santa Fé, NM: Red Crane Books.

Elder, B. (1998) *Blood on the Wattle*, Sydney: New Holland.

Escobar, A. (1995) *Encountering Development: The Making and Unmaking of the Third World*, Princeton, NJ: Princeton University Press.

Fredericks, L. and Schanche Hodge, F. (1998) 'Traditional approaches to health care among American Indians and Alaska Natives', in R.M. Huff and M.V. Kline (eds), *Promoting Health in Multicultural Populations: A Handbook for Practitioners*, Thousand Oaks, CA: Sage.

Freidson, E. (1970) *Profession of Medicine*, New York: Dodd, Mead and Co.

Gostin, O. and Chong, A. (1998) 'Living wisdom: Aborigines and the environment', in C. Bourke, E. Bourke and B. Edwards (eds), *Aboriginal Australia: An Introductory Reader in Aboriginal Studies*, St. Lucia: University of Queensland Press.

Goudie, A. (1997) *The Human Impact Reader: Readings and Case Studies*, Oxford: Blackwell.

Gray, A. (1991) 'The impact of biodiversity conservation on indigenous peoples', in V. Shiva, P. Anderson, H. Schucking and A. Gray (eds), *Biodiversity: Social and Ecological Perspectives*, London: Zed Books.

Grinde, D.A. and Johansen, B.E. (1995) *Ecocide in Native America: Environmental Destruction of Indian Lands and People*, Santa Fé, NM: Clear Light.

Groome, H. (1998) 'Education: the search for relevance', in C. Bourke, E. Bourke and B. Edwards (eds), *Aboriginal Australia: An Introductory Reader in Aboriginal Studies*, St Lucia: University of Queensland Press.

Hill, H. (1996) *Shaking the Rattle: Healing the Trauma of Colonization*, Victoria, BC: Orca Books.

Hodgkenson, H. (1990) *The Demographics of American Indians: One Percent of the People, Fifty Percent of the Diversity*, Washington, DC: Center for Demography Policy.

Horton, D. (1994) *The Encyclopaedia of Aboriginal Australia: Aboriginal and Torres Strait Islander History, Society and Culture*, Canberra: Aboriginal Studies Press.

Human Rights and Equal Opportunity Commission (1997) *Bringing Them Home: National Inquiry into the Separation of Aboriginal and Torres Strait Islander Children from Their Families*, Canberra: Commonwealth of Australia.

Indian Health Service (1997) *Trends in Indian Health 1997*, Washington, DC: US Department of Health and Human Services, Indian Health Service.

Joe, J.R. and Young, R.S. (1994) *Diabetes as a disease of Civilization: The Impact of Culture Change on Indigenous Peoples*, Berlin/New York: Mouton de Gruyter.

Kelm, M.E. (1998) *Colonizing Bodies: Aboriginal Health and Healing in British Columbia, 1900–50*, Vancouver: University of British Columbia Press.

Koertvelyessy, A.M. (1996) *Native American Voices: Native American Health Educators Speak out*, New York: National League of Nursing.

Kuletz, V.L. (1998) *The Tainted Desert: Environmental and Social Ruin in the American West*, London/New York: Routledge.

Kunitz, S.J. (1996) *Disease and Social Diversity: The European Impact on the Health of Non-Europeans*, New York: Oxford University Press.

Lacey, L. (1993) *Micmac Medicines: Remedies and Recollections*, Halifax, NS: Nimbus Publications. See also: <http://www.nativeweb.org/NativeTech/lacey/index.html>.

Long, D. and Dickason, O.P. (1999) *Visions of the Heart: Aboriginal Issues in Canada*, Toronto: Harcourt Brace.

Lyon, W.S. (1998) *Encyclopedia of Native American Shamanism: Sacred Ceremonies of Northern America*, Santa Barbara, CA: ABC-CLIO.

Mamiwinini, W.C. (1991) Available at: <http://www.ilhawaii.net/~stony/quotes.html>.

McElroy, A. and Townsend, P.K. (1996) *Medical Anthropology in Ecological Perspective*, 3rd edn, Boulder, CO: Westview Press.

Meyer, J. (1993) 'Native American women's health', *American Indian Literary Quarterly*, 1(4): 241–2.

Molenda, M. (1991) 'A philosophical critique of the claims of constructivism', *Educational Technology*, September: 44–8.

Ramenofsky, A.F. (1987) *Vectors of Death: The Archeology of European Contact*, Albuquerque: University of New Mexico Press.

Reid, J. and Trompf, P. (1991) *The Health of Aboriginal Australia*, Sydney: Harcourt Brace.

Robinson, G. (1996) *Aboriginal Health: Social and Cultural Transitions: Proceedings of a Conference at the Northern Territory University, Darwin, 29–30 September 1995*, Darwin: NTU Press.

Romanyshyn, R.D. and Whalen, B.J. (1987) 'Depression and the American dream: the struggle with home', in D.M. Levin (ed.), *Pathologies of the Modern Self: Postmodern Studies in Narcissism, Schizophrenia, and Depression*, New York: New York University Press.

Saggers, S. and Gray, D. (1998) *Dealing with Alcohol: Indigenous Usage in Australia, New Zealand and Canada*, Cambridge: Cambridge University Press.

Sandefur, G.D., Rindfuss, R.R. and Cohen, B. (1996) *Changing Numbers, Changing Needs: American Indian Demography and Public Health*, Washington, DC: National Academy Press.

Shephard, R.J. and Rode, A. (1996) *The Health Consequences of 'Modernization': Evidence from Circumpolar Peoples*, Cambridge: Cambridge University Press.

Spector, R.E. (1996) *Cultural Diversity in Health and Illness*, Stamford, CT: Appleton and Lange.

Stephenson, P.H. (1995) *A Persistent Spirit: Towards Understanding Aboriginal Health in British Columbia*, Victoria, BC: University of Victoria Department of Geography.

Vogel, V.J. (1970) *American Indian Medicine*, Norman, OK/London: University of Oklahoma Press.

Waldram, J.B., Herring, A. and Young, T.K. (1995) *Aboriginal Health in Canada: Historical, Cultural, and Epidemiological Perspectives*, Toronto: University of Toronto Press.

Wall, S. and Arden, H. (1990) *Wisdomkeepers: Conversations with Women Elders of Native America*, Hillsborough, OR: Beyond Words Press.

Weatherford, J. (1988) *Indian Givers: How the Indians of America Transformed the World*, New York: Fawcett Books.

Wenzel, E. (1997) 'Environment, development and health: ideological metaphors of post-traditional societies?', *Health Education Research*, 12: 403–18.

WHO (1946) *Constitution of the World Health Organization* (amended May 1998), Geneva: WHO.

World Council of Indigenous Peoples (1977) Available at: <http://www.halcyon.com/pub/FWDP/International/intconv.txt>.

Young, E. (1995) *Third World in the First: Development and Indigenous Peoples*, London/New York: Routledge.

Young, T.K. (1994) *The Health of Native Americans*, New York: Oxford University Press.

12 The politics of female genital cutting in displaced communities[1]

Pascale Allotey, Lenore Manderson and Sonia Grover

Introduction

Over the past decade, national and international programmes, including those of multilateral agencies such as the World Health Organization (WHO) and non-government organisations, have expanded their operational interests in women's health to include violence against women. As defined at the Fourth World Conference on Women (Koch and Basu 1996), the term refers to 'any act of gender-based violence that results in, or is likely to result in, physical, sexual or psychological harm or suffering to women, including threats of such acts, coercion or arbitrary deprivation of liberty, whether occurring in public or private life'. Such acts may occur within the family or household, within the community, or as perpetrated or condoned by the state. Acts specified as occurring in the household include battering, sexual abuse of children, dowry-related violence, marital rape, non-spousal violence and violence related to exploitation, and 'traditional practices harmful to women'. This latter category refers to a range of practices, one of which is female genital mutilation.[2] As this chapter argues, this issue raised important concerns about how rights action can inadvertently jeopardise the rights of some communities, and cause further stereotyping, stigmatisation and marginalisation.

The international context

The debates on female genital cutting (excision, clitoridectomy and infibulation), performed predominantly for cultural reasons, are highly emotive. Typical descriptions have involved the use of expressions such as 'barbaric', 'atrocious' procedures, and 'terrible violations against all humanity, kindness, respect and love' (Harding and Thomas 1994; Sheldon and Wilkinson 1998). The strength of this sentiment has resulted in the labelling of the procedures as female genital mutilation. However, in recognition of the implied judgement and insensitivity towards women who have undergone the procedure, 'cutting' rather than 'mutilation' has increasingly been adopted as the accepted term in international documents.[3]

International programmes seeking to eliminate these procedures take as their starting point agreements under the auspices of organisations within the United Nations (UN) and other international agencies. In 1982, a Human Rights Subcommittee of the WHO assured governments of its readiness, with UNICEF (United Nations Children's Fund), to support national efforts against FGM; this was followed by further statements by the WHO in 1986, the IPPF (International Planned Parenthood Federation), and other non-government organisations (WHO 1997). The Convention on the Rights of the Child (1989: article 24 section 3), in referring to 'traditional practices prejudicial to the health of children', sets precedence for the language used in conventions and statements (UNICEF 1990). The UN Declaration on Violence against Women includes specific reference to FGM (WHO 1998), and most countries have ratified this convention.

In general the result has been more open discussion of the effects of the procedure. A number of countries where female genital cutting is practised have introduced legislation making the practice illegal (for example, Sudan and Ghana; Gruenbaum 1991). Where eradication is not legislated or is legislated but not enforced, as in Egypt, for example, there is some evidence of increased empowerment of women and men who object to the practice (Leonard 1996; Green 1999; Jones *et al.* 1999).

The other result of international efforts to eradicate female genital cutting has been an increasing interest by Western rights activists, health practitioners and governments at all levels to introduce programmes within their own non-practising countries. This interest is fuelled by current migration patterns, which have brought the issues to Australia, North America and a number of countries in Western Europe. Where the practice affects immigrant populations, the approach taken has been to protect girls from practising communities through legislation within the country.

The United Kingdom perhaps has the longest history of exposure to migrant groups from countries where female genital cutting is practised. Female circumcision in the UK is illegal under the Prohibition of Female Circumcision Act (1985) (Sheldon and Wilkinson 1998). In France, female genital cutting is covered by Article 312 of the Penal Code, related to 'grievous bodily harm to a minor under 15' (Gallard 1995). In Canada, the Criminal Code was interpreted to apply to female genital cutting in 1992 (without specifying age), with a specific amendment passed in 1993 to include any traditional practices that cause bodily harm to a Canadian citizen in another country. This allowed prosecution where a child was sent overseas for the procedure and was then brought back to Canada (Hussein 1995). Legislation exists also in Sweden, Belgium and some US states, most of which is worded to cover adult women and minors (Jones *et al.* 1997).

Measures to prevent FGM in Australia

Records from the Australian Bureau of Statistics (ABS 1996) indicate that approximately 87,000 women and girls living in Australia are from countries where some form of genital cutting is practised, including Ethiopia, Somalia, Eritrea, Sudan, Egypt and Nigeria (Olenick 1998). While women from these communities do not comprise a large proportion of the total number of immigrants to Australia, the numbers are not insubstantial. They have also tended to settle in specific geographic locations and so are visible by virtue of their spatial concentration and use of particular health services.

The Australian parliament and both federal and state health services were relatively late compared with North American and European countries to develop and implement policies specific to female genital cutting. In Australia, it is identified as a harmful practice that impinges on the rights and freedom of women. Under the Australian Legal Code, it is an offence to have the surgery performed in Australia or to arrange for the procedure to be performed on a child outside Australian jurisdiction (Australia Family Law Council 1994). In 1995, federal and state governments funded a national programme on FGM (Australian Department of Health and Aged Care 1995; Legislative Council 1998). The aim of the programme is to eliminate the practice of female genital cutting and to assist women and girls who have undergone the procedure through a two-part strategy. The first is the enforcement of the specific legislation banning the practice, and the second is a health-promotion strategy to raise awareness of its harmful effects, while enhancing community development and community education (Australian Department of Health and Aged Care 1997).

Legislation

Crimes Acts in most states in Australia have been amended to make provision for female genital cutting. In Victoria, for example, a person who performs the procedure on a child or adult is guilty of the offence punishable by a fifteen-year imprisonment term. A similar penalty is imposed on a person who takes a child from the state with the intention of having the procedure performed (Legislative Council 1998). The Act also states, 'It is not a defence to a charge . . . to prove that the person on whom the act which is the subject of the charge was performed, or the parents or guardian of that person, consented to the performance of that act' (Legislative Council 1998: 28). The exceptions to the offence are if the procedure is necessary to the health of the person and performed by a medical practitioner; necessary during labour and birth to relieve symptoms associated with labour and performed by a medical practitioner or midwife; or is a sexual reassignment procedure performed by a medical practitioner (Legislative Council 1998). The determination of the necessity of the operation is based on issues relevant to the medical welfare or the relief of physical symptoms of the person (Legislative Council 1998). The implications will be discussed later in the chapter.

Health promotion

The aims of the national programme on FGM were to prevent the occurrence of female genital cutting in Australia, and to promote the development of a consistent holistic health approach to facilitate support and access to health services for women and girls affected by or at risk of the practice (Australian Department of Health and Aged Care 1995; RACOG 1997a and b). The national goals remain the same across states and relate to all women who have had or might be subject to circumcision or associated procedures, including therefore women from much of Africa and most of the Islamic world,[4] including Indonesia and Malaysia. The programme also recognises women's rights as health consumers to be treated with dignity, in an environment which provides for privacy, informed consent and confidentiality (Australian Department of Health and Aged Care 1995). The programme focuses on those women who have traditionally been subject to the most extreme forms of the procedure and in practice most women involved in the programme, or who are the targets of legislation and interventions, are from the Horn of Africa countries of Eritrea, Somalia and Ethiopia, or from Sudan or Nigeria. In addition, the emphasis is on female genital cutting rather than the broader issues of health rights.

The operating framework for the programme involves several activities, ranging from education and community development/health promotion to the use of community-based bicultural workers trained by the health services to conduct education sessions on topics identified through consultation with the communities or by the health services and the use of interpreters trained in issues relating to female genital cutting with emphasis on confidentiality and sensitivity, acknowledging their own attitudes towards female genital cutting (Australian Department of Health and Aged Care 1997). To support the programme, the federal government also provided funding to the Royal Australian College of Obstetricians and Gynaecologists (RACOG) to develop medical resources to assist health professionals to give appropriate care to women and girls who have undergone female genital cutting.

Different specific approaches have been taken by the various states. In New South Wales, there is greater emphasis on education, targeted at both the specific communities and at the general public, with the aim of protecting girls who may be at risk from undergoing the procedure (Nkrumah 1995). Programmes in Queensland, South Australia and Western Australia have a stronger focus on health services, educating providers on the care of women who have undergone the procedure. The Victorian programme has the community as its primary focus in order to contextualise activities within the broader reproductive health issues of women in the community. This approach appears to be the most acceptable to the community (Nkrumah 1999).

Policy to practice: effects on community in Victoria

The strategy has had important implications for various aspects of the lives of women from the target communities. Although the national FGM programme in Australia presumes to represent the rights and interests of women who have undergone female genital cutting (Family Law Council 1994), there have been problems in its implementation that have raised concerns in the target communities over media coverage of female genital cutting, genital surgery in adult women and perceptions of racism. These are discussed *seriatim*, based upon findings from a study on the reproductive health needs of migrant women from Sahel Africa and the Middle East resident in Victoria (Manderson and Allotey 2003a and b).

Media coverage

The passing of legislation in 1994 and the launch of the programme in 1995 occurred around the same time as a series of graphic documentaries on commercial television, including 'The cruellest cut', a *60 Minutes* interview of Somali fashion model Aman, who had undergone the procedure and was campaigning against it. This broadcast was followed closely by her visit to Australia, demonstrating her commitment to the international eradication of the practice. National public radio also carried news of the Australian government's response with the opportunity for the public to provide feedback. Ideas about genital cutting, including excision and infibulation, for most Australians derive from these sources (Nkrumah 1995) and from popular paperback books sold in newsagents' and bookstores. These events emphasised the commitment to open debate and the desire to curtail the suffering of women who were seemingly powerless to protect themselves. However, there were some adverse consequences within the community.

One of these adverse effects is a perception by the target community that health professionals and the general public assume that all black African women are excised or infibulated. Women from Horn of Africa communities complained about the open discussion of their 'private parts', with total disregard for cultural sensitivities or notions of privacy. Programmes in some states produced and/or promoted graphic educational materials (Nkrumah 1999) that reduced women from affected communities to describing themselves as 'walking around with their vulval status on their foreheads' (interview 1999). One woman reported that she had consulted her general practitioner about upper respiratory symptoms and became distressed when, in taking her history, he wanted to know which type of genital cutting she had undergone. These reports are consistent with other studies. Horowitz and Jackson (1997), for instance, refer to women's discomfort in physicians' interest in their genital status. They note, too, that clinicians' views and attitudes were influenced by perceptions of female genital cutting as 'barbaric' and 'primitive', and that these views were implicit in clinical settings such that women felt that they did not get optimal healthcare.

Genital surgery in adult women

Data from our research demonstrate that there is a high degree of understanding and acceptance of the legislation against female genital cutting in young girls. A few women expressed concern that uncircumcised girls would lose an important aspect of their cultural heritage, would have 'ugly' and 'unclean' genitalia, and would not be protected from external pressures (i.e., safe from rape). However, it is clear to them that the practice is illegal in Australia and that it would be near impossible to find a practitioner to perform the surgery on a child without clear medical indications.

Major concerns associated with procedures and regulations around genital cutting involve de-infibulation, usually before marriage or childbirth, and re-suturing or re-infibulation following childbirth, all procedures for consenting adult women.

De-infibulation before marriage is offered to young women and this reduces possible trauma at first intercourse. Problems that have arisen from this are based on lack of information from family and other women within the community of what to expect following the de-infibulation procedure. Women report an increase in vaginal discharge because of a larger vaginal opening that they had not experienced prior to de-infibulation. They also report acute embarrassment from the sound of urine in a toilet bowl, an unfamiliar experience prior to de-infibulation, when micturition occurs much more slowly (focus group 1999). These changes often make it difficult for women to differentiate what is normal or requires medical attention. However, de-infibulation prior to marriage is usually elective, and as long as health professionals provide the necessary counselling and follow-up, women have been reasonably satisfied with the procedure.

When de-infibulation is performed prior to childbirth to assist the birth process, however, more problems have arisen. Several women have expressed a preference for re-suturing to what they perceive as their normal state prior to de-infibulation. Women speak of their desire to be re-infibulated after childbirth in the context of feeling embarrassed about being exposed (having an 'open hole' or 'gaping'). This is supported by researchers who have also argued that the most compelling rationale for the endurance of the practice of female genital cutting in some cultures is that it has been practised for so long that reduced or infibulated genitals are simply considered normal (Lane and Rubinstein 1996). Under RACOG guidelines, however, re-suturing to the infibulated state should be discouraged by health professionals (RACOG 1997b). Little is known of the outcomes for women who have been de-infibulated in terms of their satisfaction with the procedure, their ability to accommodate bodily changes, the psychological and social effects of the bodily change, or the impact of de-infibulation on sexual pleasure. In addition, the vaginal opening and other vulval tissue are highly sensitive after de-infibulation, causing some women distress. It is also not clear, for women who have not experienced any genital cutting-related complications, whether being de-infibulated has any health benefits.[5] At the same time, women are not unanimous in their views, and the primary point of contention is not surgery performed on children, but the right of women already infibulated to be re-infibulated after childbirth.

Institutionalised racism

Following from the above example of the issue of re-infibulation, for some women, the reluctance of medical practitioners to re-suture is perceived by immigrant women as institutionalised racism within the health services and the application of double standards in the interpretation of the legislation related to female genital cutting. Women in our study cited clitoral piercing as an example of a practice that was not considered illegal. They also referred to other procedures performed on the genitals of white Australian women that could similarly be considered cultural or 'not really medical'.

In order to explore these claims further and to contextualise de-infibulation and requests for re-infibulation, we reviewed a sample of labioplasties performed in a hospital in Victoria. Labioplasty (plastic surgery on the labia) was chosen because this is the administrative classification for de-infibulation and is therefore considered an equivalent procedure. Medical labioplasties may be performed for women who have vulval cancer, pre-cancerous skin changes, vestibulitis, revision of episiotomy scars, and lesions as a result of fistulae. Over a five-year period (1994–8), a total of 165 procedures coded as labioplasty were reviewed, 108 of which were associated with an underlying medical condition. These 108 cases were excluded. Of the further fifty-seven, forty-four were performed on women from African countries and represented de-infibulation. The remaining thirteen cases with no associated medical pathology were classified as 'vulval deformity', 'labial reduction' and 'reduction labioplasty'. The age range of the women undergoing these procedures was sixteen–forty-nine years. Although very little information was presented in the case notes, descriptions of symptoms included 'discomfort in jeans' and 'asymmetry of labia'. There was no documented evidence of specific complications or problems arising as a consequence of the stated labial shape or size. Thus, most of these procedures can be described as cosmetic. It is worth noting that these data are from a public hospital and that most cosmetic surgery is performed in private hospitals. The numbers presented here are therefore an underestimation of women undergoing surgery to change the appearance of their genitals.

Cosmetic surgery is plastic surgery with the primary aim of changing the appearance of the client, when the procedures are not performed to have an impact on the functional or physical health of the patient. Arguments for cosmetic labio-plasties – like those for breast augmentation and reduction, rhinoplasties and related surgery, for instance – typically appeal primarily to the importance of belonging, self-perception, taking control of one's life, and (in this case) making the genitals aesthetic (Hodgkinson and Hait 1983; Davis 1991). The pressure to conform has been described as mainly indirect, based on the need to belong to a social group with deep-rooted internalised social expectations (Slack 1988). Similar arguments could be made by adult women (as opposed to children) who undergo female genital cutting and certainly by those who request re-stitching following childbirth.

On the basis of the hospital data, the perception by women from the Horn of Africa of double standards is somewhat justified. Sheldon and Wilkinson (1998) and Kerin (1998) comment on the peculiar lack of critical reflection in arguments of Western writers who condemn female genital cutting while failing to consider the implications of local cultural practices such as cosmetic surgery and tattooing. While the absolute number of cosmetically related labial operations presented here is low, these are only a proportion of similar operations performed in both public and private hospitals in Australia. Logically, the operations are merely an extension of other procedures designed either to draw attention to female genitals (as is the case with genital jewellery, and hence rings for labia and clitoral hoods) or to render invisible signs of secondary sexual development, of which the laser removal of pubic hair is the most prevalent example. In this context, the 'trimming' of visible labia minora for young women or for adult women who feel that their labial have become less 'ladylike' with childbearing is part of a continuum. While labia reduction is not a well-known procedure, hair removal products and procedures are common.

Further, while genital piercing is not as accessible as ear, nose, eyebrow and navel piercing, there are plenty of tattoo and piercing parlours throughout Melbourne that advertise regularly in conventional and free newspapers.

Given that labial cosmetic surgery continues to be performed despite the legislation, one could interpret re-infibulation as falling under the exceptions in the legislation: it is necessary to the health of the person and is performed by a medical practitioner. A further argument supporting the perception of different rules is that while there has been some concern about the proliferation of practitioners offering various forms of cosmetic surgery, there has never been any suggestion that women who seek cosmetic surgery need to be protected from themselves through legislation (Sheldon and Wilkinson 1998). However, in the law that governs female genital cutting, women's vulnerability to 'culture' is seen as sufficient reason to invoke and act upon legislation. There is the assumption that adult African migrant women lack agency, and are particularly vulnerable to social and familial pressures, and to authoritative, patriarchal belief systems (Hayes 1975).

Conclusion

It is inevitable that an attempt to eradicate a cultural practice that in one society plays a role in defining femininity and womanhood and in another is considered barbaric and atrocious would not be easy. Some change has been achieved in countries where the practice is traditional, and the process has been empowering for women under those circumstances. Conversely, in countries such as Australia, where practising communities are a visible minority, the process has been disempowering. While this paper does not seek to present arguments in favour of female genital cutting, it does seek to highlight the inconsistencies in approaches to health services for different ethnic groups within Australia and possibly in other developed countries seeking to represent the rights of women who are perceived, due to their cultural backgrounds, as unable to represent themselves.

The use of multiple approaches to address the government's position on the practice is in theory an effective technique in health promotion. However, legislation, policy and practice undoubtedly occur within the context of the dominant culture and there is a real risk of marginalising minority ethnic groups. The Australian Legislative Council explicitly stated on 21 February 1994: 'Migrant settlement is a process of give and take. If Australia finds a certain folk custom repulsive, a migrant has the duty to give this custom away. This is the price to pay for our common good' (cited in Fraser 1995: 351).

Ethicists such as Sheldon (Sheldon and Wilkinson 1998), however, argue the importance for interventions such as this legislation, which limit individuals' freedom, to be justified and applied fairly across cultures. While well meaning, the legislation does appear specifically to target the culture, leaving open the possibility of a racially discriminatory interpretation.

The indirect costs to immigrant African women's health have been reports of discrimination within the health services, women's reluctance to present for antenatal care, non-use of gynaecological services and lack of treatment for urinary and reproductive tract infections (Maggi 1995). This is unfortunately borne out in the many case histories that have been collected for the current ongoing research project with African communities (Manderson and Allotey 2003a and b).

Acknowledgements

The authors would like to acknowledge the work of Samia Baho and Lourice Demian in the collection of data from women within the community, the community advisory group of the project, and, in particular, Mmaskepe Sejoe for many stimulating discussions.

Notes

1   This chapter was first published as Allotey, P., Manderson, L. and Grover, S. (2001) 'The politics of female genital surgery in displaced communities', *Critical Public Health*, 11: 189–201.
2   Female genital mutilation, or its acronym FGM, is used in the paper when referring to instrumentality but otherwise we use the term 'cutting' rather than 'mutilation' to avoid the value judgement implicit in the use of the latter term.
3   See: <http://www.un.org/popin/unfpa/dispatches/mar96.html>.
4   The prevalence of FGM has been associated with Islam, and although many Muslims in practising countries believed that genital modification in women was required by their faith, it is now clear that this is not the case (CSAAMA 1995; Olenick 1998).
5   There is a general presumption that female genital cutting of various types has a heavy morbidity rate and contributes substantially to female mortality, and that the procedures dramatically inhibit female sexual response. However, Obermeyer (1999: 92–4) draws attention to the poor epidemiology from which extrapolations are made. Published studies show surprisingly low rates of complications (Knight *et al.* 1999) and the few studies undertaken that enquire about sexual pleasure and response suggest less damage to physiological (as well as psychological) response than might be expected (Obermeyer 1999: 94–6).

References

ABS (1996) *Basic Community Profile Series*, Report No. Catalogue 2020.2, Canberra: Australian Bureau of Statistics.

Australia Family Law Council (1994) *Female Genital Mutilation: A Report to the Attorney General*, Barton, ACT: Council of Family Law.

Australian Department of Health and Aged Care (1995) *National Education Program on Female Genital Mutilation*, Australia: Australian Department of Health and Aged Care.

—— (1997) *Operating Framework for the National Education Program on Female Genital Mutilation*, Australia: Australian Department of Health and Aged Care, Population Health Division.

Council on Scientific Affairs, American Medical Association (CSAAMA) (1995) 'Female genital mutilation', *Journal of the American Medical Association*, 274: 1714–16.

Davis, K. (1991) 'Remaking the she-devil: a critical look at feminist approaches to beauty', *Hypatia*, 6: 21–43.

Family Law Council (1994) *Female Genital Mutilation: A Report to the Attorney General Prepared by the Family Law Council*, Canberra: Commonwealth of Australia.

Fraser, D. (1995) 'The first cut is (not) the deepest: deconstructing female genital mutilation and the criminalization of the other', *Dalhousie Law Journal*, 2: 310–79.

Gallard, C. (1995) 'Female genital mutilation in France', *British Medical Journal*, 310: 1592–3.

Green, D. (1999) *Gender Violence in Africa: African Women's Responses*, New York: St Martin's Press.

Gruenbaum, E. (1991) 'The Islamic movement, development and health sector education: recent changes in the health of rural women in central Sudan', *Social Science and Medicine*, 33: 637–45.

Harding, R. and Thomas, T. (1994) 'Cruel cuts', *Bulletin*, 116: 38.

Hayes, R. (1975) 'Female genital mutilation, fertility control, women's roles and the patrilineage in modern Sudan: a functional analysis', *American Ethnologist*, 2: 617–633.

Hodgkinson, D. and Hait, G. (1983) 'Aesthetic vaginal labioplasty', *Plastic and Reconstructive Surgery*, 74: 414–16.

Horowitz, C.R. and Jackson, J.C. (1997) 'Female "circumcision": African women confront American medicine', *Journal of General Internal Medicine*, 12: 491–9.

Hussein, L. (1995) *Report on the Ottawa Consultations on Female Genital Mutilation Held for Representatives of the Somali Community*, Ottawa: Canada Department of Justice.

Jones, H., Diop, N., Askew, I. and Kabore, I. (1999) 'Female genital cutting practices in Burkina Faso and Mali and their negative health outcomes', *Studies in Family Planning*, 30: 219–30.

Jones, W.K., Smith, J., Kieke, B. Jr. and Wilcox, L. (1997) 'Female genital mutilation/ female circumcision: who is at risk in the United States?', *Public Health Reports*, 112: 368–77.

Kerin, J. (1998) 'Double standards: principled or arbitrary', *Bioethics*, 12: iii–vii.

Knight, R., Hotchin, A., Bayly, C. and Grover, S. (1999) 'Female genital mutilation: experience of the Royal Women's Hospital, Melbourne', *Australia and New Zealand Journal of Obstetrics and Gynaecology*, 39: 50–4.

Koch, S.J. and Basu L. (1996) 'Beyond Beijing – the UN Fourth World Conference on Women: implications for health education practitioners', *Journal of Health Education*, 27: 187–9.

Lane, S.D. and Rubinstein, R.A. (1996) 'Judging the other: responding to traditional female genital surgeries', *Hastings Center Report*, 26: 31–40.

Legislative Council and the Legislative Assembly of Victoria (1998) *Crimes Act, 1958*, Act of Parliament, Report No./Act No. 6231/1958, Melbourne: Legislative Council and the Legislative Assembly of Victoria (last amended, 1 July 1998).

Leonard, L. (1996) 'Female circumcision in southern Chad: origins, meaning and current practice', *Social Science and Medicine*, 43: 255–63.

Maggi, A. (1995) *Beyond the Tradition: Female Genital Circumcision: Responding to the Health Needs of Women*, unpublished report, Melbourne: Northern Women's Health Service.

Manderson, L. and Allotey, P. (2003a) 'Story telling, marginality and community in Australia: how immigrants position their differences in health care settings', *Medical Anthropology*, 22: 1–21.

—— (2003b) 'The cultural politics of competence in Australian health services', *Anthropology in Medicine*, 10: 70–85.

Nkrumah, J. (1995) 'Breaking the silence', *Infocus*, 18: 17.

—— (1999) 'Unuttered screams: the psychological effects of female genital mutilation', in B. Ferguson and E. Pittaway (eds), *Nobody Wants to Talk About It – Refugee Women's Mental Health*, Sydney: Transcultural Mental Health Centre.

Obermeyer, C. (1999) 'Female genital surgeries: the known, the unknown and the unknowable', *Medical Anthropology Quarterly*, 13: 79–106.

Olenick, I. (1998) 'Female circumcision is nearly universal in Egypt, Eritrea, Mali and Sudan', *International Family Planning Perspectives*, 24: 47–9.

RACOG (1997a) *Female Genital Mutilation: A Pamphlet for Health Professionals*, East Melbourne: Royal Australian College of Obstetricians and Gynaecologists.

—— (1997b) *Female Genital Mutilation: Information for Australian Health Professionals*, East Melbourne: Royal Australian College of Obstetricians and Gynaecologists.

Sheldon, S. and Wilkinson, S. (1998) 'Female genital mutilation and cosmetic surgery: regulating non-therapeutic body modification', *Bioethics*, 12: 263–85.

Slack, A. (1988) 'Female circumcision: a critical appraisal', *Human Rights Quarterly*, 10: 437–86.

UNICEF (1990) *First Call for Children: World Declaration and Plan of Action from the World Summit for Children: Convention on the Rights of the Child*, New York: United Nations Children's Fund.

WHO (1997) *Female Genital Mutilation: A Joint WHO/UNICEF/UNFPA Statement*, Geneva: WHO.

—— (1998) 'A priority health issue (physical, psychological and sexual violence on women)', *World Health*, 51: 15.

Part IV

Edgy spaces: technology, the environment and public health

Introduction

Judith Green

Since the mid-twentieth century John Snow, the nineteenth-century anaesthetist and pioneer of epidemiology, has been an iconic figure in the history that public health tells of its own origins (Vandenbroucke *et al.* 1991). Indeed, Snow has been a remarkably adaptable icon, and the story of how he solved the mystery of the Broad Street cholera epidemic, and advised removal of the handle from the offending local water pump, has been a fertile one for illustrating some of public health's core values. Snow's early use of statistical mapping to uncover the cause of cholera outbreaks (Snow 1855), and his activism in stopping the disease at source have been utilised to symbolise the dual role of public health practitioners as simultaneously rational scientists and passionate advocates for health. Like the modern speciality of public health, Snow was at once an establishment insider, as an anaesthetist to Queen Victoria, and an outsider, with his unorthodox (but ultimately legitimated) views of water-borne cholera transmission.

Such stories, as Nancy Krieger (1992) has noted, are of course to a large extent self-serving historiography. They are told to justify the present, and seek antecedents that fit with contemporary preoccupations. The story of Snow's empiricism in uncovering the environmental cause of disease certainly risks presenting the 'truth' as the triumph of progressive science, rather than as contingent, and subject to the social and political determinants of shifts in scientific understanding. However, Snow-as-metaphor has been so serviceable for public health, we might be forgiven perhaps for utilising the elements of the story yet again for exploring some recurring themes in the relationships between environments, technologies and public health.

First, the story of the pump handle illustrates some of the difficulties public health has with regard to the broader environmental determinants of health. Like the contaminated water feeding the Broad Street pump, the causes of ill-health are beyond the direct control of health services. They arise from the material and social environments in which people live, and their amelioration lies largely outside the jurisdiction of health professionals, who have little control over housing, water or air quality. The account of Snow's actions marks not medicine's belated *recognition* of these environmental influences on health, but rather the beginning of legitimacy for medicine's intervention in, and later colonisation of, them. In early nineteenth-century Britain, the sanitary reform movement that led to the 1848 Public Health

Act was not a medical one, but arose from the campaigning of reformers such as Edwin Chadwick around inadequate housing, drainage and foul air.

What justified the professionalisation of such concerns as specifically 'medical' was the science, as public health adopted epidemiology to provide the esoteric base of its particular medical contribution. Of all the continuities and discontinuities that mark the history of public health, it is perhaps the special claim to the uniqueness of its 'scientific' contribution that has endured the most: this is what distinguishes Public Health as a professional specialty from the myriad activities that constitute public health as practice. Public health as practice is everybody's business, from contributing local taxes to maintain sewers to controlling infections in the household and workplace. The professionalisation of Public Health, and its location within the medical academy rather than (or as well as) within local government, relies on the continued profession of a specialised knowledge base. The technologies of public health (the statistical techniques of epidemiology, methods for establishing cost effectiveness, the development of systematic literature reviewing and meta-analysis) have become ever more rationalised and elaborate.

One resulting tension that persists through the history of public health is that of what to do with lay knowledge. This is vital as a contributor to an understanding of what keeps communities healthy, but also, it seems, vital (at least discursively) as a foil for expert knowledge. Snow's analysis, for instance, was essentially inductive detective work. He identified cholera cases in outlying districts, and discovered that these people were ex-residents of the locality so fond of the Broad Street water that they had it transported in bottles. He discovered that local brewery workers unaffected by cholera were drinking beer, not water. These methods could be framed as demonstrating the virtues of lay epidemiology, and the necessity of respect for local knowledge about environmental hazards, rather than the beginnings of a rigorous epidemiology based on hypothesis testing. The people's knowledge is valorised, but also suspect, being located in the specifics of political and social spaces of individual communities, whereas epidemiological knowledge can present itself as somehow neutral and beyond ideology. In contemporary public health practice, these problematic gaps (between the social and environmental causes of disease and the reach of health services; between public health as medical speciality and as 'everybody's business'; between the profession of special, scientific expertise and the valorisation of public knowledge) persist. They are particularly evident when public health confronts hazardous environments: those spaces and technologies which generate risks for the public health.

It is, for instance, around environmental concerns over industrial technologies, such as the toxic contamination of housing at Love Canal in New York (Levine 1982), or industrial air pollution in the north of England (Phillimore and Moffatt 1994), that clashes between lay epidemiology and expert knowledges are often at their most acute. As Phil Brown (1992: 268) notes, 'community activists repeatedly differ with scientists and government officials on matters of problem definition, study design, interpretation of findings and policy applications'. Drawing on a case study of how families in Woburn, Massachusetts, attempted to identify whether industrial toxins in their water supply were causing a local leukaemia cluster,

Brown coined the term 'popular epidemiology' to delineate the logics of community action around health. In the activism of communities affected by environmental hazards he saw a broader approach than that of traditional epidemiology, one that recognised structural factors in disease causation, and was orientated towards action as well as explanation, using judicial and political solutions as needed. Brown suggested that the challenges these new social movements present to traditional epidemiology may be more easily accepted as interest in environmental degradation grows. In recent years, there has been a growing concern with the environment, and the interrelationships between human action, the environment and social justice have indeed moved on to the mainstream public health agenda.

What is meant by 'the environment' has, though, shifted considerably over time in public health discourse. To some extent this reflects the changing risks that environmental epidemiologists identify in different stages of development, from those arising essentially from the household in the least affluent countries, to community-based exposures (such as urban air pollution) in middle-income countries, to the global environmental risks that are generated largely by affluent counties, but imposed on the least affluent (Smith and Ezzati 2005). The salience of the environment to the public health agenda in general has also waxed and waned. Anthony Kessel (2006) has argued that the 'environment' was at its peak in the early nineteenth century, with first the recognition that the overcrowded urban environments resulting from the rapid industrialisation of Europe were creating poor health and then, by the end of the century, with the identification of specific toxins, linked to specific outcomes. With the growing relative importance of non-communicable disease in the early twentieth century, the environment, and indeed public health itself, waned in terms of its influence. The emergence of the new public health may have been tied to a renewed acknowledgement of the role of both social and material environments but, in affluent societies, the key questions of health were those of inequality, and how relative social and economic inequalities were related to differential health outcomes. The 'old' public health concerns with polluted physical environments drifted from the public health agenda in developed counties, of interest only to environmental epidemiologists until recently, when the environment began to figure as a global referent, rather than a local one.

This most recent conception of the environment is holistic, encompassing the entire planet as an ecosystem, across which local actions (transport choices, energy use) are considered in terms of their distant impacts on global climate change, and the associated direct and indirect health impacts. The focus has shifted from a narrow one of the health impacts of single pollutants on identifiable outcomes to one that ties up global environmental change with environmental justice. Those that are most likely to suffer from the effects of climate change are likely to be those who have done least to contribute to it (Smith and Ezzati 2005). Carbon dioxide emissions leading to global warming have been predicted to have dire direct effects, through the impacts of increasing temperatures on human health, and the anticipated broader spread of infectious and parasitic disease those greater temperatures will bring (Kovats *et al.* 1999). Even more difficult to calculate will be the indirect effects on health through the environmental degradation that will affect communities far from those who are generating most of those emissions. For many, climate change represents the most serious threat to the public health, yet (as with environmental challenges of the nineteenth century) the solutions lie in political action, not within the health sector. Once again, there have been calls for public health professionals to act as good examples, in moving towards low carbon living (Roberts 2006), and as activists, in campaigning for environmentally friendly policies (Stott 2006).

A global perspective on the environment obliges us to consider health in its broadest sense. Transport is one arena in which critical voices have long argued for a shift away from focusing on single outcomes (such as injuries) and towards a more integrated perspective on how systems shape the kinds of environment which promote or inhibit health. This entails thinking through our reliance on high levels of energy consumption in terms of such diverse outcomes as the destruction of liveable communities, in which large roads reduce our access to social networks (Appleyard and Lintell 1972), and the increasing potential for war, as global conflict over energy resources intensifies (Roberts 2004). When Sonja Hunt (1992) identified private car use as a public health issue that had been largely ignored, she noted that most research had focused on individualised behavioural risks, for instance those associated with drinking and driving or not using a seat belt. She called for a more critical approach to the problem, which recognised the disproportionate burden of injury on the most deprived sections of society, the impact of increased atmospheric pollution, and the more diffuse health effects, such as those from the stress of driving itself and the disincentives to healthier modes of travel. Since then, there has been a surge of interest in how urban environments, in particular, militate against physical, mental and social health.

The reading from Peter Freund and George Martin (Chapter 15) is in this tradition, carefully unpicking some of the effects of a 'pro-car ideology' which normalises private car transport. Their analysis of the social organisation of car-centred transport goes beyond a concern with immediate health effects and offers a more sophisticated understanding of how car dependence organises space and time in ways which are profoundly unhealthy. The effects are not only those of pollution, injury and lack of exercise, but more systemic, shaping urban space in ways that particularly disadvantage the young, the elderly and the impaired. Car-dominated environments demand, they argue, a state of constant alertness, leaving little room for other subjective states – playfulness, daydreaming or drunkenness. This is a useful critical reminder that public health too easily adopts the values of dominant cultures, asking questions about how we can increase alertness, or reduce drunkenness, rather than asking why these states should be so valorised. It is also a reminder of the need to look at both technologies and environments from the broadest perspective possible, asking not only how specific risks might impact on single health outcomes, but how entire systems shape the ways in which we live, interact and feel, and how they might influence our social as well as individual health.

If the environment has had a shifting position on the agenda of public health, that of technology has, until recently, remained firmly on the sidelines. In the battles over environmental degradation and pollution, industrial progress is positioned as a risk-generator, but the actual technologies generating the risks have rarely been objects of analysis in themselves. Similarly, health technologies have traditionally been marginalised as a topic of enquiry for public health, being associated with the curative medical approach, and conceptualised as part of the problem of an overmedicalised healthcare system. As Charlotte Humphrey reminds us in Chapter 13, these arguments follow the legacy of Ivan Illich, and the rejection of diagnostic and therapeutic technologies as evidence of 'progress'. Taking the case of antibiotic resistance as a test of the contemporary application of Illich's arguments, Humphrey analyses those strategies which were proposed for controlling resistance in terms of the interplay between technological possibilities, policy responses and the likely impacts on professional working. Her argument is a prompt to consider the complex relationships between technological change and organisational change. New therapies require new organisational forms, which in turn impact on how technologies are used in practice, by whom and with what effects. The protocols and guidelines likely to be introduced to control antibiotic resistance, for instance, are likely to have implications beyond those that relate to antibiotic use, in terms of how they shape professional behaviours and cultures. Mundane technologies (such as new recording and accounting systems) as well as the more dramatic developments in diagnostic or therapeutic technologies, also have profound impacts on organisational practice, and the kinds of healthcare relationships that are possible. There has been an increased interest in the role of information and communication technologies in the practice of health (Heath *et al.* 2003), but this has largely focused on direct healthcare, and the interactions of health professionals in primary and secondary care. With few exceptions (see, e.g., Berg and Mol 1998), there has been little that has explicitly examined the role of mundane technologies on the practice of public health itself.

The focus on iatrogenesis, on the negative effects of technological progress, has clearly been an invaluable one for public health, and critical voices have had a key role in uncovering the structures of power embedded in such health technology advances as psychotropic drugs. In their analysis of rising rates of methylphenidate prescriptions for young people with attention deficit disorders, for instance, Steve Baldwin and Rebecca Anderson (2000) point to the role of pharmaceutical companies in creating and expanding a market, and medicalising the troubles of children and teenagers. These political analyses of the role of 'big pharma', and the medical control of social problems, have been a recurrent and necessary part of a critique of medicalisation, and essential for addressing questions about who benefits, and who is at risk, from medical innovation. However, they leave technologies themselves relatively under-explored, in that the analysis has been of the social uses and abuses of those technologies, rather than of the material technologies themselves and how they interact with the social environment.

Therapeutic technologies clearly affect the public health in ways beyond their obvious impacts on those individuals utilising them, in terms of the ways in which they impinge on identity, social relationships and cultural norms. One example is the shifting cultural and behavioural responses to the risks of HIV/AIDS that have been documented in the wake of the development of anti-retroviral treatments. In

Australia, for instance, the possibilities of better prognosis for people living with HIV from the mid-1990s heralded what Paul van de Ven and colleagues (2004: 362) describe as a period in which 'gay social and sexual relations were reassessed'. Van de Ven *et al.* discuss shifting patterns of behaviour, such as increases in what had earlier been seen as 'risky' practices, such as unprotected anal intercourse. However, they suggest that this has been accompanied by the development of other risk minimisation strategies to protect sexual health. Their point is that the introduction of new therapeutic technologies (improved anti-retrovirals) did not in any simplistic way *cause* changes in behaviour, but it is one element in an evolving community, which is also affected by contemporaneous changes, such as changing patterns of community activism and a growing use of the internet to contact partners. Thus, although technologies do not drive behaviour change in a unidimensional way, they do have a real, and important, role to play; and important questions arise about how technologies are used in action, as well as the likely impacts in terms of social control.

Taking technology seriously, as being part of a social system rather than just an external influence on it, entails a more nuanced approach than that of simply categorising technological advances as 'risks' for the public health. Two particular theoretical traditions have influenced critical attempts to do this. The first is a Foucauldian approach, evident in the chapter by Robin Bunton and Alan Petersen on genetic governance (Chapter 14). Within this perspective, questions focus on the role technologies have to play in shaping subjectivities. Developments in technologies of health such as risk assessment, screening and psychotherapy do not have implications only for therapeutic efficacy or iatrogenesis but for governance: how the population, and individuals within it, are managed, and manage themselves. Following on from the arguments of Michel Foucault on the exercise of power in modern societies, these approaches look at the role of technologies in the development of particular subjectivities. David Armstrong (1993), in his historical review of different regimes in public health, explored the role of hygienic rules of separation in early social medicine in opening up a 'psychosocial space' in which the body became associated with such characteristics as attitudes and instincts. This space was expanded, he argues, with the new public health, with its focus on ever-present dangers and the need for surveillance. The practice of public health (its emerging technologies, the socio-material spaces it created) was part of the systems of governance of modern states that enabled the emergence of the concept of an 'identity', the notion of a self that was aware of the risks they faced, motivated towards their own health, and responsible for managing those risks. To engage in the practices of contemporary public health requires self-awareness, subjectivity. The 'risky self' (Nettleton 1997) is aware of their own agency, self-reliant and enterprising in the pursuit of health and mental well-being. The growth in technologies of screening, for instance, obliges us all to be risk-aware and responsible in managing our own health risks in order to behave as reasonable, autonomous adults. Such technologies have a role, then, in shaping identities in late modern societies, and the kinds of active citizens who are the subjects of health policy. Bunton and Petersen review the implications of technological developments in genetics, including biobank projects and new diagnostic tests, and argue for an analysis of their role in public health. This requires careful analysis of the technologies in action as well as their failures, successes and how they are understood by various stakeholders, including scientists, public health professionals, patients and the wider public. It also requires a critical approach to the role public health plays in governance, which is often hidden, or obscured by a focus on narrow ethical issues such as consent and confidentiality.

The second set of perspectives that have provided some purchase on conceptualising these complex relationships between technologies and society are those from the sociology of science. These have moved away from the traditional polarities of technological determinism, on the one hand, in which technology is seen as driving social change, and the social constructivism of much sociology, on the other, in which the material world is conceptualised purely as an artefact of social and political process. One fruitful contribution from the sociology of science has been actor–network theory. The basis of this theory is that the division of the world into 'nature' and 'society' is unsustainable. We live in a world of what Bruno Latour (1991) calls 'hybrids': conglomerations of the human and non-human world. The material and the social co-produce each other, as organisations and technologies come to be stabilised as networks, through the ordering of heterogeneous materials, including craft skills, machines and knowledges (Law 1992). Networks are not simply constructed from social relations, but through material artefacts, which in themselves shape the social. Thus technologies and social relations are conceptualised as being 'co-produced', rather than one determining the other. Joost Van Loon's chapter (Chapter 16) is a nice example of this kind of approach, in his reflections on 'epidemic space'. Given the social significance of contemporary concerns about infectious diseases such as SARS, avian influenza and BSE, understanding the networks that produce virulent pathogens and the 'panics' that can spiral out of control around them is important. Van Loon examines what makes epidemic spaces stable or not, in terms of networks which include materials (pathogens, vectors, medical equipment), technologies (epidemiological techniques), human actors and assemblages, such as those of the military or medicine. Taking these kinds of theoretical development on board means we can no longer ignore material technologies as irrelevant to an analysis for public health, or 'black-box' them as taken for granted and external to the social fabric. Instead, we have to pay close attention to how technologies, environments and social actors interrelate, each shaping the other.

In his work on how environmental hazards produce disease, Snow could isolate single causes for epidemic outbreaks in bounded geographic localities, in which flows in and out (of water, or people) could relatively easily be tracked as additional risk factors. Today, public health confronts globalised spaces, across which complex flows of people, material things and ideas destabilise any simplistic notion of a single 'population' within a material environment. The environment has been an enduring core concern for public health, but a critical approach needs first to deconstruct traditional notions of pollution, risk and space and the causal relationships between them. It must then reconstruct these as complex networks, and bring to these nuanced analyses that draw widely on lay and expert knowledges from a range of approaches and disciplines. Taking into account a more global concept of the environment, and a more interactive model of the interplays between technologies and society, requires new theories and methods. The readings in this part are not intended to be a comprehensive overview of the work in this area. They do, however, give some flavour of the kinds of approach that have been utilised in critical public health to make sense of the edgy spaces we inhabit, and how they can either promote or threaten our health.

References

Appleyard, D. and Lintell, M. (1972) 'The environmental quality of city streets: the residents' viewpoint', *American Institute of Planners Journal*, 38: 84–101.

Armstrong, D. (1993) 'Public health spaces and the fabrication of identity', *Sociology*, 27: 393–410.

Baldwin, S. and Anderson, R. (2000) 'The cult of methylphenidate: clinical update', *Critical Public Health*, 10: 81–6.

Berg, M. and Mol, A. (1998) *Differences in Medicine: Unravelling Practices, Technologies and Bodies*, Durham, NC: Duke University Press.

Brown, P. (1992) 'Popular epidemiology and toxic waste contamination: lay and professional ways of knowing', *Journal of Health and Social Behavior*, 33: 267–81.

Heath, C., Luff, P. and Sanchez Svensson, M. (2003) 'Technology and medical practice', *Sociology of Health and Illness*, 25: 75–96.

Hunt, S. (1992) 'The public health implications of private cars', in C.J. Martin and D.V. McQueen (eds), *Readings for a New Public Health*, Edinburgh: Edinburgh University Press.

Kessel, A. (2006) *Air, the Environment and Public Health*, Cambridge: Cambridge University Press.

Kovats, R.S., Haines, A., Stanwell-Smith, R. *et al.* (1999) 'Climate change and human health in Europe', *British Medical Journal*, 318: 1682–5.

Krieger, N. (1992) 'Re: who made John Snow a hero?', *American Journal of Epidemiology*, 135: 450–1 (letter).

Latour, B. (1991) *We Have Never Been Modern*, Harlow: Pearson Education.

Law, J. (1992) 'Notes on the theory of the actor–network: ordering, strategy and heterogeneity', *Systems Practice*, 5: 379–93.

Levine, A. (1982) *Love Canal: Science, Politics and People*, Lexington, KY: Lexington Books.

Nettleton, S. (1997) 'Governing the risky self: how to become healthy, wealthy and wise', in A. Petersen and R. Bunton (eds), *Foucault: Health and Medicine*, London: Routledge.

Phillimore, P. and Moffatt, S. (1994) 'Discounted knowledge: local experience, environmental pollution and health', in J. Popay and G. Williams (eds), *Researching the People's Health*, London: Routledge.

Roberts, I. (2004) 'Injury and globalisation', *Injury Prevention*, 10: 65–6.

—— (2006) 'When doctors learned to speak carbon', *British Medical Journal*, 332: 497.

Smith, K.R. and Ezzati, M. (2005) 'How environmental health risks change with development: the epidemiologic and environmental risk transitions revisited', *Annual Review of Environmental Resources*, 30: 291–333.

Snow, J. (1855) *On the Mode of Communication of Cholera*, London: John Churchill.

Stott, R. (2006) 'Healthy responses to climate change', *British Medical Journal*, 332: 1385–7.

van de Ven, P., Murphy, D., Hull, P., Prestage, G., Batrouney, C. and Kippax, S. (2004) 'Risk management and harm reduction among gay men in Sydney', *Critical Public Health*, 14: 361–76.

Vandenbroucke, J.P., Eelkman Rooda, H.M. and Beukers, H. (1991) 'Who made John Snow a hero?', *American Journal of Epidemiology*, 133: 967–3.

13 Antibiotic resistance

An exemplary case of medical nemesis[1]

Charlotte Humphrey

Introduction

Thirty years ago, as part of a general assault on professional dominance, Ivan Illich published a searing critique of the 'health denying' effects of modern medical practice (Illich 1974). He suggested that professional overconfidence in therapies of sometimes dubious value was leading to serious problems, not only of clinical iatrogenesis but of social dependence in a 'medicalised' society, characterised and disabled by excessive faith in doctors. To explain these problems, Illich invoked the Greek concept of nemesis, or divine vengeance, visited by the gods on ordinary mortals who overreached themselves by meddling with unearthly powers and trying to become heroes. One significant offender in ancient times was Aesclapius – since regarded by many as the founder of modern medicine – who angered the gods by taking the ability to cure disease away from them and giving it to mankind. Aesclapius became so skilled in surgery and the use of medicinal plants that he could even restore the dead. Hades, ruler of the dead, became alarmed at this and complained to Zeus, who killed Aesclapius with a thunderbolt.

Illich regarded the growing problems of social and clinical iatrogenesis as contemporary manifestations of medical nemesis brought about by the escalating and misplaced arrogance of modern medicine. In his view, these problems clearly could not be solved by further 'progress' in the same direction and were, indeed, more likely to become compounded:

> The unwanted physiological, social and psychological by-products of diagnostic and therapeutic progress have become resistant to medical remedies. New devices, approaches and organizational arrangements, which are conceived as remedies for clinical and social iatrogenesis, themselves tend to become pathogens contributing to the new epidemic.
>
> (Illich 1976: 34)

Rather, Illich suggested, recovery would depend on judicious retreat. Specifically he argued that the power of medicine should be reduced by limiting the professional monopoly of physicians, challenging the techno-rationalist values underpinning scientific progress and industrial growth and, above all, recovering the will to self-care.

Illich's writings were widely criticised for both style and content, but his basic thesis nevertheless caused a considerable stir because it provided a focus for increasing doubts about the wisdom of the mechanistic philosophy of healthcare and chimed with a range of wider concerns about the effectiveness and fallibility of medicine (Fox 1977; Dollery 1978). Reviewed in the *Lancet*, he was seen, at the least, as offering a timely caution against excessive optimism (Cohen and Backett 1974).

Ironically, the introduction of antibiotics was one of the very few medical advances which Illich regarded as clearly beneficial (though he recognised the potential problem of resistance) and which he therefore explicitly exempted from his general critique (Illich 1976). And yet, in many ways, the present problems associated with antibiotic misuse may be seen as a classic example of the type of hazard with which he was concerned. This paper explores the relevance of Illich's ideas to contemporary concerns about these problems and how they should be dealt with, particularly those associated with the development of resistant bacteria. It is based on analysis of recommendations made in reports on antibiotic resistance from a number of sources, including the House of Lords Select Committee on Science and Technology (1998), the Standing Medical Advisory Committee (1998) and the Invitational EU Conference on the Microbial Threat held in Copenhagen in 1998 (MHFAF 1998).

The antibiotic age

When antibiotics were first introduced in the 1940s, they were hailed as the proverbial 'magic bullet' – a naturally occurring substance which would kill invading bacteria without harming the host – for which chemists had been searching since the nineteenth century (Levy 1992). The success of this new class of drugs in transforming the outcome of infectious disease dramatically diminished the risks associated with other forms of treatment, such as surgery, thereby enabling the development of increasingly complex and heroic interventions on sicker patients. It also encouraged exaggerated belief in their power as a benign and general cure which led, in turn, to incautious and excessive use. In the half century since penicillin was first introduced, consumption of antibiotics has rocketed, especially in industrialised countries. By the end of the twentieth century in the UK over fifty million prescriptions were being issued every year. It is estimated that about half of all human use of antibiotics is inappropriate (SMAC 1998).

The medical and social iatrogenic consequences of this behaviour are now well recognised. For individual patients, inappropriate treatment with antibiotics may result in unnecessary side-effects, super infections, ineffective treatment, delayed recovery, inappropriate expectations and dependence on medical care. For the healthcare system, inappropriate use of antibiotics and the associated development and spread of antibiotic-resistant organisms both lead to greater costs, slower throughput and decreased ability to treat. In medicine, the development of resistance threatens to wipe out the very advances in clinical practice which the introduction of antibiotics first made possible. In the words of the Standing Medical Advisory Committee, the spread of pathogens resistant to all antibiotics 'threatens a return to darker times when surgery was restricted to simple operations on the otherwise healthy, and when organ transplants, joint replacements and immunosuppressive therapies were unthinkable' (SMAC 1998: 14). For society as a whole the consequences are increased vulnerability to disease and less protection from it when encountered.

Looked at through Illich's eyes, resistance can be seen as the Aesclapian thunderbolt – the inevitable dark side of the miraculous treatment, hastened in its release by the medical profession's misuse of the antibiotic miracle. When presented at the 1998 Invitational EU Conference on the Microbial Threat – albeit in more secular terms as the payback for doctors having 'screwed up' by squandering a 'wonderful gift' – such an analysis appears to have been widely shared (Smith 1998).

Strategies for dealing with the problems of resistance

The problems associated with developing antibiotic resistance can be approached in different ways. First, they may be outrun by the continual introduction of new agents to which resistance has not yet developed. This is the way in which resistance problems have been dealt with in the past, but no new class of antimicrobial agents has been licensed in the last fifteen years. The SMAC report identifies a number of promising factors in the search for new agents, including the new science of 'genomics' which may help in the identification of new families of agents, more efficient methods of synthesising new candidate drugs and improved methods of screening antimicrobial activity which speed up the testing of new compounds. However, even if new agents are identified in the future, this seems likely to take some time and 'it is virtually certain' that resistance will develop to these new compounds also.

A second approach to dealing with resistance is to avoid the problems by preventing the occurrence of infectious disease through vaccination or treating diseases in ways that do not involve the use of antibiotics. Some major diseases have been eradicated by vaccination and good progress is being made against others, but the SMAC report cites a number of key pathogens, such as tuberculosis, where the development of good vaccines 'remains a major challenge'. The report is similarly cautious about the prospects for success with a variety of unconventional approaches to the treatment of infectious disease, commenting that it would be unwise to anticipate swift results or broad applications.

The third approach is to control the development and spread of resistance by ensuring more prudent use of antibiotics and better methods of infection control. Much attention is currently being given to identifying effective ways to achieve these aims. Recommended strategies to reduce misuse include: better education of both patients and clinicians; improved organisational support in the form of guidelines, protocols, antibacterial policies, decision support and faster testing to identify infectious agents; and action in relation to the development, licensing and marketing of antibiotics. Suggestions for controlling the spread of infection include isolation and cohorting of patients and improved ward design, handwashing, bed occupancy and admissions policies (SCST 1998; SMAC 1998; MHFAF 1998). The aim here is a limited one: not to beat or dispose of the problem of resistance, but to stave it off for as long as possible and perhaps buy time for another, more fundamental answer to be found.

Prospects of success

To the extent that Illich's ideas on iatrogenesis provide a helpful framework for reflecting on the causes and consequences of antibiotic misuse, it is worth considering how he might view the current thinking about the problems of resistance and proposals for addressing them.

In the various reports referred to earlier, antibiotic resistance is not regarded as an exemplary manifestation – albeit with exceptionally serious iatrogenic effects – of a generic problem with medical culture (as Illich would see it), but rather as a unique scientific problem arising from the exceptional biological properties of antibiotics and the bacteria they are used to treat. The activities and behaviours which lead to antibiotic misuse are not understood as products of the values and social relations which create the environment in which they occur (as Illich would do), but rather as organisational and individual errors caused by technical shortcomings, inefficient systems and information deficits. The policies proposed are not intended (as Illich recommends) to challenge professional monopolies or techno-rationalist values, or to encourage the will to self-care in general terms. Rather, they have the focused and specific aim of cutting antibiotic use and strengthening effective infection control to enable medicine to continue to advance, unhindered by the problems of resistance for as long as possible.

In short, the approach being taken is much of the kind that Illich counsels against as doomed to failure. Both the framing of the problem and proposed solutions reflect and reinforce the aims and values of the system within which the difficulties have arisen, rather than reflecting on or challenging that system. As such, he would say, they can only contribute to worsening iatrogenesis in the longer term.

However, it could be argued that the proposed strategies for controlling resistance, if introduced successfully, might actually help – however unintentionally – to bring about some of the broader changes that Illich would like to see. Successful negotiation of prescribing and infection control policies would involve better communication and collaboration on a more equal basis between medicine and other health professions. Successful introduction of guidelines and protocols would mean that clinical practice was more explicit, better justified, and less influenced by the idiosyncrasies, habits and traditional prejudices of unaccountable professions. Successful intervention to control the distribution and marketing of new drugs would mean departments, governments and international organisations working together at an economic and political level to moderate the pharmaceutical industry's imperative for development. Successful professional education and public information campaigns would mean a better-informed and more self-reliant public, less dependent on doctors and medicines to deal with problems for which these are not appropriate.

If it were possible to bring about such changes in respect of antibiotic management and infection control alone, they could at least provide a model for new ways of working and relating in other areas of healthcare also. But it is well recognised that the process of changing professional activities in order to reduce antimicrobial resistance 'cannot be undertaken in isolation [and] the overall culture and organisation in which professionals work has to be addressed' (SMAC 1998: 109). The very process of attempting to introduce control strategies in this particular arena requires – and could generate – much wider change.

Since the 1970s, when Illich published his critique, concerns about medical dominance and accountability and the wider hazards associated with scientific advances and global industrial development have become widespread. There was even a call for an Illich Collaboration (along the lines of the Cochrane Collaboration) 'to make readily available objective evidence of harms of medical care' (Edwards 1999: 58). Over the same period, growing experience of attempts to change public, professional and organisational behaviour has generated an increasingly sophisticated appreciation of the complexities of bringing about change as well as some knowledge of what does and does not work. The evidence is that while change is possible, it certainly is not easily achieved.

But here, the severity of the problem of antibiotic resistance might just become its saving grace. The fact that it strikes so profoundly at the core of medical progress (and undermines an advance so important that even Illich turned a blind eye to its hazards) provides an exceptional imperative and commitment to make the control strategies work. In a commentary on the matter, after laying out the scale of the intersectoral and international collaboration required to deal with what he described as 'health care's version of global warming', the editor of the *British Medical Journal* concluded: 'Unusually, I'm optimistic' (Smith 1998: 764). It would be a fine paradox if this most extreme case of medical nemesis proved to be the stimulus required to begin a general reversal of medicine's 'health-denying' effects.

Note

1 This chapter was first published as a paper in *Critical Public Health* (2000) 10: 354–8.

References

Cohen, N.S. and Backett, E.M. (1974) 'Medical nemesis', *Lancet*, 2(ii): 1503–4.
Danish Ministries of Health and Food, Agriculture and Fisheries (MHFAF) (1998) 'The Copenhagen recommendations: report from the Invitational EU Conference on the Microbial Threat', in Secretary of State for Health, *Government Response to the House of Lords Select Committee on Science and Technology Report: Resistance to Antibiotics and Other Antimicrobial Agents*, CM 4172, London: Stationery Office.
Department of Health Standing Medical Advisory Committee (SMAC) (1998) *The Path of Least Resistance*, London: Department of Health.
Dollery, C. (1978) *The End of an Age of Optimism*, London: Nuffield Provincial Hospitals Trust.

Edwards, R. (1999) 'Is it time for an Illich Collaboration to make available information on the harms of medical care?', *British Medical Journal*, 318: 58 (letter).

Fox, R.C. (1977) 'The medicalisation and demedicalisation of American society', *Proceedings of the American Academy of Arts and Sciences*, 106: 9–22.

House of Lords Select Committee on Science and Technology (SCST) (1998) *Resistance to Antibiotics and Other Antimicrobial Agents*, London: Stationery Office.

Illich, I. (1974) 'Medical nemesis', *Lancet* (i): 918–21.

—— (1976) *Limits to Medicine*, London: Calder and Boyers.

Levy, S.B. (1992) *The Antibiotic Paradox: How Miracle Drugs are Destroying the Miracle*, New York: Plenum Press.

Smith, R. (1998) 'Action on antimicrobial resistance', *British Medical Journal*, 317: 764.

14 Genetics, governance and ethics[1]

Robin Bunton and Alan Petersen

Developments in genetic research have dominated recent public and professional debate about public health. One feature of this debate is the promise of the social and scientific transformation of public health. There have been calls for engagement with the 'new' genetics and an updating of concerns, sometimes to extend more traditional approaches, at other times presenting new ways of working and new problems. Developments in the field have been rapid and far reaching and have raised a wide range of social, political and ethical issues that we discuss here as issues of *genetic governance*.

At one level, there has been a call for public health to take account of insights generated from molecular biology and genetic studies in the last twenty years or so. Public health has traditionally focused on modifiable risk factors for disease, more usually apparent in adolescence and later life and focusing preventative interventions on these periods. Genetic testing and screening offer opportunities to extend these sites to well before the onset of clinically recognised disease (Holtzman 1997). Such a focus has long been evident in attempts to identify single-gene disorders such as sickle cell disease and phenylketonuria and has informed interventions such as pre-natal counselling. With improved detection and surveillance facilities, there are now opportunities to extend concerns to the 'genetic basis' of common, adult-onset disorders and more mainstream public health disease targets (Coughlin 1999). Public health should, it is recommended, explore the complex interactions between genetic and environmental factors, 'Particularly how environmental factors and human behaviour might have differential effects on disease risk by virtue of the genetic susceptibility of particular individuals' (Zimmern 1999: 136). Genetic testing for childhood asthma may improve predictive assessment of the risk of exposure to environmental allergens such as cigarette smoke, for example (Khoury 1996). The new genetic knowledge and techniques allow opportunities to extend risk surveillance and intervention.

At another level, the recent discourse on the new genetics (its techniques and promises of therapeutic interventions) poses fundamental epistemological and ethical questions for public health. We have explored such issues elsewhere (Petersen and Bunton 2002), arguing that fundamental assumptions about public health as a field of knowledge and domain of practice are brought into question by the new genetic technologies. Working concepts of the environment, the host and the agent in public health become destabilised when genetic technologies subject each to human manipulation and choice. Genetic technologies promise increased choice over the types of body and mind we have, the types of agricultural environment we live and work in, as well as the types of contagion we are exposed to. As such, the new genetics represents a change in the ways in which we think about our bodies, ourselves, our society and our physical world, and raises questions about what it means to be human and what constitutes the natural world.

The new genetic knowledge, highlighted by prestigious international projects such as the Human Genome Project (HGP), promises a new era of technological optimism and control over the forces of nature, chance and fate and seemingly extends the modern ideal of the rational control of life. The new genetic technologies, in combination with information technologies, facilitate the surveillance of populations in ways not previously possible, enabling the construction of nation-wide datasets, such as the Icelandic Health Sector Database.

In 1998, Iceland began a controversial project to build a public/private electronic database using the near total Icelandic population as its biological sample in order to study genetic aspects of common diseases, drawing upon genetic samples, medical records and genealogical records. The Iceland Biobanks Bill of 2000 immediately generated intense public debate among scientific and clinical communities about the ethics of developing large-scale DNA banks and of the increasing commercialisation of genetic knowledge. Public and professional fears of the 'brave new world' consequences of the new genetics led to newspaper stories claiming, 'Iceland sells its people's genome', and 'Selling the family secrets'. The Bill came under criticism from data protection experts and brought to the fore a number of social and ethical concerns. Members of Europe's Data Protection Commission considered that the draft Bill would violate several European treaties, including the European Convention on Human Rights (Rose 2001).

The Icelandic case focused broader academic interest on the social and moral issues involved in large biological sample collections (Martin and Kaye 2000). In the UK, the collection of such samples has been the subject of a House of Lords Select Committee and the deliberations of a Human Genetics Commission. Some of this debate relates to the potential of the new genetics to commodify nature and the human body and to transfer what are considered collective, family or personal qualities into the hands of corporate ownership. A fusion of biotechnology and informatics enables genetic information to become a marketable commodity (Rose 2001).

Public understanding of such ventures has demonstrated an ambivalence characteristic of life in late-modern societies, in which risks and uncertainty are generated by technological and scientific developments. Life in such societies has a critical or 'reflexive' quality and mistrust of technical and scientific developments such as genetics is common (Kerr and Cunningham-Burley 2000). The question of how best to re-establish trust, whether through legislation, the development of new ethical guidelines, improved participatory mechanisms or other mechanisms, has become prominent in recent debates among sociologists and other social scientists. Efforts thus far, including participatory 'experiments' such as citizens' juries, have fallen short of ideals in a number of respects (Dunkerley and Glasner 1998), and raise questions about how best to facilitate public input into decisions and develop people's confidence that new technologies will benefit the general community.

Issues of governance lie at the heart of public participation in the development of gene technologies, and we argue here that we need to address these centrally in developing a perspective and critique of developments in genetics and their take-up in public health. Like many widely used terms, the concept of governance is imbued with diverse meanings. 'Clinical governance' has emerged as a feature of UK health policy, for example, indicating local needs for regulation and standard-isation. At an international level the need for good governance for health has been identified by cross-national bodies linking social and economic development with health (Lavis and Sullivan 1999; WHO 1998). All concepts of governance acknowledge the accomplishments of a network of agencies or system of regulation, not simply the actions of individual agencies or nation-states.

Our work in the field of genetics as applied to public health has drawn extensively on Michel Foucault's concept of governmentality. Understood by Foucault as 'the conduct of conduct' or the rationality of government, governmentality refers to something including, but far exceeding, the technologies of state govern-ment institutions. It refers to all forms of the regulation of wealth and resources, territory and means of subsistence, climate, irrigation, fertility as well as social relationships and customs, habits, and ways of acting and thinking (Foucault 1991). In this broad sense, governance can also refer to techniques or organising tech-nologies. Forms of expert knowledge, the professions, disciplines and the practices surrounding them, are particularly important in establishing the governability of the social and physical environment. Public health and other medical practices have developed a wide range of technologies for regulating the environment and behaviour in the name of health from early development of the *cordon sanitaire* and the environmental health measures encapsulated in nineteenth-century public health legislation through to the large-scale screening programmes of the twentieth century. The new genetic technologies of health supplement this arsenal of public health regulation and represent new opportunities for governance. A new body of knowledge carries with it potential for new forms of power, regulation and surveillance. Professing to offer new ways to reproduce and 'improve' our bodies, our minds and our environments, such techniques raise new questions about the nature of human existence and the types of social relationship we want to perpetuate. It is this sense of governance that is our concern here.

Foucauldian work on governmentality, such as that of Nicholas Rose (1999), provides critique of the unforeseen and unintended consequences of new, particularly neoliberal, forms of governance. Malpas and Wickham (1997), for example, have argued that governance has effects even in failure, which is a common feature of governance strategies. Governance concerns the ways that divergent preferences of citizens and other non-state actors are translated into policy choices. There are emerging structures of governance in the field of genomics that have followed its rise from scientific dream to large-scale socio-technical project. Important here are the ways in which genomic research has been supported and regulated by governmental agencies as well as the genomics industry, which acts as a powerful force in the network.

Social compromise and binding decisions often feature in policy aims, yet there are a great many obstacles to achieving such consensus and gaining public support for policies. Despite opposition to agricultural biotechnology, there are signs of public support for the various medical applications of genomics, such as genetic testing and pharmaceutical intervention. There is an unprecedented dynamic coalition of government, industry and big science interests in developments in genomics which has far-reaching consequences for research and policy decisions on patenting rights, for example. The traditional roles of government, industry and science in scientific–technological development are being redefined as newer systems of governance are sought. Debate about whether these new mechanisms are adequate and democratic enough for the task in hand are central to public health concerns.

Public health's involvement in governance is not always transparent, and is not always apparent to, or acknowledged by, public health practitioners. The new genetics is routinely involved in small acts of governance, enacted in relation to, for example, parental genetic counselling, the construction of national genetic databases and the messages of health education campaigns. Issues of governance do not feature largely in debate concerning the new genetic knowledge and techniques. Rather, debate is largely framed in terms of 'ethical' concerns. Foucault highlighted the close relationship between ethics and governance. Within his schema, questions of conduct are inextricably linked to questions of ethics. He showed the various ways, from classical Greece to the present, that ethical judgement was implicated in the formation of the self and citizenship. Individuals, he argued, govern themselves through forms of self-care, self-examination and self-discipline, training and exercise. The development of the self and ethical living in relation to sexual morality, for example, depends upon daily practices, routines or techniques for living promoted by the Christian Church in Europe but also by modern secular institutions, such as the family, the school and the clinic (Foucault 1977). Medical and public health institutions similarly promoted ethics of self-care by promoting a particular 'political anatomy of the body' (Armstrong 1983, 1995). Foucault's concern with ethical conduct can be contrasted with the philosophical and religious focus on morality – a general system of imposed or suggested rules or guides for conduct – and with how the former may provide the basis for breaking with the 'normalising' tendencies in modern societies. When used in contemporary debates about genetic technologies and other new technologies, however, the term 'ethics' tends to equate with the latter, thus limiting debate about the profound implications of new technologies for how we think about the self and social relations. Thus, the exploration of the 'ethical' implications of the new genetics is often restricted to concerns about confidentiality, informed consent, people's 'right to know or right not to know'. Meanwhile, fundamental questions about how people might best relate, and how to nurture 'desirable' forms of self-conduct and a society that is just and more equitable, remain unaddressed.

It is perhaps not surprising, then, that much of the debate surrounding the emergence of the new genetics has focused on what are seen as ethical dilemmas.

A number of critical studies have concentrated on the ways in which medical ethics became a feature of genetic screening, counselling work (Jallinoja 2002) and reproduction (Ettorre 2002), which has developed within a framework of medical ethics, ethics committees and formalised codes of ethics, and the often hidden assumptions contained within the take-up of new techniques. The discourse on screening has similarly focused on individualised risk assessment rather than on broader issues of governance and technological advance and what has been referred to elsewhere as 'governance by freedom' (Rose 1999; Poutanen 2002). The imperatives that newer technologies bring with them often reflect the social and ideological circumstances of their creation. It has frequently been noted that public health problems with multiple causes can be conveniently reframed as matters of individual responsibility, thereby avoiding difficult macro-political issues. This is also apparent with the new biotechnologies which can invite us to focus on individual or familial susceptibility to cancers, for example, rather than to their environmental cause (Willis 2002). Genetic technologies can reduce potentially complex social, political issues to simple technological solutions.

Further, as Lemke (2002) argues, the increasing uptake of genetic technologies may contribute to the 'apparatuses of insecurity'. The increased prophylactic possibilities engendered by the new genetics, just like those of the proceeding 'older' eugenic movement, have far-reaching implications for consumers of healthcare. Research on genetics in public health is often unwittingly involved in the regulation of identity by perpetuating broader cultural notions of 'collective genetic affinities' (Ellison and Rees-Jones 2002). Assumptions about social identities are perpetuated in public health research on genetics by processes of 'essentialism', and 'naturalisation'. Classifications of social identity often have limited external and internal validity and produce misleading information on the distribution of genetic variation and gene–gene and gene–environment interactions. Such 'identity work' in research can have far-reaching implications for public health, such as increasing demands for dedicated services to address heightened genetic risk.

Screening and surveillance are given greater power with the aid of biotechnologies in relation to broader populations and sub-groups, such as classes, people with disabilities or groups identified by ethnicity. Such surveillance can also be focused by locale on specific communities, or in the workplace, for example. The potential for social regulation and discrimination against those carrying particular genes raises some familiar moral and social issues in public health and it is incumbent on public health practitioners and researchers to anticipate and critique the take-up of biotechnically informed screening.

Much interest in the ethical and governance implications of the new genetics stems from the ability of genetics to transform understandings of risk. The concept of risk has become the focus of contemporary understandings of health and a fundamental organising principle for public health (Bunton *et al.* 1995; Petersen and Lupton 1996). Secular risk discourses can replace more traditional religious moralities that have categorised and governed populations. There is a tendency for risk judgements to become increasingly 'geneticised' (Lippman 1991, 1994) and form a technical rather than a social means for regulating populations, which is possibly less transparent or even hidden. Such issues have been addressed in some detail in relation to the new genetics. There is a tendency for neoliberal governance strategies to invoke the power of individuals to make informed decisions about their health, to become self-regulating citizens who become agents of their own health by taking on identities such as 'carrier', for example (Polzer *et al.* 2002). If contemporary subjects take responsibility for acquiring genetic risk information and for managing their own genetic risk by modifying their health behaviour in self and family surveillance for conditions such as skin cancer, for instance, then they contribute to a broader social management of risk strategy whereby knowing one's genetic risk is a type of public duty.

While the social surveillance implications of new genetic developments have been highlighted by recent social science work, no less important is the potential for the creation or reinforcement of social inequalities. Certain discourses have coupled the 'genetic burden' of society with particular groups, such as those based on social class and disability (Kelly 2002). The idea of a 'genetic underclass' or an economically segregated, biologically inferior, marginalised group, separated from the benefits of genetic enhancement, presents a dystopian vision of a potentially troubling uptake of the newer biotechnologically informed surveillance techniques. Such geneticisation of inequality in relation to families with children with genetic disabilities is in need of scrutiny. People with learning difficulties, for example, arguably one of the groups most affected by developments such as pre-natal testing and counselling, have, until recently, largely been absent from this public discourse, and thus excluded from full citizenship rights (Ward 2002). Routinisation of pre-natal testing is frequently assumed to be integral to 'improvements in prenatal care', despite the anticipated outcome being the selective abortion of foetuses detected as being impaired. The extension of parental choice would seem to be allied to a commitment to impairment prevention. Disability activists and scholars have long challenged the potential of genetic knowledge and technology to medicalise disability, particularly when framed in terms of pre-natal 'choice' (Bailey 1996). Such concerns raise the spectre of eugenics, from which proponents of the new genetics have sought to distance themselves. The nature of 'choice' becomes critical, as do the technological and ideological influences over such 'choices'. Shakespeare (1998) has referred to the emphasis on non-coercive choice in pre-natal genetic counselling as a type of 'weak eugenics'.

Public understanding remains a key issue in developing adequate systems of regulation. Claims that scientists have decoded life's inner workings have over-represented actual scientific developments, and such narratives of science need to be challenged. Enthusiasm for the work of the new genetics has resulted in great public interest as well as substantial venture capital, which has generated momentum. However, much genetics research has undermined the notion that genes are the keys to organic development and pathology. Many conditions are now believed to arise from the contributions of multiple genes and gene–environment interactions rather than from single gene mutations. The slow pace of associating genes with diseases combined with the poor predictive power of genetic tests and the technical challenges involved in gene modification have meant that scientists and biotechnology corporations have fallen far short of initial ambitions. There is a need for critical analysis of their record to date and resistance to genetics-based narratives of organism physiology and development. Genetics can no longer be regarded uncritically as the key to all biologically related problems. The gene is an important cultural icon and one which is able to promote a particular, one-sided view of health and public health. Critical scholars can contribute much to revealing the ideological and narrative force of the new genetics (Nelkin and Lindee 1995).

In 2002, a major report of the World Health Organization, entitled *Genomics and World Health*, was released, underlining not only the contemporary significance of the new genetics for public health at the global level but the urgent need for new tools of analysis in this area. The report noted that the public health implications of genomics are of a global order, and include developments in pharmacogenetics, gene therapy, stem cell therapy, agriculture and vector control. In the developing world, the new genetics is seen to hold great promise in the fight against infectious diseases, in enhancing the nutritional values of crop species, and in the treatment of group- or region-specific diseases, such as the thalassaemias and sickle cell disease (WHO 2002: 44). However, the report also offered a number of cautionary notes in relation to these applications, including the lack of appreciation of the complexity of many of the common diseases, ethical and organisational constraints on research, the potentially prohibitive costs of associated treatment and prevention, and the potential to exacerbate inequalities in healthcare (WHO 2002: 73–8).

Amid the hype about the potential benefits of the new genetics for 'the public's' health, we need to remain aware of the variable impacts of these developments on different publics, and of the global and local implications of applying new genetic technologies. The new genetics is rapidly changing not only public health as a body of knowledge and field of practice but conceptions of identity, health, disease and death. New genetic developments are occurring in a context where concepts of 'the natural' and 'the social' are being rethought, and where the role of the nation-state in regulating economic and social life is becoming less self-evident than in the past. Understanding the ethical and governmental implications of the new genetics at the global and local levels, therefore, calls for a multi-disciplinary approach, including the contributions of such disciplines as sociology, anthropology, politics, feminist studies, legal studies and bioethics.

In this chapter we have discussed some of the implications of the new genetic knowledge and technologies for public health. We have outlined various ways that concerns with ethics and individual 'choice' have implications for broader issues of the governance of populations. As such, these new technologies are implicated in the construction of contemporary forms of citizenship in which the self-management of health is seen as a moral duty. The new genetics brings with it new imperatives. We note that, although not always acknowledged as such, interventions such as parental genetic counselling, the creation of national genetic databases and the transmission of knowledge in health education campaigns influence and define social relationships in purposeful ways. Clearly, much critical work is needed to highlight the future moral and political issues at stake, as well as the policy and practice possibilities presented by these developments.

Note

1 This chapter was first published as two introductions to the special issues of *Critical Public Health* on 'Genetic Governance, Ethics and Public Health', 12(2) and 12(3).

References

Armstrong, D. (1983) *Political Anatomy of the Body: Medical Knowledge in Britain in the Twentieth Century*, Cambridge: Cambridge University Press.

—— (1995) 'The rise of surveillance medicine', *Sociology of Health and Illness*, 17: 393–404.

Bailey, R. (1996) 'Prenatal testing and the prevention of impairment: a woman's right to choose?', in J. Morris (ed.), *Encounters with Strangers: Feminism and Disability*, London: Women's Press.

Bunton, R., Nettleton, S. and Burrows, R. (1995) *The Sociology of Health Promotion: Critical Analyses of Consumption, Lifestyle, and Risk*, New York: Routledge.

Coughlin, S.S. (1999) 'The intersection of genetics, public health and preventative medicine', *American Journal of Preventive Medicine*, 16(2): 89–90.

Dunkerley, D. and Glasner, P. (1998) 'Empowering the public? Citizens' juries and the new genetic technologies', *Critical Public Health*, 8: 181–92.

Ellison, G.T.H. and Rees-Jones, I. (2002) 'Social identities and the "new genetics": scientific and social consequences', *Critical Public Health*, 12: 265–82.

Ettorre, E. (2002) 'A critical look at the new genetics: conceptualizing the links between reproduction, gender and bodies', *Critical Public Health*, 12: 237–50.

Foucault, M. (1977) *Discipline and Punish: The Birth of the Prison*, London: Allen Lane.

—— (1991) 'Governmentality', in G. Burchell, C. Gordon and P. Miller (eds), *The Foucault Effect: Studies in Governmentality*, Hemel Hempstead: Harvester Wheatsheaf.

Holtzman, N.A. (1997) 'Genetic screening and public health', *American Journal of Public Health*, 87: 127–57.

Jallinoja, P.J. (2002) 'Ethics of clinical genetics: the spirit of the profession and trials of suitability from 1970 to 2000', *Critical Public Health*, 12: 103–18.

Kelly, S.E. (2002) '"New" genetics meets the old underclass: findings from a study of genetic outreach services in rural Kentucky', *Critical Public Health*, 12: 169–86.

Kerr, A. and Cunningham-Burley, S. (2000) 'On ambivalence and risk: reflexive modernity and the new human genetics', *Sociology*, 34: 283–304.

Khoury, M.J. (1996) 'From genes to public health: the applications of genetic technology in diseases prevention', *American Journal of Public Health*, 86: 1717–22.

Lavis, J. and Sullivan, T. (1999) 'Governing health', in D. Drache and T. Sullivan (eds), *Health Reform: Public Success, Private Failure*, London: Routledge.

Lemke, T. (2002) 'Genetic testing, eugenics and risk', *Critical Public Health*, 12: 283–90.

Lippman, A. (1991) 'Prenatal genetic testing and screening: constructing needs and reinforcing inequities', *American Journal of Law and Medicine*, 17: 15–50.

—— (1994) 'Worrying – and worrying about – the geneticization of reproduction and health', in G. Basen, M. Eichler and A. Lippman (eds), *Misconceptions: The Social Construction of Choice and the New Reproductive and Genetic Technologies*, Prescott, Ontario: Voyageur.

Malpas, J. and Wickham, G. (1997) 'Governance and the world: from Joe Dimaggio to Michel Foucault', *UTS Review*, 3: 91–108.

Martin, P. and Kaye, J. (2000) 'The use of large biological sample collections in genetics research: issues for public policy', *New Genetics and Society*, 19: 165–91.

Nelkin, D. and Lindee, M.S. (1995) *The DNA Mystique: The Gene as a Cultural Icon*, New York: W.H. Freeman.

Petersen, A. and Bunton, R. (2002) *The New Genetics and the Public's Health*, London: Routledge.

Petersen, A. and Lupton, D. (1996) *The New Public Health: Health and Self in the Age of Risk*, London: Sage.

Polzer, J., Mercer, S.L. and Goel, V. (2002) 'Blood is thicker than water: genetic testing as citizenship through familial obligation and the management of risk', *Critical Public Health*, 12: 153–68.

Poutanen, S. (2002) 'The first genetic screening in Finland: its execution, evaluation and some possible implications for liberal government', *Critical Public Health*, 12: 251–64.

Rose, H. (2001) *The Commodification of Bioinformation: The Icelandic Health Sector Database*, London: Wellcome Trust.

Rose, N. (1999) *Powers of Freedom: Reframing Political Thought*, Cambridge: Cambridge University Press.

Shakespeare, T. (1998) 'Choices and rights: eugenics, genetics and disability equality', *Disability and Society*, 13: 665–81.

Ward, L.M. (2002) 'Whose right to choose? The "new" genetics, prenatal testing and people with learning difficulties', *Critical Public Health*, 12: 187–200.

Willis, E. (2002) 'Public health and the "new" genetics: balancing individual and collective outcomes', *Critical Public Health*, 12: 139–151.

WHO (1998) *Health 21 – Health for All in the 21st Century: An Introduction*, European Health for All Series No. 5, Copenhagen: World Health Organization.

—— (2002) *Genomics and World Health, Report of the Advisory Committee on Health Research*, Geneva: WHO.

Zimmern, R. (1999) 'Genetics', in S. Griffiths and D.J. Hunter (eds), *Perspectives in Public Health*, Oxford: Radcliffe Medical Press.

15 Moving bodies

Injury, dis-ease and the social organisation of space[1]

Peter Freund and George Martin

Introduction

As Hunt (1989) pointed out nearly two decades ago, individual lifestyle practices such as drinking, smoking, dietary habit and exercise have long been public health topics, while the public health effects of car use have been neglected as public health issues. It is not surprising that the health effects of automobility have not been seen as a systemic problem. Car transport is naturalised and embedded in everyday life – psychically, socially, culturally and materially – and a pro-car ideology minimises its troubles (Freund and Martin 1993).

Of course, 'car troubles' have been addressed as public health issues – notably traffic accidents and air pollution – since the 1960s (Schwela and Zali 1999). Pollution has been ameliorated through technological fixes such as catalytic converters, lead-free fuel, etc. Accident rates have been lowered through technological fixes as well, such as safety belts. In the case of accidents, the focus has been on individuals, who are seen as sources of risky behaviour, and interventions involve educating drivers and pedestrians. Group-level variables, including social class, gender, age, race–ethnicity and disability status, do not receive as much attention as structural factors.

Hunt's catalogue of car troubles (e.g., accidents and pollution) was important for its environmental emphasis, for raising the car as a public health issue, and for linking car troubles to social structure (Nettleton and Bunton 1995). Hunt focused on the public health implications of private car-using lifestyles, as opposed to car-centred transport systems and spaces. Her perspective on car troubles hence was not systemic, and like most social scientific analyses of behaviour and lifestyles was despatialised. The focus here is on these missing systemic and spatial aspects.

The USA, and to a lesser extent the UK, feature car-centred transport systems that are characterised by a high level of car dependence and a domination of social space by the car. The car is the centrepiece of a car-centred transport system with its material infrastructure of roadways and other accoutrements, cultural patterns of beliefs and practices, social organisation of space, and political economy of production and consumption. The relationships among the car, the environment and health revolve not only around the car as a technology but around the fact that massive numbers of automobiles are used by individuals to transport themselves to work, to play and to shop, etc. The major problem is thus neither 'the automobile' nor 'car culture' but car-centred transport systems in which alternative modes of transport are neglected and underdeveloped.

One of the significant ways in which car-centred transport affects public health is through its impact on the social organisation of space, time and motion. Car-centred spatiotemporal and motional organisation influences, first, the social production of injury (fatal and non-fatal), its intensity and frequency. Second, it affects people's experiences of transport/public space, including their perceptions of risk and feelings of security and insecurity. Third, whether or not individuals are able to use transport is related to its spatiotemporal organisation. Spaces enable some bodies while disabling others. Women, children, older people and people with disabilities are, in different ways and degrees, disenfranchised by car-hegemonic spaces.

Introducing space

It has been argued that space is neglected in sociological studies of health. For instance, Popay *et al.* (1998) argue that studies must analyse social structure and process as 'situated concretely in time and space'. While disciplines such as medical geography have long studied the spatial distribution of health and illness and its determinants, little attention has been given to the social organisation of space. As Smith *et al.* (1998) indicate, car-centred transport systems structure urban forms and lifestyles. While by no means the only cause, they contribute to fragmenting sociophysical space, dispersing and severing activity sites and influencing social relations, cohesion and community – all of which impact on public health (Freund and Martin 1993).

Car accidents are produced to a degree by the social organisation of space. For instance, in car-hegemonic space people with physical and mental impairments are marginalised and put at greater risk of injury. Thus, in examining the impact of the social organisation of car-centred space on health, it is important to move beyond biomedical discourses about injury and include experiential dimensions of space. Material deprivation (in this context, physical risk) is only one consequence of the social organisation of space. How secure or insecure actors feel in moving through sociomaterial space is also an important consideration. In turn, how ontologically secure people feel in space may influence their sense of well-being and health.

As in workplaces, in transport the organisation of space–time involves differential impacts on individuals, with some bodies being more vulnerable to injury and others secure. Spatial–temporal contexts and patterns of using technology, for example, either encourage or discourage uses of bodies in ways that promote physical fitness. Thus, Hanson (1995: 23) concludes about the USA: 'Air pollution, traffic accidents, and lack of exercise are all health problems that stem from the current configuration of urban transportation'. Elsewhere, the authors have analysed the connections between increased motoring and decreased physical fitness (Freund and Martin 2004), and between motoring and fast foods (Freund and Martin 2005).

The production of risk and the social organisation of space–time

Death by car is the most dramatic of its negative effects on health. In 2002, nearly 1.2 million people died worldwide from road accidents. More people die from traffic accidents than from any one of the following causes of death: sexually transmitted diseases; malaria; breast and prostrate cancers; cirrhosis of the liver; violence; war; or self-inflicted injuries. Road accidents are the leading cause of death for males aged fifteen to forty-four (Murray and Lopez 1996). Moreover, between twenty and fifty million people are injured or disabled each year. These fatality and injury figures are projected to increase by about 65 per cent in the next twenty years (WHO 2004).

In the developed world car and road safety has improved considerably over time. However, decreases in fatality rates have to be placed in context. The absolute number of deaths remains high because increased safety has been accompanied by increased car use. Nevertheless, safer vehicles, improved roads, quicker medical interventions, more effectively monitored and socialised drivers, and better traffic control systems have contributed to safety – especially for those in automobiles. The question raised here relates to the structural limits of such interventions. Despite all the safety improvements, the road remains one of the riskiest locales in daily life.

Additionally, the aggregated and decontextualised nature of the quantitative data used in epidemiological analyses of accidents provides a refracted view of macro-social patterns. Such data give little insight into the micro-social processes of traffic and the sociospatial conditions in which accidents occur. Epidemiological studies show general patterns but do not explain the meaning of those patterns and their connections to the social organisation of space–time and motion. The qualitative data needed for more detailed analyses of the sources of risk in traffic are scarce.

Agents, vehicles and the social organisation of traffic

The encounters of agents in traffic require that each monitors and acts on the other's location, intent, direction of movement, etc. To manage complex traffic conditions requires that interacting agents exercise cognitive-motoric skills, and to do so rapidly and repeatedly. It is this human agency in traffic which leads critics of car safety measures and advocates of risk compensation theory to argue that there are limits to the efficacy of safety measures like safer vehicles and roads, seat-belt laws, etc. (Davis 1993). The increased security that such measures bring may lead to more risky behaviour on the part of drivers. What is risky, and for whom, depends on the kind of traffic and the type of vehicle. Norms (such as those allowing pedestrian right of way), speed limits and other rules influence interactions in traffic. Thus, in the micro-social encounters of traffic, the agents, the vehicles and the temporal and spatial contexts in which they operate all influence what behaviour is risky and who is vulnerable.

The 'technicisation' of the routines of daily life involves intensive and extensive use of complex and potentially dangerous technologies. As individuals are socialised into a 'technological society', unprecedented levels of psychomotor and technical capabilities are developed in populations. Driving at high speeds, manoeuvring in traffic, and managing movement as a pedestrian through complex transport spaces have become everyday routines and taken-for-granted abilities. The pervasive and intensive dependence on negotiating complex spaces and technologies is a source of stress and can disenfranchise or put at risk those unwilling or unable to meet its demands. However routine participation in technologised socio-material environments is for many people, there are some who are excluded and disenfranchised (Mohan 1997). Thus, a significant latent reason for traffic accidents is the car-centred transport system itself – a system that demands a high level of human functioning.

As more and more space is appropriated by the car, as more drivers travel (and travel alone), the demand for an instrumental, diligent, wide-awake state of being is increased. This leaves less psychosocial space and time for other states of mind, including playfulness, and for altered states of consciousness, like daydreaming. This imposition of a particular kind of subjectivity while driving, walking or cycling in traffic represents one of the more subtle forms of social control that accompanies car-centred transport. The constant vigilance and self-control that driving and moving in driving space require are not the natural conditions of subjectivity. The narrow band of consciousness demanded by successful movement in car-dominated space poses problems for humans. The modes by which we transport ourselves are not unrelated to how dangerous various altered states of consciousness (e.g., drunkenness) may be. The issue of whether people should or should not get high (on substances or activities) or daydream is one issue. How safely one can do this in the context of a particular mode of transport is another issue. In the debates about drink-driving few have defended the right to get drunk or have criticised the lack of transport alternatives. That driving while drunk is dangerous and that drivers who get high are more likely to cause accidents are self-evident facts. Yet the image of the 'killer drunk' is a convenient one for it allows society to demonise particular individuals and hence to sequester the problem. What is not apparent is the taken-for-grantedness of the need for a more general sobriety in a technological society. Increasing reliance on the car makes sobriety, full wakefulness and the optimal functioning of mind–bodies unquestioned norms demanded of anyone who wishes to have full freedom of movement. While fatalities related to driving while drunk have decreased in the USA since the 1980s because of shifts in attitudes and better enforcement of laws, driving under the influence of alcohol remains a significant problem, indicating that there are systemic limits to individual interventions. Drugs (some of them prescription drugs) also contribute to impairments and thus to risky behaviour. There is, however, little discussion of this in the safety literature – despite the fact that, according to one estimate, approximately one million drivers in the UK take prescription drugs that can contribute to psychomotor impairments (Davis 1993). Such numbers may increase as the population becomes 'greyer' and as the general use of pharmaceuticals continues to increase.

What can be called 'normal distraction' (as opposed to chemically induced distraction) is an important factor in car accidents. Rothe (1987) has observed that normal emotional arousal contributes to car crashes. Recalling a fight with the boss along with other distractions (such as mobile phones) can temporarily impair drivers. Given the speeds of cars and the densities of traffic, even a momentary lapse in concentration can be calamitous. Daydreaming and the intrusion of personal troubles must be held at bay in a car-oriented subjectivity.

Unsafe and disabling spaces

Particularly vulnerable in a car-centred system are the very young, the elderly and those who have psychomotor impairment. It has been noted that 'modern landscapes seem to be designed for forty year old healthy males driving cars' (Relph 1981: 196). The hegemony of the car over contemporary social space means that space once used for other functions, such as socialising and playing, has been appropriated. Children in poorer, inner-city neighbourhoods are particularly affected by this.

Since spatial arrangements are taken for granted and children are powerless, their disadvantage in the politics of space remains uninteresting for adults. Yet the inability of children to move safely through car space and the car's appropriation of spaces in which children play are important forms of social inequity (McNeish 1997). 'In order to reduce their children's exposure to risk, many parents routinely restrict their play space' (Roberts *et al.* 1995: 87). A British study found that the space usable by children was reduced considerably between 1971 and 1990. The principal reason given by parents for the decreased independent mobility of their children was increased traffic (Hillman *et al.* 1990).

In a car-centred transport system children are to some degree made housebound by car-dominated space, as are older and disabled people. Elderly pedestrians are especially vulnerable in traffic. Because safety discourses about elderly pedestrians often blame the ageing process, risk-perception training is seen as an appropriate measure to reduce accidents. Yet, those over fifty tend to be the most cautious in travel. Elderly female pedestrians are the most aware of their traffic context but still remain at high risk for injury and death from car accidents (Harrell 1991).

The social organisation of space, time and motion is influenced by the socio-economic status of a locality. A poorer neighbourhood is likely to have fewer safe crossings, worse-maintained roads, more (and less regulated) traffic, and less access to car-free spaces for rest, play, etc. Like the effects of pollution and other health costs of car-centred transport, mortality from accidents, then, is socially distributed along class lines. For example, the Public Health Alliance (1991) found that the mortality rate from traffic accidents for British men was 84 per cent higher for classes IV and V than it was for classes I and II. Among pedestrians only, the mortality was six times higher for the lowest two social classes than it was for the highest two. Child mortality from motor vehicle accidents showed similar social class disparities. The higher mortality rate for child pedestrians of the lower social classes may be due to the probabilities that they are more dependent on walking, less likely to be accompanied by an adult caregiver, and more likely to walk in areas that are not as well organised for traffic safety (Quick 1991).

A distinction between impairment and disability is made in what in the USA is called the 'minority group', and in the UK the 'social model', approach to disability (Oliver 1996). Impairment is relatively verifiable in objective medical terms. Disability, however, is not as easily defined separate from its cultural and material contexts. The disability rights movement's focus on the relationship between the social organisation of space and moving bodies is relevant for 'bodies with impairments' but applies to healthy bodies, too. As Zola (1982) points out, we are all at best 'temporarily able bodied', subject to the vagaries of injury, old age and intermittent emotional and physical disruptions.

Contradictions between car-hegemonic space–time and healthy, secure mind–bodies manifest themselves on yet another level. Given the increased severances and dispersions among activity sites, a car-centred organisation of space–time and motion influences the opportunities to engage in activities that contribute to musculo-skeletal and cardiovascular fitness. Thus, the social organisation of time and the material environment not only influences safety and how space is experienced but has a bearing upon opportunities for using the body, as well as upon the consciousness of such opportunities.

The social organisation of public space also influences access to what some have called 'healing places' or 'therapeutic landscapes'. Increasingly, sensual, aesthetic and healing environments are removed from the context of public spaces and everyday life, existing as retreats from daily life (thus, many cities are places to escape from). Unequal access to such healing spaces may contribute to health inequalities (Curtis and Jones 1998).

Mass transit, walking and cycling are not viable options in most outlying areas for those who cannot, will not, or should not drive. These populations make up the 'new class of access-poor' (Whitelegg 1997). It is quite possible that their lack of safe and pleasurable means of access affects their health and quality of life by contributing to a sense of powerlessness. A sense of powerlessness, or what has been called a low 'sense of coherence', contributes not only to a decreased quality of life but to poor health (Antonovosky 1987).

Conclusion

In what ways do the spatial and temporal contradictions of a car-centred organisation of space–time contribute to the production of accidents? High levels of individualised car use and dependence on the car for access, as well as the car's importance as a means of self-expression and its potential as a dangerous weapon, impose a requirement for sobriety and vigilance on all those who would move in traffic. Given the myriad factors that can disrupt sobriety or encourage risky behaviour (some of which are sociocultural), it is certain that some participants will not or cannot behave safely. Heavy, high-speed vehicles that predominate in car-centred space render softer vehicles (including human bodies) more vulnerable. Any intervention to improve safety is limited, as Davis (1993: 10) points out, by a system which puts many fallible human beings in charge of many vehicles 'with an exceptionally high potential for harming others'.

The overall incidence and severity of accidents, as well as the distribution of agents and vehicles that are risky or vulnerable in traffic, are also influenced by a variety of macro-factors, for example age and sex. For instance, as populations move towards a greyer shade, tensions between the social organisation of space–time and transport technology, on the one hand, and older mind–bodies, on the other, are aggravated. The participation in traffic of people who are under economic and other pressures influences how much risky behaviour there is. One's social class bears upon the condition of the vehicle one uses; it also shapes the social organisation of space and time in a neighbourhood and consequently the level of vulnerability of its residents.

It is important to recognise that some mind–bodies are more prone than others to injury and to feeling disempowered and insecure in car-hegemonic space. As car hegemony saturates and transforms the 'microgeographies' (Dyck 1995) of everyday life, safe access becomes more problematic and a greater stressor.

Public health efforts should be attentive to the spatiotemporal contexts of social process, structure and health. As health promotion pays increasing attention to the salutogenic effects of environments, analysis of the organisation of space becomes paramount (Frohlich and Potvin 1999). The Healthy Cities movement is an example of this direction (Smith *et al.* 1998). Car-centred transport systems that structure the landscapes of developed societies (and increasingly developing ones) provide a basis for such an analysis – one that would look at the spatiotemporal contradictions of car-centred transport, its public health consequences and the ways in which consequences are mediated for individuals by social status. On a theoretical level, this means emphasising the politics of bodies and embodied experiences, and their relationships to health and well-being.

Acknowledgements

George Martin acknowledges support from the Centre for Environmental Strategy, University of Surrey, and the Sociology Department, University of California, Santa Cruz.

Note

1   This chapter is a revised version of a paper which originally appeared in *Critical Public Health* (2001) 11: 203–14.

References

Antonovsky, A. (1987) *Unraveling the Mystery of Health: How People Manage Stress and Stay Well*, San Francisco, CA: Jossey Bass.

Curtis, S. and Jones, I.R. (1998) 'Is there a place for geography in the analysis of health inequality?', *Sociology of Health and Illness*, 20: 646–54.

Davis, R. (1993) *Death on the Streets: Cars and the Mythology of Road Safety*, Hawes: Leading Edge Press.

Dyck, I. (1995) 'Hidden geographies: the changing lifeworlds of women with multiple sclerosis', *Social Science and Medicine*, 40: 307–20.

Freund, P.E.S. and Martin, G.T. (1993) *The Ecology of the Automobile*, Montreal: Black Rose Books.

—— (2004) 'Motoring and walking: fitness and the social organisation of movement', *Sociology of Health and Illness*, 26: 273–86.

—— (2005) *Fast Cars/Fast Foods: Hyperconsumption and its Health and Environmental Consequences*, 37th World Congress of International Institute of Sociology, Stockholm.

Frolich, K.L. and Potvin, L. (1999) 'Health promotion through the lens of population health: toward a salutogenic setting', *Critical Public Health*, 9: 211–22.

Hanson, S. (1995) 'Introduction', in S. Hanson (ed.), *The Geography of Urban Transportation*, New York: Guildford Press.

Harrell, A. (1991) 'Precautionary street crossings by elderly pedestrians', *International Journal of Aging and Human Development*, 32: 65–80.

Hillman, M., Adams, J. and Whitelegg, J. (1990) *One False Move – a Study of Children's Independent Mobility*, London: Policy Studies Institute.

Hunt, S. (1989) 'The public health implications of private cars', in C. Martin and D.V. McQueen (eds), *Readings for a New Public Health*, Edinburgh: Edinburgh University Press.

McNeish, D. (1997) 'Keeping children safe – toward an effective strategy', *Critical Public Health*, 7: 34–40.

Mohan, D. (1997) 'Discussion', in T. Fletcher and A.J. McMichael (eds), *Health at the Crossroads*, New York: John Wiley.

Murray, C.J.L. and Lopez, A.D. (eds) (1996) *The Global Burden of Disease*, Cambridge, MA: Harvard University Press.

Nettleton, S. and Bunton, R. (1995) 'Sociological critiques of health promotion', in R. Bunton, S. Nettleton and R. Burrows (eds), *The Sociology of Health Promotion*, London: Routledge.

Oliver, M. (1996) *Understanding Disability: From Theory to Practice*, London: Macmillan.

Popay, J., Williams, G., Thomas, C. and Gatrell, A. (1998) 'Theorising inequalities in health: the place of lay knowledge', *Sociology of Health and Illness*, 20: 619–44.

Public Health Alliance (1991) *Health on the Move*, Birmingham: Public Health Alliance.

Quick, A. (1991) *Unequal Risks: Accidents and Social Policy*, London: Socialist Health Association.

Relph, E. (1981) *Rational Landscapes and Humanistic Geography*, London: Croom Helm.

Roberts, H., Smith, S.J. and Bryce, C. (1995) *Children at Risk? Safety as a Social Value*, Buckingham: Open University Press.

Rothe, J.P. (1987) '*Erlebnis* of young drivers involved in injury producing crashes', in J.P. Rothe (ed.), *Rethinking Young Drivers*, Vancouver: Insurance Corporation of British Columbia.

Schwela, D. and Zali, O. (eds) (1999) *Urban Traffic Pollution*, London: E. and A.N. Spon.

Smith, M., Whitelegg, J. and Williams, N. (1998) *Greening the Built Environment*, London: Earthscan.

Whitelegg, J. (1997) *Critical Mass: Transport, Environment and Society in the Twenty-first Century*, London: Pluto Press.

WHO (2004) *World Report on Road Traffic Injury Prevention*, Geneva: World Health Organization.

Zola, I. (1982) *Missing Pieces*, Philadelphia, PA: Temple University Press.

16 Epidemic space[1]

Joost Van Loon

Introduction

> It was the rainy season, and the 'road' was a string of mudholes cut by running streams. Engines howling, wheels spinning, they proceeded through the forest at walking pace, in continual rain and oppressive heat. Occasionally they came to villages, and at each village they encountered a roadblock of fallen trees. Having had centuries of experience with the smallpox virus, the village elders had instituted their own methods for controlling the virus, according to the received wisdom, which was to cut their villages off from the world, to protect their people from a raging plague. It was reversed quarantine, an ancient practice in Africa, where a village bars itself from strangers during a time of disease, and drives away outsiders who appear.
>
> (Preston 1995: 132)

Buried beneath the semiotic rubble of the second Gulf War which flooded the mediascape in the first few months of 2003, there was a small piece of seemingly unimportant news. It concerned an outbreak of ebola haemorrhagic fever in the Republic of the Congo, where the Ministry of Health had reported 140 cases, including 123 deaths (WHO 2003). A mortality rate of 88 per cent is common for ebola. Compared with the heightened media attention to the 'newly discovered' virus of SARS, whose mortality rate is significantly lower (6–12 per cent), the relative indifference with which the globalised world of news responded to this outbreak of ebola warrants at least some critical reflection.

Considering the question of why some diseases receive more attention than others, we need to emphasise the temporo-spatialisation of infectious diseases. Rather than prioritising the way in which public health is constructed symbolically, this chapter seeks to argue – by invoking actor–network theory – that the disease (or, to be more exact, the virulent pathogen causing it) is itself an active agent in the ordering of its own 'epidemic space'. Epidemic space is not merely a 'figure of speech', but an essential linchpin in the continuous iteration between the microphysics of infection and the macrophysics of epidemics (Van Loon 1998). It is the site where various actors meet, including virulent pathogens, medical experts, politicians and journalists; it is there where sense-making condenses into specific realities.

Actor networks

In *Science in Action*, Bruno Latour (1987: 180) notes that:

> the word network indicates that resources are concentrated in a few places – the knots and the nodes – which are connected with one another – the links and the mesh: these connections transform the scattered resources into a net that may seem to extend everywhere.

Central to Latour's account of 'science in action' is the way in which particular statements become 'matters of fact'. He refers to this process as 'enrolment' – the 'tying in' of various sorts of resources: financial, symbolic, human, technological, spatial, etc., through cycles of credit and accreditation (Latour and Woolgar 1979). Via this extension into a network, the particular claim becomes a 'matter of fact'. The matter of fact is not as much a matter of ideological imposition or deception, but part of the structure of obviousness that constitutes the network itself. For Latour, networks are not all-powerful uncontested systemic forces but, in contrast and despite the huge concentration of resources, still rather fragile achievements, prone to collapse and disorder. It is the doubling of power and fragility. Much of the investment of technoscience goes into the recuperation of social order from potential breakdowns and instability.

Latour's main proposition – that humans, technologies and gods constitute 'actor networks' – has important spatial implications as networks are themselves first and foremost spatial forms. Moreover, it forces us to take into account the particular functions and operations of (medical) science and technology as something that generates particular mediated contexts that in turn function as self-referential enclosures of 'reality'. Pathogen flows are central to understanding concepts such as enrolment and induction. They constitute the materiality of specific network relationships.

Epidemic can be contrasted with *endemic* (the Greek word en means 'in'), which refers to a condition that is or has become part of the people. The notion of epidemic thus implies a difference between the 'normal' state of being (the order of things) and what it refers to as 'externally imposed'. Epidemic must remain outside the ordinary; it is a turbulence that is expected to disappear. This is vital for understanding our relationship to infectious diseases. Nearly all diseases have a history of ascendance, disappearance and reappearance (McNeill 1976; Ryan 1996; Wills 1996). Once diseases have become endemic, their problematic nature tends to fade away as a 'matter of fact'. Central to epidemic space is thus its extra-ordinariness. In other words, in epidemic space pathogen virulence is an 'odd' element in the actor network: one that disturbs its smooth functioning, challenges its integrity and undermines its coherence.

The macro-physics of epidemics

Epidemiology is principally concerned with describing and explaining diseases as they occur in populations. In terms of descriptions, it uses a triad of place, time and people; in terms of (causal) explanations, it refers to etiological agent, host and environment (Lilienfeld and Stolley 1994). The latter is of crucial significance here as it is the intersection between the macro- and micro-physics of infectious diseases. The intersecting of these two different scales is the principal work of 'flows' (Shields 1997) which thus induce epidemic space.

In terms of micro-physics, contamination entails the relationship between host and parasite; it is the violation of a (seemingly) discrete and integral unity by 'pathogen' information. It thus focuses on discrete and different entities. In contrast, contagion could be represented with an arrow, from host A to host B. The 'content' of the arrow is the pathogen information (virus, bacteria). The hosts are seen as similar, and the arrow as a mode of connecting or enrolment. The focus shifts from the infected body to the infectious body. Rather than a parasite whose eradication is seen as central to the overcoming of the disease, the infectious body is seen as ambivalent – both *a risk* and *at risk*. This ambivalence is highlighted in the organisation of the modern hospital, which 'processes' at once risky and at-risk bodies, in a complex series of dualisms of 'isolation' (sterilisation) and 'care'. The infectious body, however, is never seen as discrete, but always as 'open'. This enables not only a removal of obstacles for medical intervention but a label of 'endangerment' being associated with the body itself.

In epidemiology, the mode of passing on (flow) is called a vector. Vectors can occupy different roles in flows of infection. They can be simple transmitters, receptors, or more complex reservoirs and incubators. Through the usage of vectors, one could draw up an 'abstract space' of a particular contagion as it 'moves'. As it moves, it spatialises the epidemic, constructing an epidemic space. When comparing the etiology of different diseases it becomes apparent that different pathogens use different 'vectors'. Influenza, for example, is largely airborne and travels without the aid of any other organism or body substance; ebola travels through blood particles and nearly all forms of bodily excreta; HIV through blood and semen; and malaria through mosquitoes. Understanding the vectors of particular diseases is a fundamental part of the diagnostic mapping of an infectious disease.

Cultural vectors: attendant-borne transmissions

During the build-up to the second Gulf War another piece of unobtrusive news failed to gain much publicity. In the publication of a series of studies on the epidemiology of HIV in the *International Journal of STD and AIDS* (Brewster *et al.* 2003; Gisselchrist and Potterat 2003; Gisselchrist *et al.* 2003), it was revealed how, since the 1980s, AIDS experts have systematically overexaggerated the role of heterosexual transmission in the spread of HIV/AIDS in Africa. Questioning the sexual hypothesis, the authors argue that 'epidemiological evidence from field studies completed through 1988 allowed that health care transmission was not only significant, but might well have been responsible for more HIV than heterosexual transmission' (Gisselchrist *et al.* 2003: 151). For example, whereas the high incidence of HIV among prostitutes is generally explained in terms of the centrality of frequent sexual activity with multiple partners as part of their profession, it is equally remarkable that all of them had been exposed to injections, immunisations and other medical interventions (such as surgical abortions) that pose potential risks regarding HIV transmission (Gisselchrist *et al.* 2003: 154). Additionally,

> Rapid HIV transmission in Africa has often occurred in countries with good access to medical care like Botswana, Zimbabwe and South Africa . . . It is difficult to understand how improved access to health care, with its offers of public health messages, free condoms, and preventative services would be associated with increased HIV transmission.
>
> (Brewster *et al.* 2003: 145)

This anomaly seems unintelligible if the majority of HIV transmissions are due to heterosexual intercourse. However, if one associates HIV transmission with medical care itself – including improper sterilisation of medical equipment and (method and/or user-related) contraceptive failures – the anomaly disappears. Suddenly, it becomes clear why in urban areas – where people have much greater access to medical care – HIV incidence increases far more rapidly than in rural areas. It also explains why in southern Africa HIV is particularly prevalent among groups of higher socioeconomic strata (Brewster *et al.* 2003: 146).

The idea that medical care itself plays a significant role in the development of epidemics is well known (Ewald 1994). For example, in the aforementioned case of ebola, syringe transmission was identified as one of the key vectors in the spreading of the disease, which, together with the concentration of people and poor hygienic environments, turned medical centres such as clinics and hospitals into 'hot zones' of infection (Peters *et al.* 1993).

> One room in the hospital had not been cleaned up. No one, not even the nuns, had had the courage to enter the obstetrics ward . . . The room had been abandoned in the middle of childbirths, where dying mothers had aborted fetuses infected with Ebola. The team had discovered the red chamber of the virus queen at the end of the earth, where the life form had amplified through mothers and their unborn children.
>
> (Preston 1995: 133)

The hospital ward is an ideal epidemic space and conducive to the development of increased pathogen virulence (Ewald 1994). Cultural vectors such as medical attendants are connected to technological devices such as syringes giving optimal opportunities for opportunistic infections to prey on already vulnerable human beings, whose immunity is likely to have been already compromised by whatever brought them to seek medical attention in the first place. Although Ewald (1994) links this process to the widespread use of antibiotics, which effectively encourage increased pathogen virulence, he stresses that, even without antibiotics, pathogen virulence tends to increase with the frequency of attendant-borne transmissions. Using evolutionary biology, his conclusion is that attendant-borne pathogens favour increased pathogen virulence.

In other words, the cultural vector hypothesis emphasises that humans, technologies and pathogens engage in networks by bringing together their own singularities of engagement. An epidemic space emerges around a set of flows that often amplify each other. The motivation of pathogen virulence, for example, forms an alliance with the motivations of medical care, even though both may have completely oppositional intentions. Flows of pathogen virulence effectively appropriate the technical infrastructure of modern medical care and for human beings the consequences are often detrimental. For epidemiologists, mapping an epidemic space therefore requires a wide-ranging and open-ended scope in which a multiplicity of vectors and flows is included.

Tracing epidemic space: index and vortex

A focus on vectors enables one to map the complex connectivity of epidemic space. However, epidemic space also incorporates a 'temporal dimension'. This involves a tracing of origins, causes and effects over time. Epidemiologists call the first identified case of an epidemic the 'index case' (Anderson 1983: 133). Especially in analyses of (vertical) contagion, tracing the index is of enormous importance since it supplies a wealth of information on possible causes of the disease and possible vectors of infection. By tracing the index case backwards the epidemic space is subsequently mapped and traced to its alleged 'origin'. Indeed, one could argue that a central part of the epidemiological endeavour to map a disease is also to understand its 'indexicality'. Space is marked not only by what is visible and present but by what is *virtual* – a potentiality of coming into being that is nevertheless more restricted than 'the possible', because it is already being indexed. In this sense, epidemiology is like cultural geography – a form of sense-making through mapping indexicalities – the context-particular tracing of affectivity of spatial forms and relationships (see Eyles and Woods 1983).

However, equally important is the subsequent link with *abstraction*. It is through abstraction that 'logos' is added to epidemic. Transforming the local and lived indexicalities (traces) into a more general framework of understanding flows of infection requires representations of space that are discursively regulated. Space becomes a site of regulation, governance and control. To obtain a higher level of generality than that of the particular incident, epidemiologists use population statistics as well as laboratory and clinical experiments to decontextualise a particular outbreak and reconfigure it within an abstracted space of flows (Latour 1988). This includes both knowledge about the general condition of the population at stake, including the environmental as well as medical factors that characterise it, and knowledge about the possible pathogens, their genetic structures, vectors and natural habitat.

Alongside mapping indexicality of epidemic space as a virtuality, followed by its abstraction into a decontextualised account that can be replicated within laboratory tests and clinical trials, the epidemiological rationale has a third dimension. This is related to what might be called 'epistemic politics' and is mainly framed within the wider logic of modern medical science, whose 'will to know' is directly coupled with the biopolitics of individual bodies and populations (Foucault 1979). The main public ethos of the scientific concern of epidemiology is the 'prevention of diseases' (Anderson 1983; Lilienfeld and Stolley 1994). That is to say, as a technoscience, epidemiology is not merely concerned with tracing the origin of a disease, mapping its trajectories or explaining its patterns and regularities; it also feeds into public health management, and it is here where epidemic space is above all a space of risk flows.

Epidemiologic technoscience effectively operates between the space of flows of abstracted knowledge and the immediate lived (but virtual) epidemic space of infectious diseases. It thereby complicates the dualism between abstract knowledge and embodied concern. Alongside vector and index, this third dimension of epidemic space operates as a *vortex*, bringing together the trajectories of seemingly unconnected events that constitute the complexity of cosmic rhythms and flows. Vortexicality is set to work by an initial disturbance or discontinuity, and leads to a more or less volatile intensification of speed of flows. Hence, the role of the Yambuku missionary hospital in the spreading of ebola and the role of the Kinshasa highway and sexual health clinics as main arteries of HIV transmission in Africa are cases of vortexicality in which 'hot zones' are constructed by the very same technoscientific practices that were designed to contain them.

Hot zones are particular intensified epidemic spaces that are at once abstract and lived. They call forth a range of technoscientific concerns, often enforced by the state's policing apparatuses. Quarantined zones of containment are such extraordinary places because normality, indeed the very logic of modernity, is suspended; the boundaries are often regulated by brute force rather than consent. The status of those inside suddenly changes as civic entitlements (e.g., liberty, equality and brotherhood) are suspended. When vortexicality becomes visible, panic strikes because modern technoscience is no longer 'in control'. This is the case, for example, when media engage in a rhetoric of endangerment (Ungar 1998). When the cosmic order rearranges itself and 'man' is (temporarily) displaced from the centre of the universe, and more importantly the myth of the human-centred universe is being displaced, it may only be a temporary event but it is one that deeply upsets the institutional logic of modern world society. It is this induction of hot zones into other domains (e.g., political, military, economic and symbolic) that makes 'epidemic space' never just an issue of biomedical containment.

Hence, whereas indexicality maintains an ideal of determinability of origin, vortexicality only operates in relation to the whole; it induces a complexity in which traces are always already multiplied and diffused. Instead of a linear tracing of origins, it requires an induction of new forms (hence transformation). It is the technoscientific intervention between the abstracted and lived epidemic spaces that engenders these new vortexical forms.

The instability of epidemic space

Latour's actor–network theory provides a means by which we can come to terms with the 'stabilisation' of specific sociotechnical settings. Although it is not

242 Joost Van Loon

really a 'theory' in terms of a relatively coherent body of assumptions, hypotheses, explanations and predictions, it does generate an analytical and conceptual framework with which we can understand the formation of specific social practices.

Epidemic space could be understood as a specific framing of 'actor networks', one which is governed by a multiplicity of flows that can be comprehended in terms of vector, index and vortex. A virus is a major actor in this network-engendered epidemic space. Between living and non-living matter, viruses exist only in becoming. Their networks are highly temporalised and fragmented. The fragility of the virus is intensified with an inability to sustain itself. The point to make here is that whereas all networks are fragile, it is their ability to adjust the 'currency flows' to newly emerging environmental complexities that allows them to sustain themselves. In other words, if the technoscience of epidemiology is to be successful, it has to be able to translate the highly intensive but also highly temporal force of epidemic space (set to work by viral infections) into more enduring flows of financial, symbolic, human, technological and spiritual matter/energy. Indeed, only virulent assemblages are capable of becoming actor networks.

Alongside the matter-specific micro-physical framing of pathogen virulence, the focus on epidemic space also allows for a more situation-specific understanding of risk society and risk culture. It enables us to extend concerns over identification and embodiment in risk cultures with notions of 'movement' (vectors), 'speed' (virulence) and 'tenacity' (incubation) that cannot be analysed at the level of 'individual bodies', but force us to take into account the relational-contextual framework of actor networks.

> The smallest AIDS virus takes you from sex to the unconscious, then to Africa, tissue culture, DNA and San Francisco, but the analysts, thinkers, journalists and decision-makers will slice the delicate network traced by the virus for you into tidy compartments where you will find only science, only economy, only social phenomena, only local news, only sentiment, only sex.
>
> (Latour 1993: 2)

The compartmentalisation of epidemic space is the main job of the medical techno-sciences such as clinical virology, immunology and epidemiology, which – often with the aid of governance and commerce – create specific 'zones' within networks that appear to operate autonomously from other particle flows. Identifying a limited number of vectors and indices indeed enables a 'tracing' that is also a reduction of complexity (see Christie 1987). Vortexicality is thus written out of the script of the disease etiology – that is until its fractal movements start to affect other parts of social organisation seriously.

Vortexicality, however, does not sit comfortably within actor–network theory. As the latter is more concerned with ordering and stabilisation, it does not really enable us to come to terms with the extraordinariness of epidemic space. It focuses on routines, alliances and representation. As a result, it runs the risk of neglecting those bits that do not fit (Van Loon 2002).

Conclusion

In this chapter, I have argued that epidemic space operates at the intersections between the micro-physics of infection and the macro-physics of public health. I have tried to show that infection can be theorised as a particular form of sociation, one that immediately brings to the fore the risk-laden and especially contagious nature of the social. At the same time, it enables us to see the social as a constellation of flows, as shifting perspectives and positions, and thus as inherently unstable.

The 'subject' of modern democratic politics is equally problematic when considering epidemic space, as the sheer otherness of the pathogen that forms constellations with the human body inherently problematises the latter's alleged integrity. Instead, bodies are 'opened up', that is 'disclosed' by pathogen flows, and are – as a result – doubled: as infected and infectious.

This doubling creates an ambivalence operating at the centre of public health: to whom is it to be responsive, the sick or the healthy? Most would say both, yet one must acknowledge that they do not add up. As a result all strategies of risk management are 'corrupted' by ambivalence. By using the concept of vortexicality, I suggest that this ambivalence is the primary engine of a growing sense of loss of control, paired with an emergent apocalyptic anxiety as expressed, for example, in popular cultural narrations of medico-military conspiracies.

If we understand epidemic space as both a trope for the organisation of anomalous space and a materialisation of a particular assemblage of forces that integrate embodied immune systems with wider sociocultural and politico-economic constellations, we are perhaps able to make more sense out of the way in which infectious diseases operate upon society and culture. As a form of expression (trope), epidemic space is a particular symbolic organisation dominated by – but not exclusively consisting of – biomedical discursive formations. As a form of content, epidemic space is constituted by the clashing forces of regularity, ordinary practices, normalised routines and habits, on the one hand, and those of ontological extraordinariness, abnormality, irregularity and deviance, on the other. Crucial here is the regularity of irregularity or epidemic space, which has allowed the creation of expert systems of epidemic management that operate upon the monadic logic that every contingency is to be colonised.

For social and cultural analysts, epidemic space relates to the very core of their respective domains: the social and 'sense-making'. Epidemic space allows for the understanding of infections, immunity and epidemics as social and cultural phenomena. However, likewise, a sociocultural sensibility towards epidemic space also engages the biomedical sciences. It is well known that the representatives of these so-called 'hard scientists' have been less than inviting to the humanities and social sciences as far as mutual engagement of knowledge is concerned. However, their monopoly on understanding infectious disease has in effect been eradicated by the failures of technoscience to live up to its grandiose predictions. In a risk society, technoscience itself faces a crisis of legitimisation. This legitimacy crisis is directly related to the displacement of the basis of agency from the integral subject to the infected/infectious body, which itself is situated in complex of flows of contagion. It calls into question the very justification of regimes of regulation and the nature of decision-making that is often obscured by the subpolitics of expertise (Beck 1997).

Viruses are enrolled in actor networks that stretch far beyond the clinic and the laboratory. Government agencies, often allied with judicial, political and military institutions, media organisations and commercial enterprises, all have a stake in the management and control of epidemic space. Indeed, one could argue that, if taken to its logical limit, epidemic space is rapidly becoming the public sphere of the risk society. As epidemic spaces are produced and reproduced by an ambivalent constellation of forces, they are therefore not contained by the physical properties of quarantine and may mobilise concerns. These concerns operate as energisers of possible actor networks that involve, apart from scientists and engineers, policy-makers, journalists, entrepreneurs and lawyers, to name but a few. It is vital, therefore, that the notion of epidemic space should not be colonised by the technosciences of epidemiology, virology and immunology for exactly the same reasons that the management of a nuclear plant should not be seen as an exclusively nuclear-physical issue. Cultural analysis could provide a modest contribution to understanding the sociocultural embedding of both the indexicality and the vortexicality of infections and epidemics.

Note

1   This chapter is a revised version of a paper first published in *Critical Public Health* (2005) 15: 39–52.

References

Anderson, M. (1983) *An Introduction to Epidemiology*, 2nd edn, London: Macmillan.

Beck, U. (1997) *The Reinvention of Politics*, Cambridge: Polity.

—— (2000) 'Risk society revisited: theory, politics, critiques and research programs', in B. Adam, U. Beck and J. Van Loon (eds), *The Risk Society and beyond: Critical Issues for Social Theory*, London: Sage.

Brewster, D.D., Brody, S., Drucker, E., Gisselchrist, D., Minkin, S.F., Potterat, J.J., Rothenberg, R.B. and Vachon, F. (2003) 'Mounting anomalies in the epidemiology of HIV in Africa: cry the beloved paradigm', *International Journal of STD and AIDS*, 14: 144–7.

Christie, A.B. (1987) *Infectious Diseases*, Vol. 1., 4th edn, London: Longman.

Ewald, P. (1994) *Evolutions of Infectious Disease*, Oxford: Oxford University Press.

Eyles, J. and Woods, K.J. (1983) *The Social Geography of Medicine and Health*, London: Croom Helm.

Foucault, M. (1979) *The History of Sexuality*, Vol. 1: *The Will to Know*, New York: Vintage.

Gisselchrist, D. and Potterat, J.J. (2003) 'Heterosexual transmission of HIV in Africa: an empiric estimate', *International Journal of STD and AIDS*, 14: 162–73.

Gisselchrist, D., Potterat, J.J., Brody, S. and Vachon, F. (2003) 'Let it be sexual: how health care transmission of AIDS in Africa was ignored', *International Journal of STD and AIDS*, 14: 148–61.

Latour, B. (1987) *Science in Action: How to Follow Scientists and Engineers through Society*, Milton Keynes: Open University Press.

—— (1988) *The Pasteurization of France*, Cambridge, MA: Harvard University Press.

—— (1993) *We Have Never Been Modern*, trans. C. Porter, Hemel Hempstead: Harvester Wheatsheaf.

Latour, B. and Woolgar, S. (1979) *Laboratory Life: The Social Construction of Scientific Facts*, London: Sage.

Lilienfeld, D.A. and Stolley, P.D. (1994) *Foundations of Epidemiology*, 3rd edn, Oxford: Oxford University Press.

McNeill, W.H. (1976) *Plagues and Peoples*, Harmondsworth: Penguin.

Peters, C.J., Johnson, E.D., Jahrling, P.B., Ksiazek, T.G., Rollin, P.E., White, J., Hall, W., Trotter, R. and Jaax, N. (1993) 'Filoviruses', in S. Morse (ed.), *Emerging Viruses*, New York: Oxford University Press.

Preston, R. (1995) *The Hot Zone*, London: Transworld.

Rothschild, H., Allison, F. and Howe, C. (eds) (1978) *Human Diseases Caused by Viruses*, New York: Oxford University Press.

Ryan, F. (1996) *Virus X: Understanding the Real Threat of Pandemic Plagues*, London: Harper-Collins.

Shields, R. (1997) 'Flow', *Space and Culture*, 1: 1–7.

Ungar, S. (1998) 'Hot crises and media reassurance: a comparison of emerging diseases and ebola Zaire', *British Journal of Sociology*, 49(1): 36–56.

Van Loon, J. (1998) 'The end of antibiotics: notes towards an investigation', *Space and Culture*, 2: 127–48.

—— (2002) *Risk and Technological Culture: Towards a Sociology of Virulence*, London: Routledge.

Wills, C. (1996) *Yellow Fever Black Goddess: The Coevolution of People and Plagues*, New York: Addison-Wesley.

World Health Organization (2003) 'Ebola haemorrhagic fever in the Republic of the Congo – Update 11', Communicable Diseases Surveillance and Response (CSR). Available at: <http://www.who.int/csr/don/2003_04_14/en> (accessed 17 May 2003).

Index